Health Care Evaluation Using Computer Simulation

Boris Sobolev • Victor Sanchez • Lisa Kuramoto

Health Care Evaluation Using Computer Simulation

Concepts, Methods, and Applications

Springer

Boris Sobolev
University of British Columbia
828 West 10th Avenue
Vancouver, BC, Canada

Victor Sanchez
Electrical Engineering
and Computer Sciences
University of California, Berkeley
253 Cory Hall
Berkeley, CA, USA

Lisa Kuramoto
Centre for Clinical Epidemiology
and Evaluation
Vancouver Coastal Health
Research Institute
828 West 10th Avenue
Vancouver, BC, Canada

ISBN 978-1-4614-2232-7 ISBN 978-1-4614-2233-4 (eBook)
DOI 10.1007/978-1-4614-2233-4
Springer New York Heidelberg Dordrecht London

Library of Congress Control Number: 2012938238

Printed on acid-free paper

Springer is part of Springer Science+Business Media (www.springer.com)

Foreword

I am honored to have been asked to write this foreword for the new book by Professor Sobolev and his colleagues. At first, I was hesitant, partly because I had a busy schedule at the time and partly because I did not consider myself a health services researcher (HSR), although I am part of the UK health Operational Research (OR) community.

In the UK, the recent international review of the status of operational research commissioned by the Engineering and Physical Sciences Research Council found that health OR was "one of the unique selling points of significant strength within the British OR research, from an international perspective", and that it can serve as "bridges between 'hard' areas like mathematics and more qualitative areas such as human resources management, knowledge management and social and behavioural sciences."

Despite this recognized research strength and the general recognition of the benefits of modeling by managers and clinicians, academic reviews of the state of simulation and modeling in health care have consistently found that there is a lack of evidence of successful implementation, probably due to a lack of communication between the relevant stakeholders. This has led in the UK to the formation of MASHnet (www.mashnet.info), the UK healthcare modeling and simulation network, and more recently, the Cumberland Initiative (www.cumberland-initiative.org), a consortia of over 15 UK universities working toward a center for system modeling and service science in health care.

I first met Professor Sobolev at a symposium on "Modeling Healthcare Systems," which he had organized at the University of British Columbia (UBC) a few years ago, not long after the establishment of MASHnet, which I chaired at the time. Professor Sobolev's vision was to bring the use of simulation modeling approaches into health services research (HSR) and, more specifically, health care intervention evaluation. The symposium brought together prominent international researchers in the field of HSR, OR, and indeed Computer Science to explore and exploit the benefits of the different disciplines, which coexist in parallel worlds. Such initiatives that attempt to break silos ought to be applauded.

Indeed, how far apart are HSR and health OR? The national OR societies in the UK and USA define OR as "the discipline of applying advanced analytical methods to help make better decisions." The definitions of HSR are equally broad. For instance, the Health Services Research Network (HSRN) in the UK defines HSR as "all research that underpins improvements in the way health services are financed, organised, planned and delivered, and includes health technology assessments and health policy research." A possible distinction is that OR focuses on modeling and simulation of processes and problem solving, while HSR focuses on evaluation of outcomes and methodologies. Whether or not there exists a strong distinction between HSR and health OR, both disciplines are ultimately about research to improve health services, and they ought to work together.

While the book is written by and for health services researchers, it has a lot to offer to those in OR as well as those in information systems and software engineering. It provides a comprehensive and systematic approach to the use of simulation in intervention research, with plenty of applications to guide the researcher through the steps of such methods.

Particular attention is given to study design, which tends to be neglected or secondary in most OR simulation books and articles, maybe because from an OR perspective, modeling is considered as a tool to assist the decision maker rather than one that provides a definite answer to what modeled system performs best. Planning and evaluation of studies at cluster and individual levels are also given wide coverage, including the number of simulation runs required for a given confidence level and extensive use of regression metamodels for intervention evaluation.

In most OR simulation texts, conceptual modeling tends to be restricted to simple flow charts or specific tools such as activity cycle diagrams. This text uses industry standard Unified Modeling Language (UML) diagrams, which are rarely seen in the OR world yet offer great potential to communicate with the wider world of information and software systems specialists. The introduction of the Statechart formalism for patient flow is also unusual yet very powerful for similar reasons.

The last seven chapters concern important applications to surgical services from appointment booking to discharge planning. The reader is taken step by step through the simulation modeling and then through the evaluation of the interventions considered.

My initial hesitance quickly disappeared and was replaced by an appetite to read this book again and explore further UML, Statecharts, and metamodeling approaches. I can recommend this book to my health OR and HSR colleagues, especially those involved in secondary care interventions, and hope it will encourage the two communities to work together. It is impressive to see this book appear only a few years after the "Modeling Healthcare Systems" workshop at UBC, and the publication of another book by the same team, which I would also recommend, "Analysis of Waiting-Time Data in Health Services Research."

University of Westminster, London Thierry Chaussalet

Preface

Over the past several decades, health services research has informed policy decisions about the most effective options for improving the delivery of medical care. However, the link between the organization and the outcomes of health services is rarely tested empirically because of ethical and methodological constraints on conducting experimental research in the patient care setting. As a result, the current state of knowledge offers limited insights into how changes in the organization and management of a health care system may affect the quality of the health services provided. Increasingly, health services researchers are seeking new approaches for evaluating the effects of proposed changes before they are implemented in health care systems. One innovation is the use of computer simulation to identify the likely outcomes of quality improvement initiatives.

The purpose of this book is to place computer simulation studies within the paradigm of intervention research that is concerned with comparing the outcomes of health care delivered under different policies. We adopt the perspective of economist James Joseph Heckman that a major use of policy analysis is to determine the effects of policy alternatives. In the ensuing chapters, therefore, we focus on evaluation rather than optimization. We present computer simulation as a tool for testing various policy alternatives that have been developed by decision makers within health care systems. This approach differs from the use of computer simulation in operations research, where simulation helps determine the configurations of a system that will allow it to function optimally.

Although simulation of health care processes is not new, few health care systems have used simulations as a basis for re-engineering the delivery of health services. There is growing appreciation that the complexity of health care processes exceeds the capacity of individual disciplines—health services research, health economics, or operations research—to guide health care reform. At a recent conference entitled "Modeling Healthcare Systems," sponsored by the Peter Wall Institute for Advanced Studies at the University of British Columbia, an international group of scholars provided convincing evidence that a new interdisciplinary approach, one that incorporates the simulation of health system operations into the evaluation of policy initiatives, is required. In this book, we focus on bringing the methodological rigor of evaluative studies to the design and analysis of such simulation studies.

Providing care to a patient population requires the coordinated effort of numerous specialists. A typical example is surgical care, which involves a variety of treatments in the preadmission clinic, an inpatient surgical unit, the operating room, the postanesthetic care unit, and the intensive care unit. Modeling patient flow is considered a powerful approach in assessing the likely response of a health care system to changes in organization, management, and policy. The underlying premise is that simulated care paths collectively represent the delivery of health services to a patient population. The simulation of patient flow improves understanding of the interactions between clinical and managerial activities by revealing the chronology of events and changes in the volume and types of patients. Examples of simulation modeling in surgical care include evaluating policies for admitting patients to hospital, for scheduling appointments, for planning capacity, for improving patient flow, and for managing wait lists. The flow of patients in surgical care settings is a recurring example in this book.

We suggest two uses for this book. First, it is intended as a reference for health services researchers. We offer a comprehensive description of the methodology of conducting simulation studies in evaluation of service alternatives in surgical care using discrete-event models, including the steps for identifying the clinical and managerial activities of the perioperative process, determining the model requirements, implementing simulation models, designing simulation experiments and analyzing the experimental data, and interpreting and reporting results. Second, the book offers examples of specific aspects of conducting simulation experiments: how to determine the number of runs needed to estimate the effect of implementing a health care policy, how to allocate the number of runs to study groups in simulation experiments aiming to evaluate policy or management alternatives, and how to use statistical analysis to estimate, interpret, and report effect sizes.

The book is divided into 19 chapters, grouped in three parts. Part I is largely introductory, setting out the main concepts of health care evaluation, outlining the role of simulation experiments, and presenting the process of surgical care in a fashion suitable for simulation modeling. Chapter 1 provides a broad introduction to intervention research. In particular, it describes the analytical framework and designs of evaluative studies within the context of health services research. Chapter 2 examines the role of simulation experiments through the prism of intervention research. Chapter 3 presents a taxonomy of the activities of surgical care and develops a perspective of health care as a reactive system. Whereas Chap. 2 offers an overview of simulation research, the last three chapters of Part I discuss the software engineering concepts of computer simulation. Chapter 4 reviews approaches for constructing simulation models of health care processes, highlighting the differences among them in terms of assumptions, system requirements, and input and output data. Chapter 5 introduces Unified Modeling Language diagrams as a means to represent functioning of the health care system. This chapter includes examples of use case diagrams for the activities of surgical care, activity diagrams for the flow of patients through care activities, sequence diagrams for the interactions of patients and care activities arranged in a time sequence, and Statechart diagrams for concurrent care activities. Chapter 6 focuses on discrete-event simulation of patient flow and goes into greater detail regarding the specifications of discrete-event models based on the Statecharts visual formalism.

Part II is concerned with issues arising in the planning and evaluation of simulation experiments. In Chap. 7, we show how to apply the methodology of intervention research to the design of a computer simulation study. In particular, we develop the analytical framework of the simulation experiment, describe how to determine the number of simulation runs and how to allocate the runs in a cluster randomized study design, and outline a plan for analyzing output data from a simulation experiment. Chapter 8 describes the performance measures suitable for evaluating the effect of an intervention at the cluster level, the experimental data necessary to derive those measures, and the corresponding measures of effect for comparing experimental groups. In Chap. 9, we further describe experimental planning from the perspective of individual-level outcomes. We present a variety of performance measures suitable for evaluating the effect of an intervention at the individual level, along with the required experimental data and the corresponding measures of effect. Part II comprises two additional topics in applying the methods of intervention research to simulation experiments: analysis and reporting of results. Chapter 10 sets out the requirements for clear and complete reporting of a simulation study to help the reader of the report to understand the study, interpret its results, and evaluate the quality of its findings. In particular, we review the principles of reporting developed by the CONSORT group. Chapter 11 presents methods for evaluating policy alternatives when the unit of randomization and the unit of analysis is the cluster, and Chap. 12 presents techniques for analyzing simulation experiments at the level of the individual. In particular, we discuss how to compare individual-level measures using methods that adjust for similarities between outcomes among patients who are served in the same hospital, and how to adjust for potential confounding factors using regression methods.

Part III presents examples of computer simulation studies in which the goal is to evaluate the effect of changes in the organization and management of surgical care. We focus on cardiac surgical care because this type of care is well structured and is thus amenable to study and improvement. Chapter 13 serves as an introduction to these case studies, presenting a thorough description of the simulation model of patient flow that we developed for the evaluations discussed in Chaps. 14–16. In particular, we describe the modeled process, the requirements of the model, and details about its implementation. For these case studies, we used experiments with a cluster randomized design, in which the unit of allocation was the hospital and the units of analysis were both the hospital and the patient. In Chap. 14, we compare several methods of booking surgical consultation appointments in a surgical service with several specialists. The simulation suggests that clearance times will be shorter in hospitals where patients wait for clinic appointments in a single queue and that within each week, a larger proportion of patients are likely to have an appointment if they are in a single queue. In Chap. 15, we compare two methods of screening patients for surgery: screening all patients or screening only some patients before admission to hospital. The simulation results suggest that the proportion of procedures that are canceled is smaller in hospitals that screen all patients before admission and that the weekly likelihood of patients undergoing their operation from the wait list is lower at hospitals screening all patients. In Chap. 16, we compare two methods of booking elective surgery: booking from a wait list and advance booking at the time of the decision to operate. The simulation results suggest that the number of surgical cancellations is smaller and the number of operations from the wait list is larger with advance booking of surgery dates.

At the end of Part III, we discuss three planned simulation studies, the first for evaluating methods of booking anesthesiology consultations (Chap. 17), the second for evaluating the management of postoperative care (Chap. 18), and the third for evaluating methods of discharge planning (Chap. 19). In Chap. 17, we describe the design of a simulation study and the plan of analysis for evaluating the effect of adopting a pooled-list method for booking anesthesiology consultations in terms of the proportion of hospitals with delay of elective procedures and proportion of patients undergoing surgery after the recommended time. In Chap. 18, we describe the design of a simulation study and the plan of analysis for comparing the effect of diverting patients to a different hospital if no intensive care unit bed is available for postsurgical recovery relative to the effect of postponing the surgery. In Chap. 19, we describe the design of a simulation study and the plan of analysis for comparing a policy in which discharge planning is performed for all patients before their admission to hospital with a policy in which discharge planning is performed for only some patients.

The writing of this book was made possible, in part, by funding from the Canada Research Chairs Program. We gratefully acknowledge the support of the Centre for Clinical Epidemiology and Evaluation at the Vancouver Coastal Health Research Institute, where most of the research was undertaken, as well as the generous advice of Dr. Guy Fradet and Dr. Robert Hayden, the scientific editing of Peggy Robinson, the able assistance of Taina Immonen in preparing the manuscript, and the contribution of Kaitlyn Tsuruda to Chap. 19.

Vancouver, British Columbia

Boris Sobolev
Victor Sanchez
Lisa Kuramoto

Contents

Part I Concepts

List of Tables

List of Figures

List of Boxes

List of Boxes

Part I
Concepts

Chapter 1
Intervention Research in Health Care

In this introductory chapter, we provide a broad overview of the evaluation of complex interventions aimed to improve the quality of health care. In particular, we outline the analytical framework and designs for evaluative studies within the context of health services research. We then describe the types of questions that commonly arise in the evaluation of management alternatives for perioperative processes. We conclude with a brief discussion about the transition from posing a study question to identifying the level of analysis and the summary measure of the outcome variable.

1.1 Intervention Studies

Intervention studies constitute the branch of health services research concerned with generating evidence about the effectiveness of health care interventions. Throughout this book, the term *intervention* is used in a broad sense. An intervention could be a policy, a quality improvement initiative, a management system, a set of practice guidelines, a prevention program, a scheduling method, or a service model, or it might refer to a new treatment, medical device, or product. The purpose of an intervention study is to compare outcomes of health services delivered under different policies. If the occurrence of the outcome differs between the policies, researchers conclude that changing the policy affected the delivery of care.

The evaluation of health care interventions involves statistical analysis to infer the effect size. In a simple case, researchers compare two groups of study participants in terms of a measure summarizing observations of the outcome. When expressed in some quantity, the difference in the summary measure between the groups is interpreted as the effect size. By convention, the study groups are called control, for existing policy, and intervention or comparison, for the proposed alternative. If multiple policies are being compared, the study groups are called intervention groups and one group is labeled as the reference group.

B. Sobolev et al., *Health Care Evaluation Using Computer Simulation: Concepts, Methods, and Applications*, DOI 10.1007/978-1-4614-2233-4_1,

Studies that evaluate the effects of a new program are the most common type of intervention study in health services research. In one example of a controlled intervention study, the effect of teaching nursing students how to lift and transfer patients was evaluated after 2 years of follow-up by comparing the incidence of one or more episodes of back pain between the two study groups [107]. A meta-analysis of studies evaluating the effect of discharge planning coupled with postdischarge support for patients with congestive heart failure showed reductions in the rate of readmission [123]. Intervention studies have been used to determine the efficacy of a falls prevention program involving short lengths of stay in geriatric care wards [43], to evaluate the effectiveness of educational outreach visits in improving physicians' reporting of adverse drug reactions [56], and to investigate whether a nurse-coordinated, family-based preventive cardiology program improved the quality of care in routine clinical practice [161]. Using the results of these planned experiments, researchers were able to obtain evidence that helped them to draw conclusions as to whether the proposed changes in management would improve patients' outcomes.

Some interventions, such as efficiency improvement initiatives, can be designed to improve outcomes at both the individual and the organizational level. For example, advanced access is a scheduling method that offers a patient the choice between a same-day appointment with any physician available or a potentially delayed appointment with a preferred physician or at a convenient time [114]. Several studies have documented benefits for both patient and service arising from implementation of the advanced access method in a specialist clinic, specifically, shorter time to appointment and decreased no-show rates [115]. In recent years, however, there has been growing recognition that some initiatives may have differential effects on patient and service outcomes. In particular, some management solutions in surgical services may improve patient flow but compromise the service quality [143].

1.2 Causal Perspective

Ideally, an intervention study is a planned experiment conducted to test a hypothesis about a causal relation between changing policy and outcomes. Causal reasoning in science relies on the premise that for each observed phenomenon, there exists an underlying mechanism that links cause and effect. In health services research, the description of such a mechanism involves specification of the structures, processes, and outcomes of medical care, as exemplified by the works of Avedis Donabedian (1919–2000) [48]. Donabedian held that the structures of care are the facilities, equipment, services, and human resources needed to provide care, as well as the qualifications of the care providers. The processes of care are the clinical and managerial activities, steps, and procedures involved in the provision of treatment within the defined structures of care. Finally, the outcomes of care are the results of the activities through which medical care is provided. Therefore, within the Donabedian triad, causal mechanisms should explain at least two sets of dependencies: those between structures and processes and those between processes and outcomes.

Operations research conducted in the second half of the twentieth century was instrumental in revealing the links between structures and processes in various social and industrial systems. The paradigm and analytic approaches of the field gradually came to be included in the Methods sections of articles in the health services research literature concerned with improving the quality of care. At the same time came the realization that processes of health care differ from those of manufacturing, variability in patients and reliance on expert judgment were cited among the most significant differences [119]. The link between a clinical process and treatment outcomes has proven the most challenging for operations analysis because of uncertainties inherent in diagnosis and choice of treatment, as well as the stochastic nature of the response to treatment exhibited by many medical conditions.

During the same period, health services research created a solid foundation for empirical analysis of the outcomes of care delivered to patient populations. First, clinical evaluative studies have documented wide variations in treatments and outcomes in most health care systems. For example, it has been reported that 20% of surgical procedures performed have no clear benefit for patients; conversely, a substantial number of patients do not receive treatments that could improve their condition [16, 162]. Second, it has been established that even in cases where there is an indication for a specific treatment and patients receive the treatment and experience the anticipated benefit, the particular response may differ from one patient to another. In specialties such as surgery and oncology, this individual-level variation may also be related to the potential harm of treatment, such as complications or death. The next natural milestone was establishing factors that influence the outcomes of care. For example, researchers investigating the link between postoperative processes and outcomes have shown that lack of improvement in a patient's condition might result from factors related to either the condition or the clinical process, or both [136].

The structure–process–outcome model provides a convenient idealization in evaluations of complex interventions in health care. Usually, such interventions constitute changes in one or more significant aspects of care delivery. Within the model, interventions could be thought of as replacements of one configuration of the structure and process of care with another. Replacing a configuration could be further viewed as modifying some parameters of the structure, such as procedural volume, or the process, such as time from hospital arrival to angioplasty. To illustrate this idea, suppose the variable Z characterizes the structure and process of care, so that Z_0 and Z_1 represent configurations set by policy 0 and 1. The effect of replacing policy 0 with policy 1 could be then evaluated by comparing the outcomes of care corresponding to values of Z set by each policy. Within the Donabedian model, health care evaluation therefore constitutes the effort to answer the following question, *What would be the change in outcome if variable Z is forced to change from Z_0 to Z_1?*

1.3 Analytical Framework

The most common question in health services research is *What effect will this intervention have?* To answer this question with empirical data necessitates specification of study variables, outcome variables, a summary measure of the outcome, and a measure of the effect. Evaluating interventions has at its core the notion that the intervention will force the study variable to change from one value to another. The outcome variables can be expected to respond to the changes in the study variable, subject to random variability in the response. Inferences can be made about interventions by comparing changes in a summary measure of the outcome according to levels of the study variable, for example, to draw conclusions about the relation between the intervention and the outcome. The change that the intervention produces in the summary measure of the outcome represents the effect of the intervention. The size of the effect is usually expressed as the relative or absolute value of the change.

1.3.1 Study Variable

Attributing an observed change to a particular intervention involves comparing the study participants exposed to the intervention with those not exposed or with those exposed to an alternative intervention. In intervention research concerned with patient care, the study participants are sampled from a larger population that is under investigation, such as patients who have been referred for elective surgery. The participants are then divided into two study groups, intervention and control, according to the intervention to which they will be exposed. Often, the study groups are naturally defined by management alternatives, practice guidelines, prevention programs, service and health system models, or quality improvement initiatives. In this situation, the study variable is assigned different categorical values to represent the intervention alternatives. In a study with two groups, it is common to use a binary study variable, which takes the value 0 to represent the control group and 1 to represent the intervention group. Although it may seem to be an artificial construct, the notion of a study variable operationalizes the causal link between intervention and outcome. In simple terms, the researcher intervenes in the study variable to test for changes in the outcome variable.

1.3.2 Outcome Variable

The outcome is an end point of interest in care delivery, public policy, or evaluation of services. In general, three types of outcomes are studied in health care evaluations: those related to patients, those related to treatments, and those related to the system. Patient-related outcomes represent the effects of delivering care in a particular system on the patient's ability for self-care, physical function and mobility, emotional and intellectual performance, and self-perception of health. Treatment-related outcomes represent biological and physiological changes in the patient's condition occurring as a result of administering therapy within the health-care system. System-related outcomes represent the effect on the health care system produced by the provision of medical services to a patient population. Examples of the outcomes studied in health services research include performance benchmarks, requirements for pain medication, length of hospital stay, waiting times, frequency of readmission, and frequency and severity of secondary health complications.

In some studies, the outcome variable is an indicator of occurrence of an event. It takes the value 1 if the event under study occurs and 0 otherwise. In other studies, the outcome variable could be continuous, for example, if the end point is time, the result of a laboratory test, or a measurement of vital status. The inherent complexities of health care, such as the diverse expertise of health care professionals, the variety of organizational arrangements, the array of treatment protocols available, and the myriad interactions between managerial and clinical activities, may necessitate that multiple outcome variables be integrated in evaluating the effects of an intervention at the level of patient, treatment, or health care system.

1.3.3 Summary Measure of the Outcome

It is a fundamental property of patient populations that the same treatment of the same condition offered by the same physician produces different results in individual patients. This property is acknowledged by the standard qualifier that the Food and Drug Administration mandates for drug advertising in the United States: "Individual results may vary." When the occurrence and timing of an outcome vary, summary measures of the outcome variable are used to contrast the study groups. For example, the distribution function for time between referral and consultation appointment characterizes the probability that a patient will see a specialist within a certain time after referral. Statistical methods of time-to-event analysis can be used to compare appointment probabilities across intervention groups with different appointment systems to identify the system with the shortest time to appointment [23]. The summary measure could be the average time to appointment, the median time to appointment, the probability of an appointment within one month, the weekly odds of the appointment being scheduled, or even an entire appointment probability function.

1.3.4 Measure of Effect Size

Changes in the summary outcome measure μ considered across levels of the study variable can be used to estimate the size of the effect. For example, the effect of replacing policy 0 with policy 1 could be defined as the change from μ_0 to μ_1 in corresponding summary measures. The change is measured in terms of the difference in summary measures between the two groups, $\mu_1 - \mu_0$, the ratio of summary measures, μ_1/μ_0, or the difference in the logarithm of summary measures, $\log \mu_1 - \log \mu_0$, if μ is strictly positive. The magnitude of the change defines the strength of the effect. If the change is negligible, then the intervention is deemed to have produced no effect.

1.4 Study Designs

Health services research employs two types of studies for measuring the effect of interventions: randomized trials and observational studies. A randomized trial is a controlled experiment concerned with the general question: *What would be the change in outcome if intervention A is applied instead of intervention B?* A typical observational study is primarily concerned with a different question: *What is the difference in outcome between patients who happen to have been exposed to intervention A and those who happen to have been exposed to intervention B?* Randomized trials compare study participants who were randomly assigned by the researcher to one of the alternative interventions. By contrast, observational studies compare participants for whom the researcher recorded what happened during the delivery of care, without any action on the part of the researcher to control factors involved in choosing the intervention.

This distinction matters, because researchers will not necessarily be able to reproduce observed differences in outcomes between two groups that happen to have been exposed to different circumstances by deliberately setting those circumstances. For example, if clinical outcomes were found to improve when health care spending happened to decrease, it cannot be concluded that deliberate decrease in spending will improve outcomes. Therefore, a deliberate application of alternative interventions by the researcher constitutes the primary approach used to estimate the causal effect of interventions.

1.4.1 Randomized Trials

The purpose of random assignment of study participants to study groups is to balance the groups in terms of both known and unknown factors that might independently affect the outcome of interest. In other words, the study groups should be as similar as possible in all respects except exposure to the intervention. It is assumed that randomization ensures this required similarity, in that all factors that might lead to a lack of comparability between the groups are likely to be distributed similarly in groups to which participants have been randomly assigned. It is further assumed that comparison of study groups in randomized experiments will produce unbiased estimates of the effect size. As a result, the differences in outcomes observed between the groups can more confidently be ascribed to the intervention rather than to other factors. In contrast, observational studies allow no such deliberate management of who receives the intervention. As such, known and unknown factors may be distributed unevenly within the study groups. If the assignment of interventions produces an imbalance in the distribution of factors related to the outcome across the groups, the resulting estimates of effect size may be biased, and adjustment for the factors may be required. However, such adjustment may be impossible if some factors are unmeasured.

1.4.2 Cluster Randomized Trials

When health care interventions are implemented at the service level, the researcher may consider random assignment of health care services rather than random assignment of patients. For example, in studies of the effect of modifying service operations, it may be necessary to assign hospitals, physician practices, or surgical services, rather than individual patients, to the control and intervention groups. Intervention studies in which randomization is done at the organizational level and data are analyzed at both the individual and the organizational level are called cluster randomized trials. Cluster randomization has implications for the design and analysis of trials. In particular, there is recognition that for interventions applied at the hospital level, the outcomes of patients served in the same hospital may be more similar than the outcomes of patients served in different hospitals, due to hospital-level factors [153]. For example, postoperative management of patients may conform more consistently with practice guidelines in one hospital than another, and therefore the similarity of outcomes in each hospital is expected because of similarities in patients' experiences with respective hospital services.

A fundamental assumption in the analysis of randomized trials is that individual outcomes are independent. In cluster randomized trials, this assumption does not hold because individuals from one cluster are more likely to have similar outcomes than individuals from different clusters. Therefore, cluster randomized trials may have lower statistical power for detecting the effect than a trial of equivalent size in which randomization occurs at the level of individuals. As such, larger group sizes are needed in a cluster randomized trial to account for potential correlation in outcomes within organizations. To account for this potential within-cluster correlation, the number of individuals in a cluster randomized trial is greater than the number that would be used in a regular randomized trial on the basis of a theoretical ratio of between-cluster variance to total variance, known as the intracluster correlation coefficient. The value of this coefficient has been reported between 0.01 and 0.15 for interventions involving implementation of evidence-based clinical guidelines across practices in the primary care setting [51]. The additional number of individuals is accomplished by increasing either the number of clusters or the number of individuals per cluster.

1.5 Statistical Reasoning

To make inferences about the effects of an intervention, it is necessary to address the randomness in observed outcomes. Whether understood as variability or as uncertainty, the concept of randomness refers to the lack of predictability of the outcome of an intervention at the level of an individual study participant. Although the Oxford English Dictionary defines *random* as "having no definite aim or purpose," in science, *random* refers to the lack of deterministic pattern in occurrence. In statistics, the concept of randomness is operationalized through notions of a random variable that takes values of the outcome with some frequency and a probability distribution function that links each possible outcome with the probability of its occurrence. This distribution function is itself deterministic, and it can be estimated from observations of the outcome variable. The effects of the intervention can be then expressed through changes in the probability distribution of the outcome observed across the study groups.

In his book *Principles of Statistical Inference*, statistician David Cox places a study question, which originates from some general problem in the subject matter, at the inception of statistical analysis [41]. In health care evaluation, the study question is often stated in the context of the social, political, organizational, behavioral, and economic theories that have influenced the design of health care systems. Data available to address the question include the study and outcome variables. It is assumed that there exists a data-generating mechanism, which can be described by a probability model. In this probability model, observed values of the outcome variable are regarded as realizations of a random variable, whereas the study variables are treated as fixed attributes of the study groups. In brief, then, the question is addressed by studying the distribution of an outcome variable that is conditional on the value of the study variable.

As mentioned above, the summary measure of the outcome distribution is used to construct a measure of the effect size, which is operationalized through the difference (or the ratio or the difference of logarithms) in the summary measures observed in the study groups that have been exposed to the intervention alternatives. The probability model for measuring the effect of an intervention includes an unknown parameter related to the effect-size measures of interest. This parameter is often represented by a regression coefficient. The choice of model and parameter links a subject-matter question and a statistical question. Statistical techniques are applied both to generate an interval of values within which the parameter is likely to lie and to assess the consistency of the data with a particular value of the parameter.

With guidance from the study question, an intervention could be evaluated at the level of both the individual participants and the cluster of participants. For example, consideration could be given to the fact that surgical patients are treated by particular specialists who perform surgery in particular hospitals. Information can be then collected on variables related to the patient (e.g., age, sex, severity of disease), to the specialist (e.g., time in practice, adherence with guidelines), and to the hospital (e.g., volume of patients, scheduling methods). In cluster-level analysis, the cluster is the unit of inference. A summary statistic is computed for each cluster (e.g., average, proportion), and standard statistical methods can be applied, because the summary statistics are considered independent across clusters. In individual-level analysis, the individual is the unit of inference. In Chap. 12, we will discuss various statistical techniques that permit potential correlation of individuals within clusters. These methods can be used to incorporate the hierarchical nature of the data into the analysis.

1.6 Types of Questions

1.6.1 Context of Surgical Care

Surgery is a medical procedure involving incision with instruments. It is performed for various reasons, such as removing diseased organs, repairing or redirecting vessels, fixing malformed or damaged anatomic structures, and implanting artificial devices. Surgical procedures may be classified by the organ, system, or tissue involved; by type of procedure; by degree of invasiveness; by equipment used; and by urgency. Examples include cardiac surgery, which is performed on the heart; gastrointestinal surgery, which is performed on the digestive tract; and orthopedic surgery, which is performed on bones. Exploratory surgery is performed to aid in diagnosis, whereas therapeutic surgery is performed to treat a diagnosed condition. Minimally invasive surgery utilizes small incisions to bring instruments to a body cavity or structure, as in laparoscopic orthopedic surgery. By contrast, a major procedure requires a large incision to access the area of interest. Laser surgery involves a laser instead of a scalpel. Some procedures require a microscope to allow surgeon to see small structures. Elective surgery is performed to treat conditions for which the risk of immediate morbidity and death is believed to be low. Urgent surgery is performed to avoid morbidity, but can be postponed for a short time. Emergency surgery is performed within hours to prevent death and disability.

Surgical care is a continuum of diagnostic, preoperative, operative, and postoperative activities [36, 42]. The diagnostic stage includes medical tests and evaluations to identify the patient's condition, and the preoperative stage includes clinical and managerial activities taking place from the decision to book the surgery to entry into the operating room. The operative stage lasts from entry into the operating room to transfer to the recovery room. The postoperative stage includes recovery care immediately after the surgery and treatment in inpatient surgical units (possibly including treatment in an intensive care unit), ending with discharge to home, to long-term care, or to rehabilitation care. In this book, we discuss in detail the evaluation of methods for improving the progress of patients through these steps of surgical care. Box 1.1 summarizes the perioperative activities considered in the policy evaluation studies described later in this volume, listing policy, and management alternatives devised in various acute care hospitals [138]. The following sections of this chapter outline activities at the individual stages of surgical care and describe the types of questions that are commonly addressed in the evaluation of the perioperative process.

Box 1.1 Examples of management alternatives for perioperative activities

Booking surgical consultation appointments in the outpatient clinic
Specialist-specific appointment lists
Pooling of all referrals on one appointment list
Offering preferred time with any surgeon or any time with preferred surgeon

Managing access to elective surgery
Specialist-specific wait lists
Centralized wait list by procedure
Unlimited, unmonitored wait lists
Regulated wait lists, with redistribution of cases
Monitored wait lists, with update of urgency
Pooling of patients for expedited admission in the network of hospitals

Presurgical screening
Assessment of patients after admission for elective surgery
Assessment of all patients awaiting elective surgery in preadmission clinic
Optimization of patients' condition before admission for elective surgery
Education of patients and their families about procedure and postoperative care

Booking anesthesiology consultations
Anesthesiologist-specific consultation lists
Anesthesiologist at consultation not necessarily service provider during surgery

Scheduling patients for surgery
Weekly booking of admission dates from wait list
Advance booking of admission dates
Confirmation of operating room schedule with surgeon's office day before surgery
Short-notice pool of patients for operating room slots that become available
Profiling of cases on basis of type of procedure
Required information for scheduling operating room time provided by surgeon office

Prioritizing patients for admission to hospital
Priority groups
Continuous urgency rating score
Dynamic prioritization (increasing priority with time spent waiting)

Rescheduling surgeries that had to be canceled
Scheduling of canceled and postponed operations for weekend
Increasing priority upon reinstatement on wait list

Managing utilization of operating rooms
Operating rooms for general assignment
Operating rooms dedicated to individual specialties
Operating rooms dedicated to emergency cases
Dedicated emergency slots within daily schedule

Sequencing patients for the operating room
Outpatient cases earlier, inpatient cases later
Similar cases grouped by surgeon, priority, or procedure
Major cases earlier, minor cases later
Longer cases earlier (to avoid overtime)

Managing postanesthesia care
Holding patients in postanesthesia unit until intensive care bed becomes available
Adjusting staffing pattern to reflect fluctuations in case mix

Planning for discharge before surgery
Identifying postoperative services before surgery
Discharge planning before admission for all patients scheduled for elective surgery

1.6.2 Outpatient Surgical Consultations

The management of outpatient surgical consultations constitutes an important aspect of planning activities in surgical services. The booking process used for surgical consultation appointments determines the appointment date for any patient who is referred for consultation about an operation [84]. Previous studies have explored various booking methods and their effect on the time to the consultation [1, 8, 30, 72, 88, 158]. Other studies have established that the length of time a patient has to wait between referral and consultation depends not only on the method of booking appointments and the number and type of referrals, but also on the availability of surgeons for appointments because these physicians may have administrative, educational, or research commitments, in addition to their clinical practice [72, 106].

The most common booking method is to place patients on the appointment list of the surgeon named in the referral, a system known as the individual-lists method. Under this system, a patient is scheduled for an appointment when the named surgeon is available and all previously referred patients, as well as those with more urgent needs, have already been scheduled [125]. For surgical services where a patient may see any one of a group of surgeons, pooling clinic referrals on a single appointment list (known as the pooled-list method) has been suggested as a way to reduce time to consultation with a specialist. The shortest-list method, whereby patients are directed to the surgeon with the shortest queue, has also been considered as a suitable alternative to the individual-lists method [52]. A potential advantage of the two alternative booking methods (pooled list and shortest lists) is that they eliminate the uneven distribution of patients across the appointment lists of individual surgeons [5], which may help to reduce variation in waiting times [85]. Both methods differ in one important respect from the individual-lists method: any particular patient may have to see a surgeon other than the one who was recommended by the referring specialist.

Few data are available about the implications of the various methods used for booking surgical consultations for access to elective surgery, particularly with regard to how the pooled-list and shortest-list methods affect time to consultation and to surgery, how the booking method affects clearance time for appointment lists, and how the pooled-list and shortest-list methods affect time to consultation across priority groups. Accordingly, the following types of questions could be answered through evaluation of policies for outpatient consultations:

- Does the method of booking surgical consultation appointments (i.e., individual lists versus pooled list versus shortest list) affect the number of patients waiting for an appointment?
- Does the method of booking surgical consultation appointments (i.e., individual lists versus pooled list versus shortest list) affect the time to appointment?
- Does the method of booking surgical consultation appointments (i.e., individual lists versus pooled list versus shortest list) affect the time to surgery?

- Does the method of booking surgical consultation appointments (i.e., individual lists versus pooled list versus shortest list) affect the clearance times for appointment lists?

1.6.3 Booking of Elective Operations

The process of booking surgery determines the day of a patient's operation and reserves the hospital resources necessary to ensure appropriate care of the patient both during and after the operation [67]. It takes into account the urgency of treatment, the availability of postoperative resources, and the number of slots available for elective and emergency cases. Booking elective patients for an operation involves three activities: allocating the amount of operating time to various surgical services [17], assigning blocks of operating time to surgeons [18], and booking patients into the operating room slots of their respective surgeons [47]. Several factors influence the assignment of blocks of operating time to surgeons [19]. Some surgical procedures require special equipment, and there may be a set of dedicated operating rooms that can be used by a certain specialty. Surgeons may not be available every day because of other activities within their respective practices, such as examining patients in their offices, teaching, performing administrative duties, and performing surgery in other hospitals where they have admitting privileges [93]. Furthermore, the allocation of time to specialties is complicated by the need to ensure that the schedule is feasible in terms of the use of postoperative resources, which usually are shared by different specialties.

Advance booking of admissions has been suggested as an alternative method for booking elective operations [66]. Instead of keeping patients on wait lists until a slot becomes available in the operating room (i.e., the wait-list booking method), the consulting surgeons prebook the operation date at the time of the decision to operate (i.e., the advance-booking method) [103]. However, little is known about the effects of advance booking on access to elective surgery, particularly in terms of the number of cancellations originating with the hospital (as opposed to the patient) and the time to surgery. Accordingly, the following types of questions could be answered through evaluation of policies for booking of elective operations:

- Does the method of booking elective operations (i.e., wait-list booking versus advance booking) affect cancellations of elective procedures?
- Does the method of booking elective operations (i.e., wait-list booking versus advance booking) affect time to the operation?

1.6.4 Presurgical Screening

Once a surgeon decides that surgery is indicated and the patient consents to the procedure, the patient undergoes preoperative assessment, which serves several purposes: determining health problems, surgical factors, and anesthetic factors that may increase the patient's risk of adverse outcomes; modifying perioperative risks through further medical tests, medical treatments, or consultations with other health care professionals; identifying medical, nursing, and social issues that may affect planning of discharge from hospital; and providing education about anesthesia and postoperative care [101, 110, 149].

In managing access to elective care, a consultation in the preadmission clinic is usually booked at the same time as the operation. A variety of methods may be used for managing presurgical screening in the preadmission clinic. For example, with the all-screened method, all patients scheduled for elective surgery are assessed in the preadmission clinic before their prebooked date of surgery. With the some-screened method, an attempt is made to screen all patients in the preadmission clinic before the prebooked date of surgery. If the attempt is not successful, electively scheduled patients may undergo the assessment after admission to hospital for the operation. Each of these methods entails some amount of waiting and inconvenience to the patient and the potential that scheduled surgery will be postponed, depending on the time of presurgical assessment. Few studies have assessed the effect of these various methods for scheduling presurgical assessments on patient-related or treatment-related outcomes [21, 121, 134, 154].

Although some evidence suggests that performing the presurgical assessment well in advance of surgery decreases cancellations of surgery relative to assessment performed on the day of surgery [21, 121], the implications of the different methods for managing presurgical screening are not well understood, particularly in terms of the number of cancellations originating with the hospital and the time to surgery. The following types of questions could be answered through evaluation of policies for presurgical screening:

- Does the method of managing presurgical screening at the preadmission clinic (some patients screened versus all patients screened) affect cancellations of elective procedures in each priority group?
- Does the method of managing presurgical screening affect time to the operation?

1.6.5 Postoperative Care

After a surgical procedure, the patient recovers in the intensive care unit, where he or she is monitored and treated for the adverse effects of anesthesia. During recovery, the patient is repeatedly reassessed against discharge goals. The management of postoperative care has a direct effect on access to elective surgery. For example, scheduled operations may be postponed or canceled when not enough beds are available in the intensive care unit. Similarly, planning for discharge before a patient is admitted for an operation may affect the postoperative length of stay.

There are no evidence-based guidelines regarding the optimal size of an intensive care unit to ensure access for all patients, including patients who have undergone

Box 1.2 Examples of questions in intervention studies of surgical care

Outpatient consultations

- Does the method of booking surgical consultation appointments affect the time to appointment?
- Does the method of booking surgical consultation appointments affect clearance times for appointment lists?

Elective operations

- Does the method of booking operations reduce cancellations of surgery?
- Does the method of booking elective operations affect time to the operation?

Presurgical screening

- Does the method of managing presurgical screening reduce cancellations of surgery?
- Does the method of managing presurgical screening reduct time to the operation

Postoperative care

- Does the method of managing postoperative care reduce cancellations of surgery?
- Does planning for discharge before admission affect the postoperative length of stay?

surgery. However, some data suggest that small intensive care units are not cost-effective [15] and that high occupancy is associated with high mortality [79]. Analytical models have been developed to plan for critical care capacity, but these have not been tested in a complex system of surgical care [38]. Given the premises outlined above, the following types of questions could be answered by evaluation of policies for postoperative care:

- Does the method of managing postoperative care (diversion to a different hospital if intensive care unit bed unavailable versus postponing surgery) reduce the number of cancellations of elective procedures?
- Does planning for discharge before admission for the operation affect the postoperative length of stay?

1.6.6 From Questions to Outcome Measures

Box 1.2 lists examples of questions that drive evaluation in the delivery of surgical care. To answer the questions of interest through an intervention study, each question must be operationalized by formulating a hypothesis, indicating the level of analysis, and determining the corresponding summary outcome measure. The unit of analysis determines the level at which conclusions about the effects of the intervention are drawn. As noted in previous sections of this chapter, the individual patient, the service, or the hospital can be the unit of analysis in trials designed to evaluate quality improvement interventions in health care. In this book,

Table 1.1 Research questions linked to hypotheses, level of evaluation, and summary measures of the outcome for studying surgical consultation appointments

Question	Hypothesis	Level	Summary measure
Effect of booking method on access to appointments?	Reduced time to appointment	Patient	Proportion of appointments after benchmark time
	More hospitals with improved access to appointments	Hospital	Proportion of hospitals with less than 10% of appointments after benchmark time

we adhere to the principle of conducting analysis at a preset level of expected generalization [152]. It requires that the estimates derived from the analysis be directly applicable to the phenomena about which we are drawing conclusions, or, in practical terms, that the unit of analysis corresponds to the level of outcome variables.

Another consideration is whether the unit of analysis will satisfy some underlying premises of the statistical methods selected. The most important premise is that the data-generating mechanism must produce independent replication of the studied phenomenon, which requires independence of observations. For common statistical tests, the assumption of independence of observations is crucial. In Chap. 7, we discuss this aspect of study design in greater detail. In an evaluation of surgical care, there are at least two levels at which evidence will be generalized: the patient and the hospital. Therefore, conclusions can be presented in terms of proportions of patients or proportions of hospitals. For example, a conclusion based on the proportion of regional hospitals that meet the policy target of providing surgery for hip fracture within 48 h set by the health authority would differ from a conclusion based on the proportion of patients who underwent the operation within the set time frame. In Chap. 8 and 9, we contrast the summary measures at the patient (individual) and hospital (cluster) levels.

Table 1.1 shows an example of linking a research question with these three elements of study design: the hypothesis, the level of analysis, and the summary outcome measure. It considers the case of different methods of booking outpatient surgical consultations and their effect on the time a patient has to wait before having an appointment. The study question can be formulated as follows: *What is the effect of the alternative method for scheduling surgical consultation appointments on the time to an appointment?* If the level of analysis is the patient, the hypothesis might state that a particular intervention reduces the time to appointment, and a possible outcome measure would be the proportion of extended waits for appointment (i.e., appointments taking place after a benchmark time). If the level of analysis is the hospital, the hypothesis might state that a particular intervention increases the proportion of hospitals with improved access to clinic appointments and a possible outcome measure would be the proportion of hospitals with less than half of patients experiencing extended waits for clinic appointments. Table A.1 in Appendix A provides more examples for research questions discussed in the previous sections of this chapter.

In this chapter, we have outlined the analytical framework, described evaluative designs, and presented the statistical reasoning of health care intervention studies. In the next chapter, we introduce the concept of applying the methods of intervention research to health care evaluations that involve computer simulation experiments.

Chapter 2
Simulation Studies

In this chapter, we merge computer simulation modeling and intervention research within one analytical framework. In particular, we consider the argument that the evaluation of organizational changes in the delivery of health services should include the simulation of health system operations. In turn, the methodological rigor of evaluative studies should be applied to the analysis of simulation experiments. We review the implications of such an approach for both the design and analysis of simulation studies. We conclude with a brief discussion of the requirements for reporting the design, methods, and results of a simulation study.

2.1 Computer Simulation Modeling

2.1.1 Purpose of Simulation Modeling

In this book, we adopt the perspective of economist James Joseph Heckman that a major use of policy analysis is to determine the effects of policy alternatives [75]. When feasible, intervention studies are conducted to compare existing and new approaches to the organization of health care delivery. However, when ethical, economic, or other reasons prevent organizational interventions, computer simulation provides an alternative method of quantifying the effects of proposed changes. In its guidance for complex interventions in health care, the UK Medical Research Council identifies modeling as a distinct phase in the evaluation of organizational or service modifications intended to improve the delivery of health care [40]. The purpose of modeling in the evaluation of complex health care interventions is to develop a better understanding of the likely effects of proposed changes. The results of the modeling phase help in the decision to implement or abandon the changes. Modeling of care processes encompasses a variety of techniques, including computer simulation and analytical models. Simulation models are commonly developed to describe the underlying mechanisms through which the interventions

B. Sobolev et al., *Health Care Evaluation Using Computer Simulation: Concepts, Methods, and Applications*, DOI 10.1007/978-1-4614-2233-4_2,

may influence the outcomes of service delivery. For example, simulation models have been used to generate performance estimates for alternative decision-making scenarios and thus to facilitate the building of consensus on resource allocation [54].

Computer simulation has been suggested as a method to identify the effects of changes in the organization of surgical services [60]. The flow of patients in surgical care settings will be a recurring example in this book. Modeling patient flow is considered a powerful approach to assessing the likely response of a health care system to changes in organization, management, and policy. Applications of the simulation approach include evaluations of policies for admitting patients to hospital, methods of scheduling appointments, planning for beds and overall capacity, patient flow, and wait-list management. Other researchers have shown that the simulation of patient flow improves understanding of the interactions between clinical and managerial activities by revealing event chronology and changes in the volume and in the mix of cases [14, 98].

It is important to contrast here the use of simulation studies in operations and intervention research. Operations researchers use computer simulation to determine configurations of a system that will allow it to function optimally, for example, to determine the method of scheduling operating room time that maximizes the number of operations performed per month. Intervention research of scheduling operating time would be concerned with estimating the effect of adopting one scheduling method rather than another. In the ensuing chapters, therefore, we focus on evaluation, rather than optimization. We present computer simulation as a tool for testing policy alternatives developed by decision-makers within health care systems. In this approach, policy alternatives come from subject-matter experts rather than from numerical optimization algorithms. For example, one source of the management alternatives studied in Part III of the book was a report on the analysis of the surgical process produced by a panel of experts in managing perioperative services [163].

2.1.2 Merging Intervention Research and Simulation Modeling

Although the simulation of health care processes is not a new approach, few health systems have used simulation experiments in reengineering the delivery of health services. However, there is growing appreciation that the complexity of health care processes exceeds the capacity of individual disciplines—health services research or operations research—to substantiate the direction of health care reform. For this book, we have used an interdisciplinary approach, which merges intervention research and simulation modeling within an analytical framework to evaluate the most probable results of quality improvement initiatives on patient-related, treatment-related, and system-related outcomes [138]. In particular, we focus on patient-level models to simulate the steps in health service delivery and the response pathways for individual patients [120, 143]. Within our framework, the use

Box 2.1 Merging intervention research and computer simulation modeling

Analytical framework for evaluating interventions
Study variables representing intervention
Outcome variables representing patient, treatment, and system responses
Summary measure representing the outcome distribution
The effect representing the difference in the summary measure between groups
Random assignment of participants to study groups
Cluster randomized design accounting for dependence among outcomes
Statistical reasoning to estimate the effect of intervention

Premises of experimental design
Other factors distributed similarly in study groups
Differences in study outcomes between groups attributed to intervention
Causal mechanism not modified by intervention

Computer simulation study
Simulation runs generating care steps and patient-level care paths
Inputs representing service, patient populations, and policy alternatives
Outputs representing response pathways
Explicit mechanism linking inputs and outputs

Premises of computer simulation
Simulated care paths representing delivery of care to a patient population
Likely response pathways under policies being evaluated

of simulation experiments for evaluating health care policy is based on two premises: first, that simulated individual care paths collectively represent the delivery of health services to a patient population, and, second, that simulation produces care paths that are likely under the policy being evaluated (see Box 2.1). Therefore, proposed changes in the organization and management of health care processes can be assessed by comparing the performance of a system under various alternatives defined in simulation experiments.

2.1.3 Understanding Simulation Experiments

The role of a simulation experiment in comparing the outcomes of two system configurations can be illustrated with the pinball box, an invention of statistician Francis Galton (1822–1911). The box is a vertical board with overlapping rows of upturned nails. Dropped from the top and collected in slots at the bottom, small ball bearings or marbles bounce either left or right when they strike the nails. Ending up in a particular slot represents an outcome of bouncing on the way down. The heights of balls in the slots form the distribution of the outcome variable. For example, with an equal chance of bouncing left or right, the slots with collected balls approximate the curve of the normal distribution (left side of Fig. 2.1). On the other hand, if the chance of bouncing left is lower, then there are more paths toward the right slots

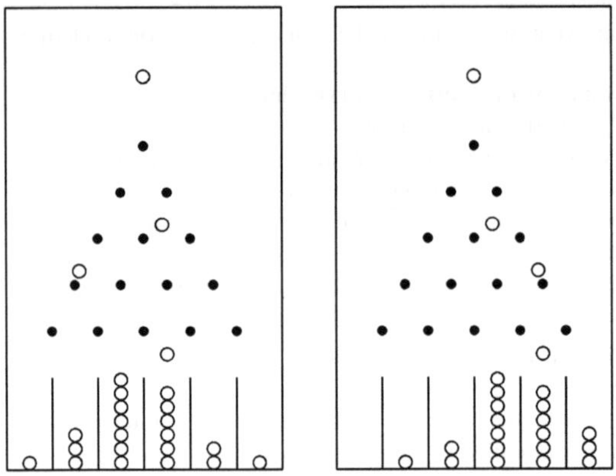

Fig. 2.1 The pinball machine of Francis Galton, designed as a board with upturned nails, creates the bell curve in marbles collected at its bottom. Here is the description of his design adopted from http://members.fortunecity.com/jonhays/quincunx.htm: "Take a board about 1 inch by 18 inches by 30 inches and box it on all sides by strips extending 1 inch above board surface; 8 inches from bottom of board, create a row of 1-inch nails, just fixed into the surface, protruding up, spaced across every inch; create similar rows of nails up toward top, stopping at least 2 inches from top of board; at bottom glue or otherwise fix slotting strips (say, 3/8 inch by 1 inch by 6 inch) on the 3/8 inch sides to collect marbles that roll down the board; finally, use board 1/2 inch by 1 inch × 18 inch, driven in, to prop up top of the nail-board. Roll, one after another, small marbles or small ball bearings from top down the board. When one strikes a nail, it either goes off to the left or to the right to collect in one of the slots at the bottom. The slot partitions prevent balls sliding to the side, leveling the bottom output. It can be shown that there are many more paths toward the middle of the board than toward the sides, so that more marbles collect between the middle slots than between those on the sides"

than toward the left slots (right side of Fig. 2.1). Therefore, the parameters of the nail configuration affect the distribution of balls in the slots. According to the analytical framework introduced in Chap. 1, some summary measure of the distribution should be used to evaluate the effect size of replacing one configuration with another.

A simulation experiment consists of multiple runs of the model with inputs representing the patient population, the health services provided, and the proposed policy alternatives. In patient-flow studies, each simulation run generates a group, or cluster, of care paths for patients served in a modeled hospital [11]. During each run, the simulation software records the occurrence and timing of simulated events for the hypothetical patient population, such as appointments, registrations, and cancellations. Experimental outcomes are then computed from patient-level records generated by the simulation runs. For example, a simulation run can produce a set of indicators, each showing whether the procedure was canceled on the day of surgery for individual simulated patients in an experimental group. Alternatively, experimental outcomes can be computed across multiple simulation runs. In that case, the simulation experiment may produce a set of indicators, each showing whether the surgical service simulated during a particular run in an experimental group met a performance benchmark. For example, this type of simulation experiment might indicate whether 90% of procedures for hip fracture in a particular surgical service were completed within the health authority's benchmark of 48 h.

2.1.4 Correlation Among Experimental Outcomes

The algorithms of generating pseudorandom numbers usually address the issue of independence across simulation runs, but in experiments that simulate care delivery, the patient-level outcomes may be correlated within each simulation run because of, for example, competition for common resources in the simulated hospital [138]. In Sect. 1.4, we introduced the idea that larger group sizes are needed for outcomes that vary more across simulation runs than within each run. Although modern computers can easily produce a large number of simulated patient care paths, the number of runs used should be sufficient to allow evaluation of the effects of multiple study factors [28]. Later in the book, we discuss how to determine the number of simulation runs and how input factors should be varied across runs (see Chap. 7). Specifically, we provide formulas for estimating the number of runs for a cluster randomized design while accounting for clustering of observations (see Chap. 9). In trials with this design, it is the simulation runs, rather than individual experimental units (i.e., patients), that are randomized to the different intervention groups. We also discuss the implications of correlated observations for testing differences between proposed management and policy alternatives by means of regression methods (see Chap. 12).

2.2 Causal Reasoning

One aspect of simulation experiments appears to be poorly understood in the previous literature on health care evaluations. This aspect is related to the *counterfactual reasoning* typically adopted in evaluating causal hypotheses in intervention research. To generate evidence about the effectiveness of a certain intervention, a hypothesis is proposed regarding the causal link between the study variables that are subject to the intervention and the outcome variables that are assumed to be related to the study variables through some material mechanism. An intervention study is used to test the hypothesis by exploring whether a change in one of the study variables results in a change in the outcome variables. The premise is that the intervention does not modify the underlying causal mechanism, that is, all functional relations remain unchanged [122].

The key concept of this causal reasoning is the construct of the *potential outcomes* of applying alternative policies to one study participant [111]. The idea, traced to philosopher John Stuart Mill (1806–1873), is to take two instances of an experimental unit (or two fully exchangeable units) and intervene with one [126].

Differences in outcomes between the two units are considered to result from the intervention. In the case of an ideal physics experiment, the experimental units would be identical or fully exchangeable, but in the real-life situation of a health care intervention, no two patients will be exactly alike. Even though each individual in a patient population will be exposed to only one of two alternative policies, and as such the outcome of only one policy can be observed for any individual, it is still possible to consider the outcomes of both policies in thought experiments. For example, in comparing the effect of advance booking and wait-list booking on time to undergo elective surgery, the potential time to surgery under a policy of wait-list scheduling could be considered for patients in a surgical service that currently employs advance booking.

Consider a thought experiment involving two policies in patient care. Each policy represents a complex intervention that will affect the outcomes of care delivery to a patient population. Suppose a researcher wants to estimate the effect of replacing policy 0 with policy 1 on outcome variable Y, where the value of this variable for patient i is y_i. If patient i is assigned to policy 0, y_i can be equated with potential outcome y_i^0; similarly, if patient i is assigned to policy 1, y_i can be equated with potential outcome y_i^1. The difference $y_i^1 - y_i^0$ can be thought of as the effect size of exposing patient i to policy 1 instead of policy 0. Although a convenient abstraction, this difference cannot be directly calculated from the data because only one of the two potential outcomes y_i^1 and y_i^0 can actually be observed for a given patient.

In real life, the responses of a single individual to the application or withholding of a treatment cannot be directly compared. Therefore, instead of studying the effect at the individual level, the researcher can attempt to compare the outcomes at the group level. The objective would be to determine the effect of replacing policy 0 with policy 1 on a summary measure of the distribution of outcomes in a group of individuals. For example, the group might consist of patients with admission for hip fracture surgery, policy 1 could be a requirement to undergo the operation within 48 h of admission, and policy 0 could be *usual* care. The summary measure μ could be the 90th percentile of the distribution of times between admission and the operation.

Suppose, then, that the summary measure μ equals μ_A^1 when policy 1 is applied to group A and that μ equals μ_A^0 when policy 0 is applied to the same group. If the same group were exposed to the two policies, the effect of replacing policy 0 with policy 1 could be thought of as the change in the value of the summary measure μ from μ_A^0 to μ_A^1. The difference $\mu_A^1 - \mu_A^0$ could be thought of as the effect size of applying policy 1 instead of policy 0. In this thought experiment, the difference between μ_A^0 and μ_A^1 is attributed to the policy change, because that is the only possible reason for a difference, given that the patient group is the same. However, the same problem arises as in the thought experiment involving individuals: only one alternative can be administered to one patient group. Therefore, if policy 1 is applied to group A, summary measure μ_A^1 is observable and μ_A^0 will be unobservable.

In real-life evaluations of health care, policy 0 is applied to a different group, group B, for which the summary outcome measure μ will equal μ_B^0. If μ_A^0 is expected to equal μ_B^0, then the difference $\mu_A^1 - \mu_B^0$ can be used to estimate the effect $\mu_A^1 - \mu_A^0$. This approach to estimating an effect has important implications for the interpretation of intervention studies in health services research. If group B differs from group A with respect to the distribution of factors affecting the summary outcome measure μ, then μ_A^0 and μ_B^0 may differ. In this case, substituting μ_B^0 for μ_A^0 will produce a measure of the association between the policy alternatives and outcomes in the two groups, A and B, which will be different from the effects of policy 1 relative to policy 0 in group A [99]. This difference would prevent an inference of causality, since the difference between μ_A^1 and μ_B^0 could be due to differences between the groups that are not related to the intervention.

In practice, researchers attempt to identify a control group B, for which μ_B^0 is known to equal μ_A^0, by using a process of chance to distribute the experimental units from a single population into the study groups. The premise is that all factors potentially responsible for differences between the control and comparison groups will be distributed within the study groups in proportion to their distribution in the population. For example, if policy alternatives are randomly assigned to individuals in a given patient population, then two samples of patients taken from the population should not differ in terms of the distributions of their characteristics. This approach is difficult to implement if the policy change targets an organization because a health care service usually accepts patients from a definitive service area. As such, comparing two service models will require sampling patients from two different populations.

These problems do not arise when computer simulation is used to test a causal hypothesis. As noted by others, simulation experiments satisfy both Mill's requirement of identical instances and the requirement of control over factors that could affect the outcome [126]. Indeed, each simulation run starts with a group of experimental units that is statistically indistinguishable, in terms of the distribution of its characteristics, from groups used in other runs. For an experiment involving two simulation runs with identical inputs, except for the intervention (which is applied to just one of the two runs), differences in outcomes will be due to the intervention. An experiment involving multiple simulation runs with various inputs that are identical for both intervention and control runs can be used to determine if the intervention has an effect in the presence of the various inputs. Therefore, computer simulation of the health care intervention will generate evidence about the net effect of the intervention in the ideal (hypothetical) case of two identical experimental groups, only one of which is subject to the intervention.

2.3 Types of Factors

Most health care interventions are characterized by a substantial number of factors, including the characteristics of patients, their conditions, their health care providers, and health care organizations. In the simulation literature, input data and model specifications that are purposely varied in an experiment to determine their influence on an outcome are called experimental factors [92]. We follow this nomenclature tradition and further classify the experimental factors into three groups: primary study factors, environmental factors, and experimental unit attributes. In simulation experiments, primary study factors represent studied interventions, environmental factors represent the setting in which an intervention is implemented, and experimental unit attributes represent the clinical and demographic characteristics of the study population (i.e., patient population).

2.3.1 Primary Study Factors

In a simulation experiment, the researcher attempts to understand differences in outcomes across experimental groups. In Sect. 1.3, we noted that in health care evaluation, study groups could be defined naturally in terms of management alternatives, practice guidelines, prevention programs, service and health care models, and quality improvement initiatives. Within the analytical framework of intervention studies, we used the notion of the study variable to represent the study groups. Similarly, in simulation experiments, we use a notion of the primary study factor to represent experimental groups. An example of the primary study factor is the method of booking surgical consultation appointments. Later in the book, we compare three booking methods: assigning patients to a pooled list, assigning them to individual lists for specific surgeons, and assigning them to the shortest available list (see Chap. 14). The purpose of this comparison is to estimate the effect of booking method on the flow of patients from referral to consultation and from consultation to surgery in the context of cardiac surgical services. The method of booking appointments could be represented by a primary study factor that takes on the value 1 for the individual lists, 2 for the pooled list, and 3 for the shortest list. It is common to use a set of two indicator variables for the primary study factor that identifies three experimental groups. These variables take a value of 0 to represent the reference group (see Sect. 7.4).

2.3.2 Environmental Factors

In general, environmental factors are input parameters for the model that contain information external to the simulated experimental units. Specifications of a simulation model usually include features of hospital operations that influence the process of care, such as allocation of operating room slots. For example, in a simple case, the slots are divided between elective and urgent procedures either daily or weekly. The model specifications may also include a set of rules controlling the sequence of activities and the progression of experimental units (patients) through care steps.

If the rules are subject to variation within the experiment, the set of rules becomes an environmental factor. This approach allows the researcher to include realistic characteristics of hospital processes, such as algorithms for scheduling consultations and booking admissions, which in turn will allow the simulation results to be applied to other surgical services. When entered in the form of environmental factors, these hospital-level variables could influence the outcome of a simulation experiment. Therefore, an analysis that accounts for variation in environmental factors would allow the estimation of the independent effect of the primary study factor. We discuss the statistical techniques of adjusting for environmental factors in Chaps. 11 and 12.

2.3.3 Attributes of Experimental Units

Patient-level factors constitute the third group of experimental factors discussed in this book. Usually, at entry into a simulation run, the experimental units representing patients are assigned attributes that would influence their progress through the process of care: age, sex, severity of disease, coexisting medical conditions, and urgency of the need for treatment [45]. As in clinical decision-making, these attributes are important for selecting the pathways of care in simulation runs. For example, they may influence the choice of treatment modality or designation of priority through a triage procedure. Patient attributes also trigger simulation events whose occurrence is modeled through random sampling rather than a fully described mechanism. Worsening of symptoms, preoperative death, need for intensive care treatment, or cancellation of a scheduled procedure occur in simulation runs with frequencies that correspond to the risk of these events, where risk is determined by the patients' attributes. For example, elderly people are at substantial risk of postoperative complications and need for intensive care.

Assessment of patients' clinical factors before surgical procedures usually accurately predicts their postoperative trajectories. For example, a variety of scoring algorithms have been developed to evaluate the risk of postoperative death among patients who undergo coronary artery bypass surgery. Surgeons use such algorithms to score the individual clinical characteristics of both the patient and the condition at the time of surgical consultation (see Table 2.1). They sum the scores to obtain the patient's total score [118]. The risk of postoperative death is then related to the total score. One scoring scale, which ranges from 0 to 18, uses a baseline of younger male patients with single-vessel disease and without major coexisting conditions (score 0, risk 0.2%). According to this scale, a patient with an intermediate score 8 would be 9 times as likely to die after the operation (risk 1.8%). In the simulation experiment, this relation between risk of death and characteristics of the patient and the disease can be used to trigger the occurrence of postoperative death.

Table 2.1 Scores for preoperative assessment of patients undergoing coronary artery bypass surgery [118]

Patient or disease characteristic	Score
Age 60–69 years	1.5
Age 70–79 years	2.5
Age ≥80 years	6.5
Female sex	2.0
Ejection fraction <40%	2.0
Three-vessel disease	1.5
Left main stenosis 50–89%	1.5
Left main stenosis ≥90%	2.0
White blood cells >12,000/μL	2.5
Myocardial infarction within a week	1.5
Urgent surgery	2.0
Emergency surgery	5.0
Prior heart surgery	2.5
Peripheral vascular disease	1.5
Diabetes mellitus	1.0
Dialysis	4.0
Creatinine >2.0 mg/dL	2.0
Chronic obstructive pulmonary disease	2.0

2.4 Types of Outcomes

In Sect. 1.3, we discussed outcome variables representing the responses of patients, treatments, and health systems to interventions. These variables provide information about the effects of an intervention that are end points of interest in health care delivery. Similarly, the output data of simulation experiments can be studied in terms of events related to simulated patients and services (see Sect. 6.7). In simulation studies conducted for health care evaluations, experimental outcomes are classified into three types: those related to the simulated patients, those related to simulated treatment, and those related to simulated systems of care delivery. Patient-related outcomes are output data that reflect the effect on simulated patients who are undergoing treatment in the simulated health care system. Treatment-related outcomes are output data that reflect the intended and unintended medical effects of the process of care. System-related outcomes are output data that reflect the effect on the health care system of delivering care to a group of simulated patients. Like experimental factors, experimental outcomes can be used to operationalize the study question for a simulation experiment into a statistical hypothesis. From a statistical perspective, an experimental outcome is a dependent variable whose distribution is conditional on the value of an experimental factor (see Sect. 1.5). Also like experimental factors, experimental outcomes can be either quantitative or qualitative. In the example of surgical consultation appointments in Sect. 2.3, the effects of the booking methods on the patient flow are evaluated in terms of clearance time for appointment lists, time to appointment, and time to surgery.

2.5 Reporting Results

Evidence-based medicine has been advanced by the development and application of standards for reporting the design and methodology of randomized trials. The rationale for an experiment, as well as its circumstances and methodological details, helps researchers to understand and interpret its findings. Indeed, without a transparent and complete description of the methods used in a particular study, it is difficult to assess the quality of evidence that it produces. In addition, inconsistency in reporting the summary outcome measure and the effect-size measure prevents placement of the reported results in the context of other findings in the field [89].

Recently, a group of scientists concerned about the lack of uniformity in the reporting of health care interventions developed the Consolidated Standards of Reporting Trials (CONSORT) [132]. They have argued that proper reporting allows the reader to understand the design, conduct, and analysis of a trial, as well as to assess the validity of its results. These standards represent a template for authors to prepare reports of trial findings, facilitating complete and transparent reporting of medical research and aiding in the critical appraisal and interpretation of such reports. The group maintains a web site where periodic updates of its recommendations are made available (www.consort-statement.org). An increasing number of journals in health services research require that submissions adhere to these standards as a way to improve the quality of reporting.

The CONSORT statement includes recommendations for reporting randomized trials, in which patients are randomly assigned to receive certain health care interventions. As discussed in Chap. 1, groups of patients in cluster randomized trials are assigned to receive interventions provided by distinct organizations (e.g., hospitals, surgical services). An extension of the recommendations for cluster randomized trials has now been developed to address the main concern related to the design, analysis, and interpretation of such trials: the discrepancy between units for allocation and units for analysis [33]. In particular, it is recommended that reports of these trials account for clustering in the rationale, study design, and evaluation; report how clustering effects are incorporated into the determination of sample size; report how clustering is incorporated into the analysis of data; and describe the flow of clusters and experimental units through the trial.

The UK Medical Research Council has suggested that reporting of simulation experiments should be included in a detailed description of health care evaluations to enable replication and evidence synthesis and to guide implementation [40]. In our experience, complete transparency in reporting on the use of computer simulation in health care evaluations helps the reader to reflect on the conceptual challenges posed by modeling a health system's operations. We present examples of what should be reported from a simulation study in relation to the health care question, the methods, and the results (see Chap. 10). Throughout the book, we use multiple case studies to illustrate how to report on the design and analysis of simulation studies comparing policy and management alternatives.

Chapter 3
Framing the Process of Care

In Chap. 1, we introduced common clinical and managerial activities involved in the delivery of surgical care. In this chapter, we describe in detail the activities occurring in tertiary care hospitals that provide cardiac surgical care to adult patients. We focus on this type of surgical care because it is well structured and is thus amenable to study and improvement. In particular, we present a taxonomy that classifies the possible variants of perioperative activities across health care facilities. We also introduce a perspective of surgical care in which the delivery of care is understood as a reactive system.

3.1 Functional View

A common approach to describing the process of care is based on the functional view of activities within the health care system. This view includes specifications of activities required to achieve the functions of the system, the inputs and outputs of those activities, and the sequences of actions within each activity. Organized in chronological order, these activities outline the steps taken in delivering surgical treatment to a patient population. For example, the process of surgical care can be described by the activities that take place during the diagnostic, preoperative, operative, and postoperative stages of care delivery.

Figure 3.1 depicts the clinical and managerial activities typically occurring in the delivery of cardiac surgical care. The primary care physician refers any patient who presents with signs and symptoms that are amenable to cardiac surgical intervention to a specialist. If, following an outpatient consultation, surgery is deemed necessary, a clerk in the surgeon's office registers the patient on an appropriate wait list and sends a request for operating room time to hospitals where the surgeon has admitting privileges.

The patient is then booked for a presurgical assessment at the preadmission clinic, where an anesthesiologist evaluates the patient's suitability for surgery and

B. Sobolev et al., *Health Care Evaluation Using Computer Simulation: Concepts, Methods, and Applications*, DOI 10.1007/978-1-4614-2233-4_3,

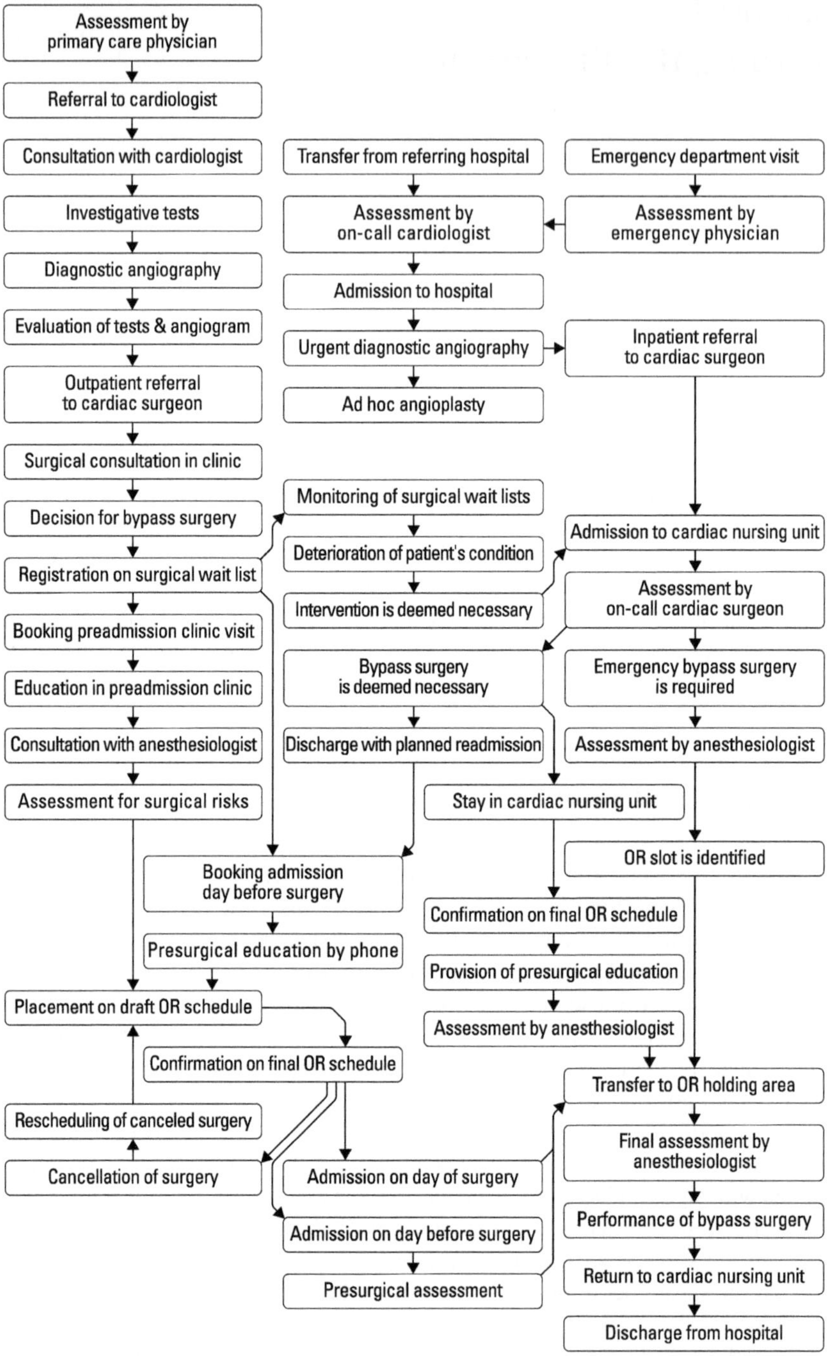

Fig. 3.1 Clinical and managerial activities constituting the process of cardiac surgical care (OR = operating room)

creates a care plan for the preoperative and postoperative stages [63]. The procedure is postponed if the patient is deemed unfit for any reason during the assessment. If necessary, the patient undergoes additional preoperative investigations for assessment of surgical risks. Clinic staff members provide education about the procedure and any preparation that will be required at home.

Each patient's access to surgery is managed through the scheduling of operating room time [20]. Patients are selected for scheduling both from hospital wards and from the surgical wait lists. Patients may be admitted to the hospital through the emergency department, the same-day admission clinic, or the admitting office. Surgical scheduling staff identify the patients who are available for time slots in the operating room that have been assigned to a particular surgeon. The staff also reserve hospital resources to ensure appropriate treatment of the patient during and after the operation [67].

The time slots in the operating room to which patients are matched during the scheduling process are determined through another process. To coordinate utilization of resources in the surgical suite, hospitals periodically release blocks of operating room time to various surgical services, including cardiac surgical services. Each service then books elective procedures, with some operative slots set aside for emergency cases [97]. Any operating time that is not booked by a particular service is made available to other services. Patients are booked for their operations on the basis of urgency, best use of allocated operating time, availability of hospital resources, and the plan for discharge from the hospital. Once set, the schedule may be changed to accommodate the needs of emergency patients, who receive preferential treatment.

3.2 Taxonomy of Activities

As is typical for a social system, the delivery of care may take various forms in different settings. A taxonomy is therefore necessary to contrast the perioperative activities within a uniform framework of knowledge. Later in this book, we use this taxonomy to develop a data model for representing the progress of patients through the perioperative process and to define requirements for simulation models (see Chap. 13). In developing our taxonomy, we identified and classified clinical and managerial activities occurring during the diagnostic, preoperative, operative, and postoperative stages of cardiac surgical care. Additionally, we identified managerial activities concerned with the allocation of resources. We focused on the three care paths following angiography that patients with established coronary artery disease are likely to experience, according to their initial presentation and subsequent decisions leading to surgery: elective, inpatient, and emergency [142]. The elective path applies to patients for whom surgical consultation and subsequent operation can safely be delayed. The inpatient path applies to patients admitted to hospital directly from the catheterization laboratory because of a need for urgent surgical

Box 3.1 Care steps in cardiac surgical care identified from the literature

1 Referral to cardiologist
2 Request for investigative tests and angiography
3 Consultation with cardiologist
4 Referral to cardiac surgeon
5 Booking of outpatient consultation appointments with cardiac surgeon
6 Investigation and ordering of tests by cardiac surgeon
7 Consultation with cardiac surgeon and decision for surgery
8 Booking of elective surgery
9 Registration of patients needing elective surgery on surgical wait list
10 Processing of inpatient referrals
11 Registration of inpatients in surgical queue
12 Preoperative assessment of patients in preadmission clinic
13 Scheduling of consultation with anesthesiologist
14 Consultation with anesthesiologist and patient education
15 Preoperative assessment of inpatients
16 Booking of operating room for elective and inpatient operations
17 Rescheduling of cancellations
18 Admission of emergency patients
19 Discharge planning
20 Surgery
21 Postoperative care in cardiac surgery intensive care unit
22 Postoperative care in hospital ward
23 Discharge from hospital

assessment; in this situation, the patient's condition may necessitate a stay in hospital to have the operation before discharge. The emergency path applies to patients requiring surgical intervention within hours to avoid unnecessary morbidity or death.

Before mapping the processes of surgical care within a cardiac service program, we searched the literature for previous descriptions of the steps in cardiac surgical care, as summarized in Box 3.1 [36, 42]. We then identified commonalities in perioperative activities, by interviewing care providers and mapping processes, at the four tertiary care hospitals that provide cardiac surgical care to adult residents of British Columbia, Canada [142]. We performed structured interviews and on-site meetings at the four hospitals to gain insight into commonalities and variations in perioperative processes. Using a standardized questionnaire, we interviewed individuals from the following groups:

- Specialists: Cardiac surgeons, cardiologists, anesthesiologists, emergency physicians
- Nurses: Clinical nurse specialists (cardiac surgery), cardiac nurses in the preadmission clinic, coordinator of the provincial patient registry
- Hospital and health care managers: Staff in the surgeon's office and the cardiac catheterization laboratory, patient care administrators, operating room clerks

We also collected and analyzed a variety of hospital documents related to the delivery of surgical care, such as practice guidelines, policies, procedures, technical documentation, flow charts, reports, planned care orders, triage and acuity scales, clinical care paths, and booking forms.

This information provided an evidence base for our taxonomy of perioperative activities. We focused on the following episodes of cardiac surgical care: referral to a specialist, booking of the surgical consultation appointment, outpatient surgical consultation, investigation and tests, decision for surgery, registration on a priority wait list, presurgical screening, anesthesiology consultation, booking of operating room time, resource allocation, cancellations, admission to hospital, final presurgical assessment, the operation, postsurgical recovery, intensive care treatment, stay and treatment in a hospital ward, discharge planning, and discharge from hospital [163].

3.3 Diagnostic Stage

The clinical and managerial activities at the diagnostic stage, including variants across care facilities, are tabulated in Table 3.1.

3.3.1 Referring Patients to a Cardiologist

General physicians or specialists refer patients to cardiologists, who request tests and assess whether a diagnostic catheterization procedure, also referred to as angiography, is required. Angiography is used to find points of narrowing or blockage of the arteries that supply blood to the heart muscle. If the patient seems to have coronary artery disease, the cardiologist orders the diagnostic catheterization, which is performed in a cardiac catheterization laboratory. Using the angiogram and the results of other tests, the cardiologist then makes the decision to refer the patient to a cardiac surgeon or to admit the patient for immediate operation by a cardiac surgeon.

3.3.2 Processing Outpatient Referrals

The elective pathway for patient care starts with referral for an appointment with a surgeon in the outpatient clinic or the hospital. The sex, age, coronary anatomy affected, and comorbidities of all referred patients are registered in the clinic's chart or in the hospital's patient information system. Referred patients join the appointment list with an appointment priority (high or low), which is assigned according to the urgency of each patient's need for consultation. During the outpatient consultation, the surgeon assesses the patient's indication for the

Table 3.1 Taxonomy of clinical and managerial activities at the diagnostic stage of cardiac surgical care

		Function	
Activity	Steps	Variant 1	Variant 2
Referring patients to a cardiologist	Request for referral	Patients are referred to cardiologist by specialist or general physician	
	Request for investigative tests	Cardiologist requests tests and assesses whether angiography is required	
	Request for diagnostic catheterization	If coronary artery disease is suspected, cardiologist requests angiography, to be performed in cardiac catheterization laboratory	
	Consultation with cardiologist	A treatment modality is recommended, and referral to a cardiac surgeon is submitted	Cardiologist makes treatment decision in cardiac catheterization laboratory and consults with an on-call cardiac surgeon in the laboratory's recovery area; if decision is to admit and operate, the cardiologist calls the cardiac regional coordinator

Processing outpatient referrals	Request for referral	Patients presenting with symptoms are sent for consultation with cardiac surgeon in outpatient clinic or office	Patients presenting with symptoms are sent for consultation with cardiac surgeon in hospital
	Receipt and documentation of referral information by fax, phone, or mail	Sex, age, coronary anatomy affected, and comorbidity of each referred patient are registered in patient chart in clinic or office	Sex, age, coronary anatomy affected, and comorbidity of each referred patient are registered in hospital's patient information system
	Registering elective patients on appointment list*	Individual appointment lists: consultations are booked with the cardiac surgeon named in the referral	Pooled appointment list: consultations are booked with the first available cardiac surgeon
	Booking elective patients for appointment	Date of an appointment is determined	
	Surgical outpatient consultation	Indication for operation is assessed, and need for further tests is determined in clinic (by cardiac surgeon)	Indication for operation is assessed, and need for further tests is determined in hospital (by cardiac surgeon)

*We identified a third variant for this step. Shortest appointment list: Patients are placed on the appointment list of the cardiac surgeon with the fewest patients waiting operation and determines if the patient needs further tests. There are three methods of booking appointments for these consultations, which take place in an outpatient clinic: The individual-list, pooled-list, and shortest-list methods. With individual appointment lists, each consultation is booked with the surgeon named in the referral. With a pooled appointment list, each consultation is scheduled with the first available surgeon. With the shortest-list method, a patient is placed on the appointment list of the surgeon with the fewest patients waiting. With all three methods, a patient with higher priority will be booked for an appointment ahead of those with lower priority. Patients with the same priority are scheduled on a first-come, first-served basis.

3.4 Preoperative Stage

The clinical and managerial activities at the preoperative stage, including variants across care facilities, are tabulated in Table 3.2.

3.4.1 Booking Elective Surgery

Once it has been determined that surgery is necessary, the surgeon registers on his or her individual surgical wait list the patients who have decided to undergo the operation. A level of priority is assigned to each patient according to the urgency of the need for surgery. There are two methods of booking patients for elective surgery: wait-list booking and advance booking. With wait-list booking, each patient is assigned a priority and is placed on the surgical list of the surgeon with whom he or she had the initial consultation appointment, without a projected date of operation. The surgical wait list stores information about the patient until the operation can be scheduled. Booking of the operation for each patient is attempted periodically until an appropriate operating room slot becomes available. Patients with higher priority for elective surgery are scheduled for operation ahead of those with lower priority, and patients with the same priority are scheduled on a first-come, first-served basis. With advance booking, patients awaiting elective surgery are registered on surgical wait lists with a projected date of operation. This date is the date of the next available operating room slot assigned to the consulting surgeon on the projected operating room schedule for the 36-week period after the clinic appointment. With this system of booking, patients are also assigned a date for a presurgical assessment at the preadmission clinic. The date of the presurgical assessment is the date of the next available preadmission clinic slot within the 3-week period before the projected date of surgery.

Table 3.2 Taxonomy of clinical and managerial activities at the preoperative stage of cardiac surgical care

		Function	
Activity	Steps	Variant 1	Variant 2
Booking elective surgery	Registration of elective patients on surgical wait list	Details of patients who require and decide to undergo the operation are registered with booking office	
	Booking patients for operation	Wait-list booking: approximate dates of operation and preoperative assessment are determined	Advance booking: committed dates of operation within the upcoming 36-week period and dates for preoperative assessment in PAC are determined
Processing of inpatient referrals	Notification of surgeons about request for inpatient referrals	Patients requiring urgent in-hospital assessment after angiography are referred to surgeon (by cardiologist); surgeon accepts referral	
	Surgical consultation with inpatients	On-call surgeon determines inpatients' suitability for surgery	
Booking inpatient referrals for surgery	Registration of inpatients on surgical queue	Details of patients who must undergo operation and who are admitted directly to hospital are registered with booking office	

(continued)

Table 3.2 (continued)

		Function	
Activity	Steps	Variant 1	Variant 2
	Booking of inpatients for operation	Committed slots for operating time within the upcoming week (or 2 weeks) are determined	
	Fast-tracking of patients who live far away	Patients who live far away from hospital are admitted for angiography, stay in hospital to undergo tests, and are booked for surgery or discharged with planned admission	
Scheduling OR slots	Weekly scheduling of OR time for the coming week by agreement among OR teams	Inpatients and elective patients waiting for operation are identified, and hospital resources are reserved, with the sickest patients being booked first	Inpatients and elective patients waiting for operation are identified, and hospital resources are reserved, with a certain percentage of elective patients being booked first
	Daily publication of OR schedule	Final OR schedule is created and published by 2 pm on the day before surgery	
	Changes to the published OR schedule	Patients requiring urgent operation are booked for procedure, and OR slots for previously scheduled patients are canceled and rebooked	

Canceling scheduled operations	Cancellation of scheduled operations by emergency arrivals	Emergency patients requiring immediate operation replace previously scheduled outpatients and inpatients in OR schedule; canceled procedures are rebooked within a couple of days	
	Cancellation of scheduled operations by inpatients	Inpatients who are too sick to go home and who require surgery replace previously scheduled outpatients in the OR schedule; canceled procedures for outpatients are rebooked in urgent slots	
	Cancellation of scheduled operations for patient-related reasons	Book operations for inpatients and outpatients are canceled because of unsuitability for surgery, "no shows," or illness	
	Cancellation of scheduled operations for hospital-related reasons	Scheduled operations are canceled because of staff shortages, unavailability of surgical equipment, or unavailability of postoperative beds	
Rebooking canceled operations	Rebooking of canceled operations	Patients who are waiting for the operation after cancellation of scheduled surgery are identified, and hospital resources are reserved	A small fraction of elective slots and a larger fraction of urgent slots absorb cancellations

(continued)

Table 3.2 (continued)

Activity	Steps	Function Variant 1	Variant 2
Assessing patient preoperatively	Preoperative assessment of patients needing elective surgery	All-screened: all patients are assessed by anesthesiologist in PAC to determine and possibly modify existing health problems and surgical and anesthetic factors that could increase patient's risk of adverse outcomes; patient receives education about the treatment and undergoes screening tests, and care is planned for before, during, and after the hospital stay	Some-screened: an attempt is made to schedule elective patients for a presurgical assessment in PAC within the 3-week period before the projected date of surgery. If this attempt is unsuccessful, patients are assessed by anesthesiologist in hospital one day before surgery to determine and possibly modify existing health problems and surgical and anesthetic factors that could increase patient's risk of adverse outcomes; patient receives education about the treatment and undergoes screening tests, and care is planned for before, during, and after the hospital stay

	In-hospital preoperative assessment of inpatients	Patients are assessed by anesthesiologist in hospital one day before surgery to determine and possibly modify existing health problems and surgical and anesthetic factors that could increase patient's risk of adverse outcomes; patient receives education about the treatment and undergoes screening tests, and care is planned for before, during, and after the hospital stay
	Discharge planning before surgery	Needed postoperative services are determined
Managing wait lists	Audit of wait lists	Names of patients who die, who became inpatients, or who are admitted on an emergency basis while waiting for the operation are removed from surgical waiting lists
	Management of unplanned emergency admissions	Patients whose condition deteriorates while they are waiting for the operation are admitted to hospital as emergency patients or inpatients
	Analysis of patients' queueing behavior	Patients decide not to enter wait list (balking) or leave wait list after being registered (reneging)

Abbreviations: PAC = preadmission clinic, OR = operating room

3.4.2 *Processing Inpatient Referrals and Booking Inpatient Referrals for Surgery*

When urgent assessment is deemed necessary, the patient is admitted to a hospital cardiac ward directly from the catheterization laboratory. If deemed fit for surgery, the patient remains in the hospital until the surgery has been performed. All such inpatients are assessed by the on-call surgeon on the day of arrival. A surgical priority (high or low) is assigned to each patient according to the urgency of his or her need for surgery. Surgery for high-priority patients is booked on the final operating room schedule; surgery for the rest is booked on the draft operating room schedule for the next period. Patients requiring urgent assessment and living far from the hospital are fast-tracked. They are admitted for angiography and stay in the hospital to undergo additional tests. Their surgery is booked in advance, or they are discharged with a planned date of admission. All inpatients undergo preoperative assessment by a hospital anesthesiologist one day before the projected date of surgery.

3.4.3 *Scheduling Operating Room Slots*

With both methods of booking surgery, wait-list booking and advance booking, a draft operating room schedule is generated every Friday and is used as the basis for the final operating room schedule that is created and published by 2 pm on the day before each day on which surgery is scheduled. The draft schedule lists the patients awaiting elective surgery who have been selected from the surgical wait lists and inpatients waiting in hospital wards. Patients placed on the draft list are removed from the surgical wait lists and the inpatient surgical queue. The final operating room schedule may be changed unexpectedly by the arrival of inpatients with more urgent needs or emergency patients, who are given preferential access to operating room slots. This causes the cancellation of previously scheduled operations.

3.4.4 *Canceling Scheduled Operations and Rebooking Canceled Operations*

For a proportion of patients with scheduled operating room time, the procedure is canceled for patient-related reasons, such as unsuitability for surgery (as determined during presurgical assessment), illness, or "no show," or for hospital-related reasons, such as staff shortages, unavailability of surgical equipment, or unavailability of postoperative beds. Scheduled operations for patients awaiting elective procedures may also be canceled by the scheduling of surgery for emergency patients or inpatients with more urgent needs. All patients whose procedures are canceled from the operating room list remain in hospital, and their surgery is rebooked on an inpatient basis.

3.4.5 Assessing Patient Preoperatively

With advance booking, elective patients are assigned a projected date of surgery and a date for presurgical assessment in the preadmission clinic. The date of the presurgical assessment is the date of the next available clinic slot within the 3-week period before the projected date of surgery. There are two methods of booking elective patients for their presurgical assessments: the all-screened method and the some-screened method. With the first of these methods, the all-screened method, all elective patients are scheduled for assessment in the preadmission clinic within the 3-week period before the projected date of surgery. If no clinic slots are available within that period, the date of the surgery is canceled on the projected operating room list and is then rebooked, so a new date for the presurgical assessment can be determined. With the second method, the some-screened method, an attempt is made to schedule elective patients for the presurgical assessment in the preadmission clinic within the 3-week period before the projected date of surgery. However, if no clinic slots are available within that period, the patients are admitted to hospital one day before the projected date of surgery for an in-hospital presurgical assessment. It is anticipated that some of the patients admitted through the some-screened method will require further tests after the in-hospital assessment. In that situation, the surgery is canceled on the final operating room list and is then rebooked to allow for an additional visit to the preadmission clinic according to the some-screened method.

With both methods, some patients awaiting elective surgery may be deemed unfit for the procedure and will require an additional visit to the preadmission clinic after the initial presurgical assessment. In this situation, the surgery is canceled on the projected operating room list and is then rebooked to allow for the additional visit to the preadmission clinic. These additional visits to the preadmission clinic are booked differently for the two methods of scheduling. With the all-screened method, if no slots are available for the additional visit to the preadmission clinic within the 3-week period before the projected date of surgery, the surgery is canceled on the projected operating room list and is then rebooked to allow for the additional visit. With the some-screened method, if no slots are available for the additional visit to the preadmission clinic within the 3-week period before the projected date of surgery, the patient is admitted to hospital one day before the projected date of surgery for an in-hospital presurgical assessment.

3.4.6 Managing Wait Lists

A certain proportion of patients in the elective pathway may decide not to join the surgical wait list. In addition, a certain proportion of patients waiting for operating room time to be scheduled for their elective procedures will be removed from the wait list because of death or deterioration of their condition or because they have decided to leave the list. Patients removed from the surgical wait list because of deterioration in their condition may be admitted to hospital on an emergency or inpatient basis. The decision to admit a patient on an emergency or inpatient basis is made by the hospital's coordinator of cardiac services. Patients originally in the elective pathway who are admitted to hospital as emergency patients are booked for surgery in the final operating room schedule after their admission, which may cause the cancellation of a previously booked case. Patients originally in the elective pathway who are admitted to hospital as inpatients are placed on the surgical wait list and are booked for surgery in the draft operating room schedule.

3.5 Operative Stage

Patients whose surgery has been booked on the final operating room schedule undergo their procedures, during which time they have access to operating room resources. After the surgery, they have access to postoperative services, which are determined and planned before the surgery takes place; see below. The clinical and managerial activities at the operative stage are tabulated in Table 3.3.

3.6 Postoperative Stage

The clinical and managerial activities at the postoperative stage, including variants across care facilities, are tabulated in Table 3.3.

3.6.1 Providing Intensive Care

After the surgery, patients are admitted to the cardiac surgery intensive care unit for recovery and for monitoring and treatment of any adverse effects of the anesthesia. This unit has a number of beds reserved for patients who have undergone cardiac surgery. In addition, a limited number of beds from the main hospital intensive care unit may be used for emergency patients who have undergone cardiac surgery, if no beds are available in the cardiac surgery intensive care unit.

3.6.2 Discharging Patients to the Ward and Managing Patients on the Ward

After recovery in the cardiac surgery intensive care unit, the patient's pain is assessed. Once the pain score has declined to an appropriate level, the patient is discharged to the ward. Patients stay on the ward to recover sufficiently to

Table 3.3 Taxonomy of clinical and managerial activities at the operative and postoperative stages of cardiac surgical care

		Function	
Activity	Steps	Variant 1	Variant 2
Operative stage			
Performing surgery	Surgical procedures	Operation is performed; patients have access to OR resources	
Postoperative stage			
Providing intensive care	Recovery of patients after surgical procedures in CS-ICU or main ICU	Patients undergo monitoring for and treatment of adverse effects of anesthesia; patients recover in the CS-ICU after operation or in a main ICU, if required	
Discharging patients to ward	Discharge of patients from ICU to ward	Assessment for acceptable parameters for transfer to the ward for further recovery	
Managing patients on ward	Further recovery on ward	Patients recover sufficiently to engage in regular daily activities	
	Discharge planning during recovery	Patients are continually reassessed against discharge goals (by multidisciplinary team)	
Discharging patients from hospital	Discharge of patients from hospital	Patients are transferred from hospital premises through pre-arranged transportation	Patients are transferred to another institution for acute care or long-term care

Abbreviations: OR = operating room, CS-ICU = cardiac surgery intensive care unit, ICU = intensive care unit be able to engage in regular daily activities. During recovery, a multidisciplinary team continually assesses patients against the discharge goals and starts discharge planning.

3.6.3 Discharging Patients from Hospital

After recovery in the ward, patients are prepared for postoperative care at home or in rehabilitation or community facilities.

3.7 Resource Allocation

The managerial activities concerned with the allocation of resources, including variants across care facilities, are tabulated in Table 3.4.

Appointment times for consultations are determined on the annual basis according to the surgeons' duty rotation and vacation schedules for the specified time horizon. Each year, the health authority revises and reassesses the annual allocation of available operating room time. The time available for surgery is determined by government funding for this procedure, which reflects population-based target rates. The available operating room slots are distributed to surgeons equally or according to the size of the surgeons' respective wait lists.

3.8 Reactive Nature of Surgical Care

As described in the preceding sections, the delivery of surgical services involves multiple concurrent activities and coordination of their outcomes. These activities entail certain functions that are accomplished through a sequence of actions. For instance, scheduling assessment of the patient before surgery requires notifying the nursing staff and the acute pain management service and ensuring the availability of the necessary equipment. Such a functional view regards the care process as a predetermined sequence of well-defined activities or tasks that transform inputs into outputs for achieving clearly defined outcomes. In computer modeling, a transformational system could be represented by a set of rules that specify how the system will evolve from one state to another. Transformational systems also allow tracking their evolution both forward and backward in time.

Some authors have pointed to difficulties with a functional view of the health care system [104]. First, it neglects the uncertainty of outcomes of treatments in patient populations. Second, functional decomposition of care processes ignores dynamic interactions among activities that could change over time or that might result from competition for resources. We also argue that describing care processes according

Table 3.4 Resource allocation activities

		Function	
Activity	Steps	Variant 1	Variant 2
Allocating resources	Annual allocation of appointment slots to surgeons	Appointment times are identified according to surgeons' duty rotation and vacation schedule for a given time horizon	
	Annual allocation of available OR time to surgeons	Available OR slots are equally distributed to surgeons within a service	Available OR slots are distributed to surgeons according to their respective queue sizes
	Revision and reassessment of annual allocation of available OR time, with available time for bypass surgery being determined by government funding, which is in turn based on population-based target rates	Planning of human resources, facilities, revenue, equipment, and supplies according to projected patient need at the hospital or hospital-unit level	

Abbreviation: OR = operating room

to the preestablished functions of agents involved in those processes cannot capture the interactions among activities and between agents and activities. Nonetheless, such a functional description is useful in understanding the structure that supports the process.

A different view of the health care system, the behavioral view, is concerned with conditions and events that trigger the system's activities and the transitions between them. When perioperative activities are autonomous, as in simple temporal sequencing, completion of one activity constitutes the start of the next activity. However, when activities are interacting, certain activities produce events that initiate or disrupt the orderly progress of actions in other concurrent activities. For example, a decision for elective surgery initiates scheduling of the presurgical assessment by an anesthesiologist and scheduling of operating room time, but cancellation of the surgery by the patient at a later stage will necessitate changes in several of these perioperative activities. Conversely, if the patient is deemed unfit for surgery during the final presurgical assessment (because of, say, a pulmonary infection), this information affects other activities, and a new series of actions commences: surgical and intensive care beds become available for another patient, the patient in question may be referred to another specialist, additional diagnostic tests may be ordered, and the operation may be rescheduled.

These examples highlight two particular features of reactive systems on which we will focus in the remainder of this book: hierarchy (i.e., subordination between activities) and interaction of concurrent activities. More specifically, the perioperative process can be abstracted as a reactive system involving various chains of transitions from one state to another. These chains of transitions are interrelated and can affect one another according to the occurrence of certain events under certain conditions such as clinical urgency and bed availability. Instead of presenting a care process as a predictable set of operations transforming inputs into outputs, health care processes can be described through possible interactions that only reveal themselves by behavior that unfolds through time. This would require the identification of events that trigger transitions between the states, the conditions that have to be met before the transitions can occur, the actions associated with the transitions, and temporal logic associated with events and conditions.

In presenting the reactive nature of health care processes, we follow the approach of computer scientist David Harel, who developed a special type of diagram, Statecharts, for describing reactive systems [71]. The Statecharts specification paradigm was originally developed for representing reactive systems by extending the formalism of finite-state machines through notions of hierarchy, parallelism, and event broadcasting. A thorough review of this type of graphical representation is provided in Chap. 5 and 6. In the context of the surgical care, hierarchy provides the means to describe steps within activities and to group related activities, parallelism provides the means to specify concurrent activities, and event broadcasting provides the means to trigger a series of actions in one activity according to transitions that occur in another activity. Combined with hierarchy and parallelism, event broadcasting offers a convenient way to describe the interaction of concurrent activities.

In Chap. 13, we apply the Statecharts formalism to describing the progress of individual patients through surgical care. We modeled the patient's pathway as a series of asynchronous updates in patient records generated in reaction to events produced by parallel finite-state machines representing concurrent clinical and managerial activities. We observe that Statecharts capture successfully the behavioral aspects of surgical care delivery by specifying the permissible chronology of events, conditions, and actions.

Chapter 4
Simulation Models

In Chap. 2, we discussed the idea of using computer simulation in evaluating the effects of proposed changes in the delivery of care before they are implemented in practice. At the core of every simulation experiment is a computer simulation model, a software program that attempts to simulate the proposed changes within a studied system. The program runs multiple times to calculate the likely outcomes for a particular system's configuration from possible histories of modeled entities. In this chapter, we briefly review approaches to constructing simulation models of health care processes, highlighting differences among them in terms of assumptions, system requirements, and input and output data.

4.1 Types of Models

Simulation models abstract the system's functioning as a set of states and transitions among those states. Modeling techniques may be classified according to the nature of the variables representing the state of the modeled process and the nature of their changes over time [92]. In terms of the state variables, simulation models may be classified as deterministic or stochastic. In deterministic models, the state variables at any given time are determined by input parameters, previous states, and a set of rules that specify how the system will evolve from a specific state. Applying these rules to initial states produces a deterministic output of the simulation program. Stochastic models, on the other hand, contain at least one random state variable, so the output is random.

In relation to time, simulation models are classified as static or dynamic. Static simulation models, such as in the Monte Carlo method, use repeated random sampling to estimate the likely state of the modeled process at a particular point in time. In contrast, dynamic simulation models represent the processes as they evolve over time. Depending on how their state variables change over time, dynamic models are further classified as involving discrete or continuous time.

B. Sobolev et al., *Health Care Evaluation Using Computer Simulation: Concepts, Methods, and Applications*, DOI 10.1007/978-1-4614-2233-4_4,

In discrete-time models, the state variables change their values only when time jumps over distinct points, whereas in continuous-time models, the state variables change continuously over time.

Dynamic simulation models may be either deterministic or stochastic. For example, the system dynamics approach represents aggregated patient flow as deterministic, continuous-time changes in the population size of a system's states. On the other hand, Markov models define aggregated patient flow by transition probabilities among states. One limitation of these two types of models is the impossibility of describing interactions involving concurrent activities [148]. It has been argued that discrete-event models are especially appropriate for simulation in health care because patients are subject to multiple concurrent processes [60]. By simulating interactions between the processes that advance patients through the health care system, these models represent reality more closely than models in which moving between states is governed by predefined deterministic or probabilistic rules.

In the discrete-event approach, the system's functioning is represented by transitions among states occurring when certain events take place [9]. In time-driven models, regular advances of the simulation clock synchronize these transitions, whereas in event-driven models, events trigger transitions asynchronously [46]. Two approaches to constructing event-driven models are common in health care applications. The first approach, known as event scheduling, identifies the moments when events occur from predefined distributions of times, whereas the second approach, called process interaction, specifies the sequence and chronology of actions associated with such events. In essence, the discrete-event approach models a process as an assemblage of concurrent activities. As a result, discrete-event models are considered especially appropriate for simulation in health care, and numerous case studies have been reported in the literature [84]. Taking it one step further, the agent-based simulation models represent processes through behavioral specifications for individual agents and the rules for their interactions across concurrent activities [135].

4.2 Monte Carlo Simulation

A Monte Carlo model is a type of static model that uses a sequence of random numbers to generate a sample of observations from a known probability distribution associated with a source of uncertainty [128]. In fact, the Monte Carlo method is a software implementation for the experiments involving the pinball box that we discuss in Chap. 2. Instead of dropping and collecting small ball bearings that bounce off a set of nails, Monte Carlo models execute computational algorithms that implement repeated random sampling to produce all possible outcomes of the modeled process under different configurations. Appropriate summary measures of the outcome distribution are then used to estimate the likely outcome and to evaluate the effect size of replacing one configuration of the process with another. The Monte Carlo simulation usually proceeds according to the following steps:

- Choice of the study outcome of the process
- Identification of configurations of input variables to the process
- Random generation of inputs according to a specified probability distribution
- Evaluation of the process by means of deterministic computation based on the inputs
- Aggregation of the results of individual computations to summarize the study outcome

In the context of health care, Monte Carlo models are frequently used to evaluate interventions when there is a need to model a large number of states whose characteristics cannot be simplified into a small number of states [116]. Examples might include evaluating a strategy for allocation of resources in operating and recovery rooms to reduce wait times [90, 131] and evaluating the effectiveness of health care strategies that require description of patients' trajectories over extended periods of time [78].

4.3 System Dynamics

System dynamics is a methodology for modeling and analyzing the behavior of complex systems over time. This methodology is based on two principles: first, that the behavior of complex systems results from the accumulation of flows into stocks and feedback and, second, that only the study of the whole system, in terms of the accumulation and feedback mechanisms, will lead to correct understanding of the system's behavior [61]. In the context of modeling, a stock is a variable that accumulates or depletes over time, and a flow is the rate of change in a stock, measured over an interval of time. Feedback refers to a situation in which the behavior of process A affects the behavior of process B, which in turn affects the behavior of process A, possibly originating a circle of cause and effect.

The system dynamics methodology consists of the following main steps:

- Identification of a problem
- Development of a diagrammatic description of the system, with a focus on the problem
- Development of a hypothesis explaining the cause of the problem
- Identification of alternative policies to solve the problem
- Development of a computer simulation model of the system, also with a focus on the problem
- Testing of the alternative policies to identify a solution
- Implementation of the solution

Two of the most important steps in creating a system dynamics model are the development of the diagrammatic description of the system, also called a system dynamics diagram, and the derivation of a set of equations describing individual mechanisms. Together, a system dynamics diagram and the corresponding set of equations aid in understanding the system's behavior in terms of feedback mechanisms, accumulation of flows into stocks, and time delays.

4.3.1 Representation of Stocks, Flows, and Feedback

In a system dynamics diagram, each stock is represented by a rectangle labeled with the variable's name, and each flow is represented by a double arrow with a valve connecting two stocks. Feedback mechanisms are represented by causal loop diagrams, which consist of nodes and arrows. The nodes represent variables within the system that change in value over time, and the arrows represent relations and interactions between and among these variables. A set of rules may be associated with each arrow to formalize these interactions. If the causal relation between variables results in a change in their values, then the relevant arrow is labeled with a plus sign (+) for an increment or a minus sign (−) for a decrement. Similarly, positive reinforcement in a loop (through an increment) is represented by a small arrow labeled R (for reinforcement), whereas negative reinforcement in a loop (through a decrement) is represented by a small arrow labeled B (for balance) [61].

4.3.2 An Example

The applications of system dynamics models in health care include modeling large and complex systems with several subsystems that interact with each other to efficiently utilize health care resources and provide on-time delivery of health care [31, 44, 76, 150]. To illustrate the use of system dynamics diagrams in modeling health care services, consider the simple process of booking surgeries for patients registered on a wait list. To keep the diagram simple, assume that only one surgeon is available to perform the surgical procedures and that no new patients can be registered on the wait list. A possible system dynamics diagram of this process is depicted in Fig. 4.1.

In this diagram, there are two stocks (patients waiting and patients whose surgery has been booked) and two nodes (the booking rate and the surgeon's workload). A series of arrows depicts the relations between stocks and nodes. The arrow labeled with a plus sign that connects the stock of patients waiting and the node for booking rate is governed by the rule `book patients` and indicates that as more patients are booked for surgery, the booking rate increases. Booking patients for surgery increases the stock of patients with surgery booked, so a double arrow with a valve (across the top of the diagram) depicts the flow of patients in the diagram: for every new patient whose surgery is booked, the stock of patients waiting declines by one and the stock of patients with surgery booked increases by one. As the stock of patients with surgery booked increases, so does the surgeon's

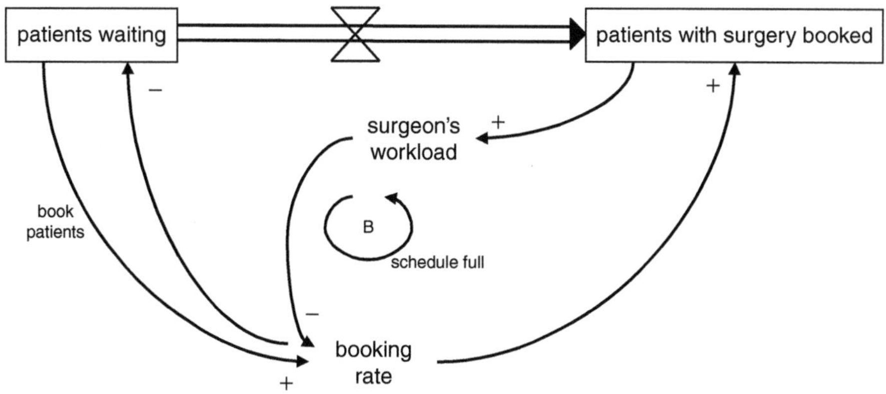

Fig. 4.1 System dynamics diagram of a process of booking surgery for patients registered on a wait list for surgery (see text in Sect. 4.3 for full explanation of the symbols used in this diagram)

workload. However, because of the surgeon's finite capacity to perform procedures, the surgeon's schedule may eventually become full, at which point the booking rate decreases. This feedback mechanism is depicted by an arrow labeled with a minus sign, which connects the nodes for surgeon's workload and booking rate. The negative reinforcement, or balance, in this loop is depicted by a smaller arrow labeled `B`, with the rule `schedule full` governing this mechanism and appearing as a nearby label. Finally, as the booking rate increases, the stock of patients waiting decreases, which is depicted by an arrow labeled with a minus sign that connects the node for booking rate and the stock of patients waiting.

4.4 Markov Models

A Markov model is a type of stochastic model that represents the various states of a system through time. Markov models are based on the concept of a Markov process, which generates random transitions among states according to certain probabilities. Markov processes are distinguished by a lack of memory, such that the conditional probability distribution of future states depends only on the present state and not on the history leading to the present state [146]. Schematically, Markov models are represented by state-transition diagrams, in which circles represent the various states of the process, arrows represent the transitions between states, and labels placed next to the arrows indicate the transition probabilities. Changes in the value of variables (or of outputs generated during the process) may also be indicated by labels placed next to the transition arrows where the change in value or output is expected to occur. The time horizon of a Markov model is usually divided into equal increments, called cycles, during which transitions from one state to another may occur.

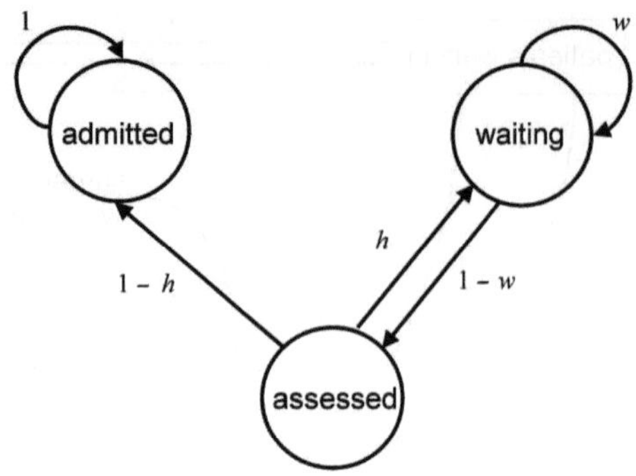

Fig. 4.2 Markov state-transition diagram of patient flow in a triage process with three states, where labels for arrows indicate transition probabilities between states (see text in Sect. 4.4 for full explanation of the symbols used in this diagram)

Mathematically, a Markov model with a discrete set of states is described by a Markov chain, which consists of the following elements [12]:

- A vector $\boldsymbol{S} = \{1, 2, 3, \ldots, M\}$ containing a set of M states
- An $M \times M$ matrix $\boldsymbol{T}$, in which entry (i, j) is the transition probability from state i to state j
- A vector $\boldsymbol{O} = \{o_1, o_2, o_3, \ldots, o_N\}$ containing a set of N possible outputs
- An $M \times N$ matrix $\boldsymbol{E}$, in which entry (i, k) is the probability of output o_k, given state i

To illustrate the application of Markov models in the health care setting, consider the flow of patients during triage in a hospital. Triage is the process by which a patient is assessed upon arrival to determine the urgency of his or her problem and to designate appropriate health care resources to address the problem [53]. Important events of a triage process include arrival, registration, initial assessment, physical examination, initial diagnostic studies, and documentation. However, many of these events can be more simply represented by one of three states: *waiting*, *assessed*, and *admitted*. This simplification of events into a reduced number of states is a characteristic feature of Markov models.

Figure 4.2 shows the state-transition diagram for patients in this triage process. In this example, only certain transitions are allowed. For example, a patient in the *assessed* state may be admitted to the hospital, at which point the patient makes a transition to the *admitted* state. However, a patient in the *admitted* state cannot make a transition to any other state. An arrow leading from one state to itself signifies that the patient may remain in that state in consecutive cycles. The labels placed next to the arrows indicate the transition probabilities. For example, a patient in the *assessed* state may make a transition to the *admitted* state with a probability of $1 - h$, or back to the *waiting* state with a probability of h. This example illustrates how Markov models represent aggregated patient flow, as the transition probabilities for specific patients do not appear in Fig. 4.2.

The Markov chain corresponding to the state-transition diagram depicted in Fig. 4.2 is defined as follows: $\boldsymbol{S} = \{1, 2, 3\}$, where state 1 = *waiting*, state 2 = *assessed*, and state 3 = *admitted*. The corresponding transition matrix is as follows:

$$\boldsymbol{T} = \begin{pmatrix} w & 1-w & 0 \\ h & 0 & 1-h \\ 0 & 0 & 1 \end{pmatrix},$$

where w and h represent the transition probabilities. Because no outputs are generated during the process depicted in Fig. 4.2, there is no vector $\boldsymbol{O}$ or matrix $\boldsymbol{E}$.

4.5 Discrete-Event Simulation

Discrete-event models represent a system's behavior in response to events that have been generated within its states or that have taken place outside of the system [9]. In such models, time advances in discrete increments rather than continuously, and transitions among states occur only at these discrete points in time. There are two main approaches to controlling the advancement of time in a discrete-event model [117]. In the first approach, the time-driven approach, time advances in preset intervals. In the second approach, the event-driven approach, time advances from event to event, with variable intervals between events. Because states remain constant between events in these models, it is not necessary to account for the inactive periods of time between events. Therefore, the event-driven approach is the most commonly used approach to control the flow of time. With this approach, once all state transitions have been completed at the point in time corresponding to a particular event, time is advanced to the point of the next event, and that event is executed. The procedure is then repeated for the duration of the simulation.

In the context of health care, discrete-event models offer the means to represent a process as an assemblage of concurrent activities involving entities (e.g., patients or caregivers) that receive actions. As a result, discrete-event models are considered especially appropriate for simulation of health care processes. For example, these models are well suited to evaluating management and policy alternatives for managing patient flow through a system [81], evaluating alternative interventions in terms of the health outcomes and costs of providing health care services to the population [34], modeling the dynamics of emergency departments and their available resources [4,7,50], studying perioperative processes [147], and comparing methods of booking surgery [10, 133].

4.5.1 *Concepts of Discrete-Event Models*

The following represent the main concepts in discrete-event modeling:

- Clock: The clock variable controls the advancement of time during the simulation.
- State: A state is the set of variables that describes the modeled system at a particular point in time.

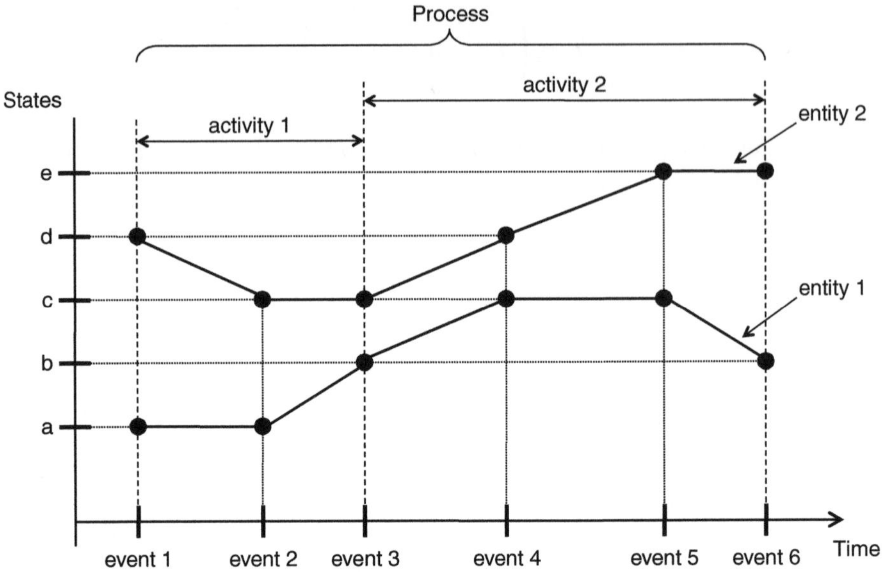

Fig. 4.3 States, entities, events, activities, and processes in a discrete-event model comprising five states, six events, two activities, and two entities

- Entity: An entity is a modeled component of the system, which has attributes; for example, age and sex are two possible attributes of a patient entity.
- Event: An event is an observed occurrence, which triggers a change in the state of the system.
- Event list: The event list contains the pending events that are to be executed. Each event in the list is connected to a specific entity or state. The list of pending events is usually sorted by the timing of events [57].
- Activity: An activity is represented by a set of transitions among states.
- Process: A process is abstracted as a sequence of events ordered in time.

To illustrate these concepts, consider a single process comprising five states, six events, two activities, and two entities (Fig. 4.3). The duration of activity 1 is delimited by events 1 and 3, whereas the duration of activity 2 is delimited by events 3 and 6. The two entities change states during each activity. The events occur at different time intervals (i.e., Fig. 4.3 illustrates the event-driven approach to controlling the flow of time). By tracking back through the set of states for an entity and the corresponding events related to changes of state, it is possible to represent the path that an entity has followed through a process.

4.5.2 Constructing Discrete-Event Models

The ways in which events, activities, and processes relate to each other within the model determine which of three approaches are used in constructing discrete-event models: the event-scheduling approach, the process-interaction approach, or the activity-scanning approach. The event-scheduling approach emphasizes events and their effect on the system. To construct a model using this approach, all events within the system must be identified, along with their occurrence in time. Events are listed in the event list, and the model represents the system as a set of snapshots captured at different time points.

In contrast, the process-interaction approach emphasizes processes and the progress of entities through the system. This approach allows representation of the path that entities follow through various processes from an initial event (usually the arrival event) to a final event (usually the departure event). Models based on this approach specify the chronology of activities associated with events [92]. The activity-scanning approach emphasizes the activities and the conditions governing their execution and termination. Models constructed with this approach advance time in equal increments, and at each time point, activities are started or terminated, provided the required conditions are satisfied [9].

4.6 Agent-Based Models

An agent-based model represents a system as a collection of autonomous decision-making entities called agents. Artificial intelligence techniques are used to allow these agents to select, according to a set of rules, the best set of actions to be performed to reach a goal [24]. Agents exhibit the following features [96]:

- Communication and interactivity: Agents can exchange information, engage in negotiations, and coordinate activities. Synchronization of and communication among agents may be organized in either a discrete-time (synchronous) or continuous-time (asynchronous) fashion.
- Adaptation: Agents can react and adapt to unexpected changes in the simulated environment. They may execute various behaviors appropriate for the system they represent.
- Autonomy: Agents have autonomous and independent behavior.
- Intelligence: Agents are given reasoning, planning, and learning capabilities through the incorporation into the model of neural networks, evolutionary algorithms, or other learning techniques.

In the context of health care, agent-based modeling is especially useful for modeling individual behavior and for implementing distributed problem-solving to tackle complex problems. Individual behavior has a stochastic nature and is characterized by thresholds, if–then rules, adaptation, learning, and memory [135].

For example, the behavior of nurses in an emergency department varies greatly depending on workload, deadlines, and experience with previous cases. The capacity for adaptation, autonomy, and intelligence in agent-based modeling offers an efficient way to model this type of behavior. In terms of problem-solving, health care systems are characterized by complex problems, such as the process of booking patients for appointments or procedures. Distributed problem-solving techniques involve the partitioning of such problems into smaller subproblems, the distribution of different tasks among agents, the exchange of information, and the combination of partial results into a final solution.

4.7 Choice of Modeling Technique

In the previous chapter, we have discussed the reactive nature of processes in health care. One of the main challenges in the simulation of reactive systems is describing the system's behavior and operation in a formal and rigorous way. Discrete-event simulation is well suited for modeling reactive systems, since this type of system (as opposed to a transformational system) is driven by events and must continuously react to external and internal stimuli [69]. We take the view that discrete-event simulation is more suitable for simulating health care systems than the other techniques because it allows the representation of interactions between the activities that advance individuals through the system. As such, this type of simulation reflects reality more closely than simulation approaches in which transitions between states are governed by predefined deterministic or probabilistic rules, such as system dynamics or Markov models [60, 84]. Discrete-event simulation represents a system as a chronological sequence of events. Each of these events, which together capture the most representative aspects of the system's behavior and operation, occurs at an instant in time and signals a change of state within the system [9]. Another advantage of discrete-event simulation for modeling health care systems is the capacity of this type of simulation to represent complex patient flows and to allow the study of different scenarios through changes to the rules and policies for patient flow [84]. In this book, we use discrete-event models based on the Statecharts formalism (see Chap. 6).

Chapter 5
UML Diagrams for the Process of Care

In this chapter, we introduce Unified Modeling Language (UML) diagrams as a means of representing health care processes. To facilitate the analysis of health care systems, health services researchers increasingly employ diagrammatic descriptions of a system's operations. Such diagrams assist researchers in analyzing complex systems in terms of their components and functionalities, as well as the interactions among components. In the context of health care evaluation, diagrammatic description is useful in two ways: first, as a tool for documenting existing policies, which will ensure a common understanding that can eventually help to identify areas for improvement, and, second, as a tool for developing specifications for the computer simulation models needed to evaluate the policies. This chapter presents examples of use case diagrams for the activities involved in surgical care, activity diagrams for the flow of patients through care activities, and sequence diagrams for the interactions of patients and care activities arranged in a time sequence.[1]

5.1 Overview of Diagrams

A variety of methods have been employed to describe health care processes by diagrams [82, 83]. Among these, flow charts have been widely used to depict the sequence of activities that constitute a care process. Other methods describe interactions between resources and individual behavior, such as input–output diagrams, process charts, and functional flow diagrams [87], as well as management practices, such as process maps, activity cycle diagrams, and stock flow diagrams [29, 124]. The success of object-oriented tools in computer engineering has increased the interest of the health services community in methods that describe complex systems

[1]In this chapter, we benefit from a literature review on the use of diagrams in the modeling of health care systems by Dr. Vasilakis and his colleagues [157].

B. Sobolev et al., *Health Care Evaluation Using Computer Simulation: Concepts, Methods, and Applications*, DOI 10.1007/978-1-4614-2233-4_5,

in terms of components (or objects) and interactions between them. Examples of these modeling methods are integrated definition [105], object-oriented modeling [129], and, more recently, UML.

The UML is a set of diagrammatic description methods for specifying, visualizing, and documenting object-oriented systems and for developing model requirements [64]. The UML, which has been under development since 1994, combines the concepts of object-oriented analysis and design [26], object-modeling techniques [129], and object-oriented software engineering [80], as well as incorporating a number of ideas from other methods and description techniques such as Harel's Statecharts [69].

UML version 2.0 defines 13 types of diagrams, which are divided into three hierarchical categories:

- Structure diagrams are used to represent static application structures (i.e., the elements of the system), which may be either conceptual or physical. This category of diagrams consists of class diagrams, object diagrams, component diagrams, composite structure diagrams, package diagrams, and deployment diagrams.
- Behavior diagrams are used to represent the behavior of the elements of the system over time and space. This category of diagrams consists of use case diagrams, activity diagrams, and state diagrams.
- Interaction diagrams, derived from the more general behavior diagrams, are used to represent the flow of data among a set of elements within a particular context. This category of diagrams consists of sequence diagrams, communication diagrams, timing diagrams, and interaction overview diagrams.

In the remainder of this chapter, we describe six basic UML diagrams, namely, the class, use case, activity, state, sequence, and timing diagrams. We focus on these six diagrammatic description methods because of their relevance for describing the structure, behavior, and interaction of health care processes. Conversely, we have omitted those diagrams that are useful only for modeling the physical structure of a system, such as the component, composite structure, and deployment diagrams. Furthermore, we concentrate here on basic concepts, omitting some of the more advanced modeling features, which are beyond the scope of this book. For a detailed description of UML version 2.0, the reader should refer to the UML documentation [27, 64].

We illustrate the basic concepts and notations of each diagrammatic description method by representing and modeling the process of cardiac surgical consultations at an outpatient clinic. In this particular setting, physicians refer patients who present with symptoms of coronary artery disease for an appointment with one of three surgeons in an outpatient clinic. These patients are kept on the appointment list with a designated priority (high or low) until an opening for a surgical consultation becomes available. The clerical staff book consultations with the surgeon named in the referrals, booking high-priority patients ahead of low-priority patients, and booking same-priority patients on a first-come, first-served basis. After the consultation, the office of the consulting surgeon registers on the surgeon's wait list those patients who require coronary revascularization and decide to undergo the operation, designating the procedure as having high, medium, or low priority, according to the affected coronary anatomy and the patient's symptoms. Patients are referred for medical treatment if the procedure is not indicated.

5.2 Class Diagrams

The class diagram is one of the most fundamental structure diagrams in UML version 2.0, since it provides the initial set of notation elements used by all of the other structure diagrams. It is a type of static structure diagram that describes the structure of a system by showing the system's *classes*, the *attributes* and *operations* of those classes, and the relations between the classes, commonly known as *associations*.

5.2.1 Classes

The core element of a class diagram is the class [64]. Classes represent entities within systems, which often relate to real-world objects or concepts. A class can be thought of as a blueprint for defining similar objects. The UML represents a class as a rectangle containing up to three compartments, stacked vertically, as shown in Fig. 5.1. The top compartment shows the name of the class. The middle and bottom compartments, which are optional, list the attributes and operations of the class, respectively.

5.2.2 Attributes

An attribute is a property of a class. The middle compartment of the rectangle for a class diagram lists each attribute of the class on a separate line. Attributes are documented in the format `name : attribute type`, where the attribute type is optional. For example, class `Patient` depicted in Fig. 5.1 contains the following attributes:

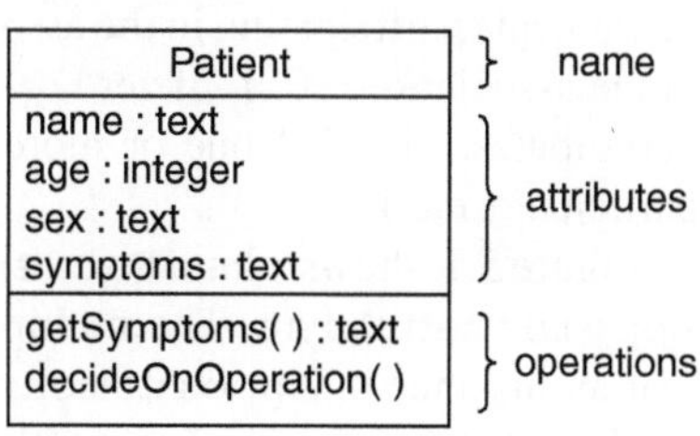

Fig. 5.1 Representation of a class in the Unified Modeling Language

```
name : text
age : integer
sex : text
symptoms : text
```

The attributes `name`, `sex`, and `symptoms` store text-based information, whereas the attribute `age` stores numeric values. The type of information stored explains the attribute type (text or integer) defined for each attribute.

5.2.3 *Operations*

An operation is a task that can be performed on the data for a class. Like attributes, operations are displayed in a list format, with a separate line for each operation. Operations are documented in the format `name(parameter list) : type of value returned`, where the parameter list and the type of value returned are optional. For example, class `Patient` depicted in Fig. 5.1 contains the following operations:

```
getSymptoms( ) : text
decideOnOperation( )
```

In this case, the operation `getSymptoms( )` requires no parameters to be executed and returns a value with type text (i.e., the patient's symptoms). The operation `decideOnOperation( )` likewise requires no parameters, and it returns no values.

5.2.4 *Associations*

The relations between classes in a class diagram are depicted by associations. Each association is represented by a solid line linking the rectangles of two class diagrams. There are two main types of associations: bidirectional and unidirectional. In the case of bidirectional associations, each of the two classes is aware of the other and of the relation between them. A multiplicity value is usually presented at each end of a bidirectional association line. The multiplicity value indicates the number of elements participating in the association ("0..*" if zero or more objects participate in the association, "0..1" if zero or one object participates, "1" if exactly one object participates, "1..*" if one or more objects participate, "2" if exactly two objects participate, etc.).

Figure 5.2 shows class `Patient` and its bidirectional association with class `AppointmentList`. The multiplicity value of "0..*" next to `Patient` means that an instance of `AppointmentList` can have no instances or more instances of class `Patient` associated with it; this reflects the fact that an appointment list

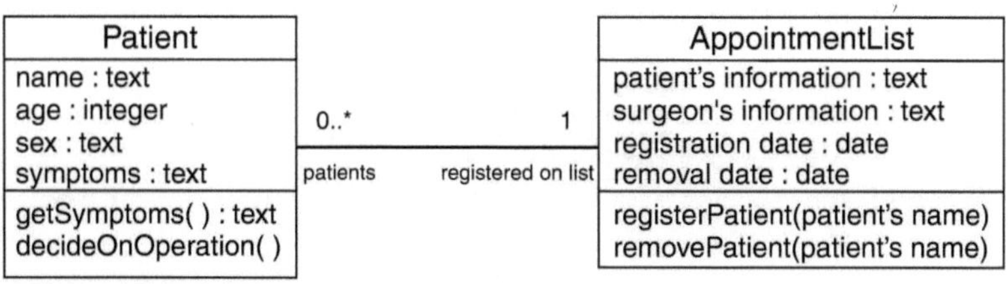

Fig. 5.2 Class diagram showing a bidirectional association between two classes

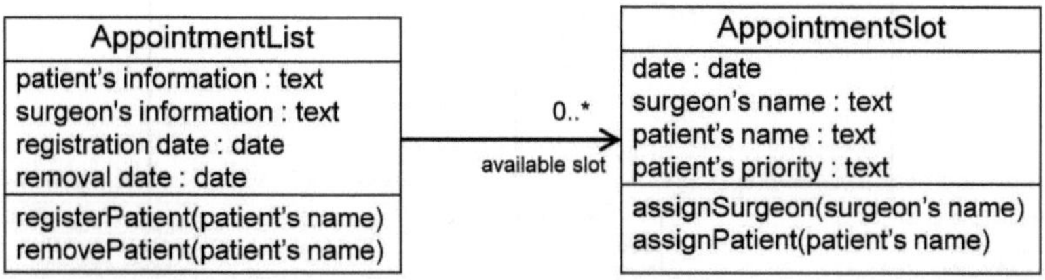

Fig. 5.3 Class diagram showing a unidirectional association between two classes

may be empty or it may contain the names of many patients. The value of "1" next to `AppointmentList` means that an instance of class `Patient` can only have one instance of class `AppointmentList` associated with it, because a patient can be registered on only one appointment list.

In the case of unidirectional association, the two classes are related, but only one class is aware of the relationship. This type of association is depicted with an arrow pointing away from the class that has knowledge of the relationship. Figure 5.3 shows `AppointmentList` class and its unidirectional relationship with `AppointmentSlot` class. In this case, `AppointmentSlot` class is not aware of its relationship with `AppointmentList` class, which makes the model more adaptive to changes; for example, more instances of `AppointmentSlot` class may be added to `AppointmentList` class without a requirement for further modifications to `AppointmentSlot`.

The multiplicity value notations used for unidirectional associations are similar to those for bidirectional associations. As such, the value next to `AppointmentSlot` class means that one instance of `AppointmentList` can have no or many instances of `AppointmentSlot` associated with it.

The full class diagram of the process of cardiac surgical consultations at an outpatient clinic is depicted in Fig. 5.4. Each appointment slot has a date, a surgeon, a patient, and the patient's priority. The appointment and surgical lists hold a patient's information, the surgeon's information, and the registration and removal dates. Because each surgeon can have only one appointment list and one surgical list, `Surgeon` class is associated with a single appointment list and a single surgical list. A patient may be associated with no appointment slots or many, whereas a single appointment slot may be associated with a maximum of one patient. Patients who are waiting for consultation are booked for an appointment by execution of

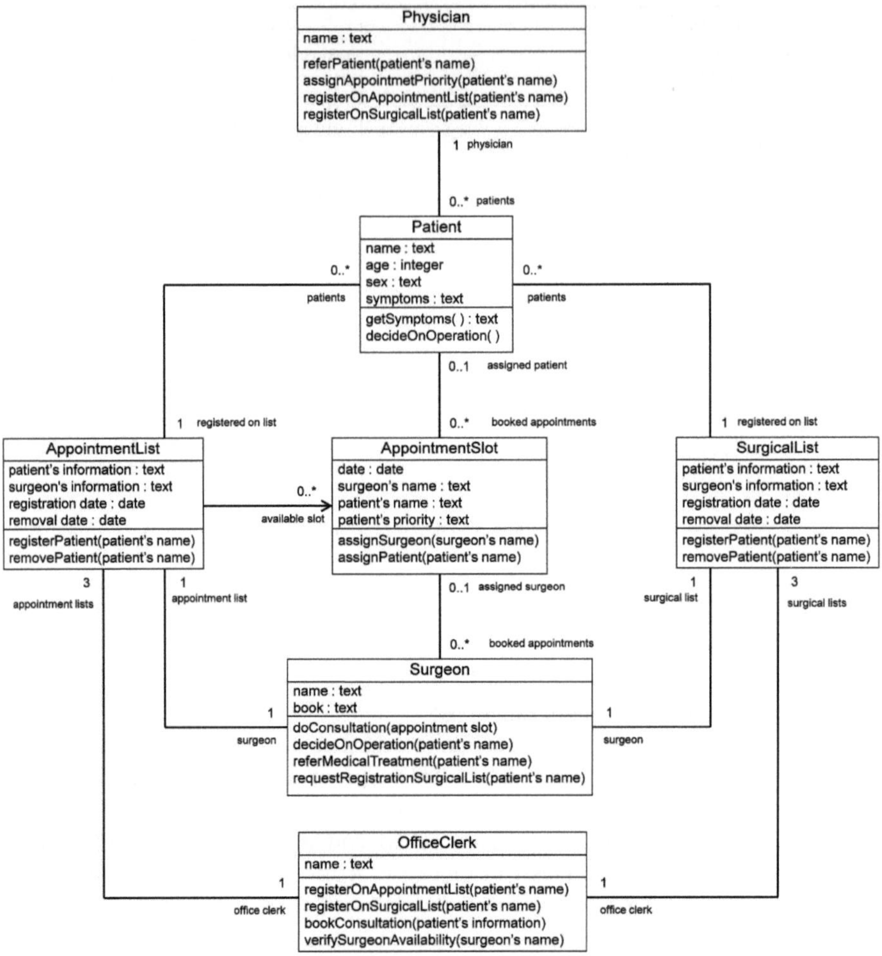

Fig. 5.4 Class diagram for the process of surgical consultations at an outpatient clinic

operation `bookConsultation(patient's information)`, which is defined in `OfficeClerk` class. Similarly, a surgeon's attendance at an appointment is accomplished by execution of operation `doConsultation(appointment slot)`, defined in class `Surgeon`.

5.3 Use Case Diagrams

Use case diagrams are a type of behavior diagram describing the functionality of a system by showing the system's actors, the scenarios to achieve the actor's goals or functions (commonly referred to as use cases), and any dependencies between the use cases [64].

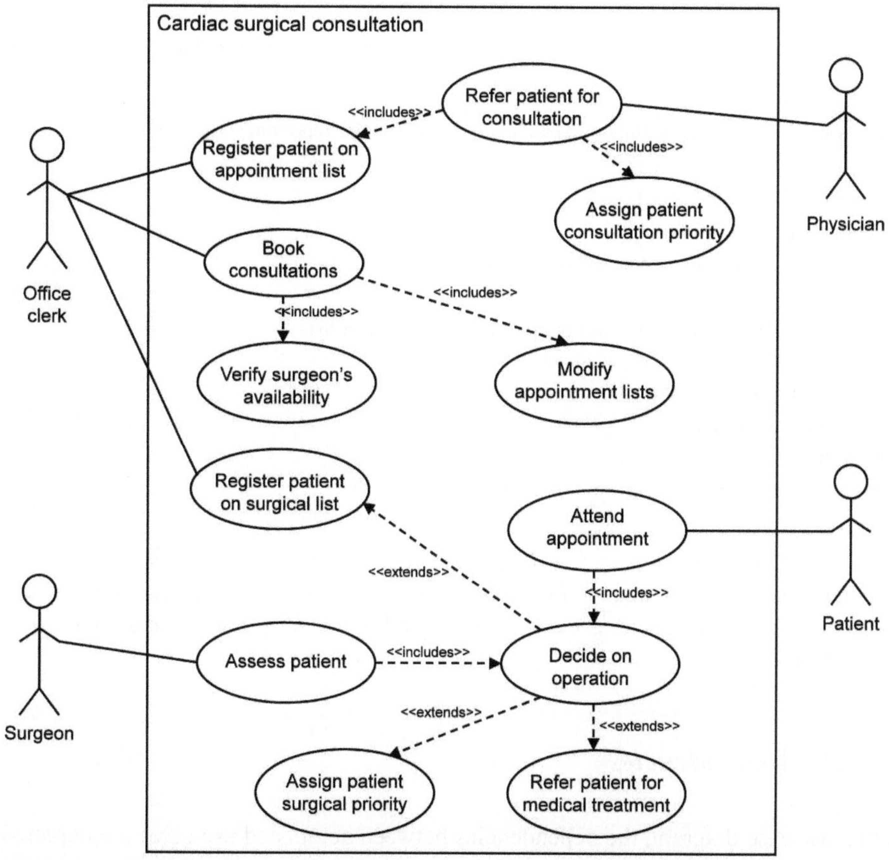

Fig. 5.5 Use case diagram for the process of surgical consultations at an outpatient clinic

5.3.1 Actors

An actor is an object that plays a role within the system. In the example of outpatient consultations, the patient, surgeon, physician, and office clerk are all actors with roles in the care process. In a use case diagram, the actors are represented as stick figures (see Fig. 5.5).

5.3.2 Use Cases

A use case is a scenario describing the interaction of the actors with a specific part of the system to achieve a goal or function. Use cases can be specified by describing the objective of the interaction, the actors, any preconditions, the steps required to achieve the objective, and any alternative actions. All of this information is then

Box 5.1 Use case for booking patients for a consultation at an outpatient clinic

Objective
Assign a date for consultation to patients registered in the appointment list

Actors
Office clerk

Preconditions
At least one patient is registered on the appointment list

Steps
1. Clerk retrieves patient's information from appointment list
2. Clerk verifies surgeon's availability
3. Clerk books appointment

Alternative actions
None

presented in tabular form, as in Box 5.1, which specifies the use case for booking patients for a surgical consultation at an outpatient clinic. In a use case diagram, the use cases are represented as ovals enclosing a brief description of the use case (see Fig. 5.5).

5.3.3 Dependencies

In a use case diagram, the dependencies between actors and use cases are depicted by connecting lines. A simple straight line shows the relation between an actor and the use cases that this actor always performs, whereas a dashed line with an arrowhead indicates the relation between any pair of use cases. There are two main types of dependencies between two use cases: directed and conditional. In a directed dependency, one use case always invokes, or makes use of, the other use case. This type of dependency is depicted by a dashed line labeled `includes`, with the arrow pointing to the use case that is always invoked. In a conditional dependency, one use case may invoke the other use case only in particular scenarios. This type of dependency is depicted by a dashed line labeled `extends`, with the arrow pointing to the use case that is occasionally invoked.

The use case diagram of the process of cardiac surgical consultations at an outpatient clinic is depicted in Fig. 5.5. In this example, the actor Physician refers a patient presenting with symptoms for a consultation. The actor Office clerk books consultations by first verifying the surgeon's availability and then modifying the appointment lists. The actor Patient attends the booked consultation. Depending on the outcome of the consultation, the actor Surgeon may refer the actor Patient for medical treatment or if the operation is deemed necessary, may assign a surgical priority to the patient.

5.4 Activity Diagrams

Activity diagrams depict a sequence of events, or activities, in a diagram resembling a flow chart [64]. This type of behavior diagram may be used to model individual use cases, a particular function, such as registering patients on an appointment list, or the flow of patients through a care process. Activity diagrams, which are based on the semantics of Petri nets, support the representation of conditional behavior and parallel execution of operations [113].

The starting point of an activity diagram is represented by a small solid circle and the end point by a bull's-eye. Activities are depicted by rounded rectangles enclosing a brief description of the activity. Transitions between activities are depicted by arrows flowing from the initial activity to the subsequent activity. Conditional behavior is represented by diamond-shaped connectors and labeled transitions, with the conditions stated in parentheses. Parallel behavior is represented by parallel horizontal bars before and after all of the activities that are executed simultaneously.

The activity diagram of the process of cardiac surgical consultations at an outpatient clinic is shown in Fig. 5.6. After referral for consultation, a patient is registered on the appointment list of the surgeon named in the referral. For the purposes of this example, consultations are booked simultaneously with verification of the surgeon's availability. After the consultation, the patient is registered on a surgical wait list only if the operation is deemed necessary and the patient decides to undergo the procedure. If the operation is deemed unnecessary, the patient is referred for medical treatment.

5.5 State Diagrams

UML state diagrams, which are based on Harel's Statecharts [69], provide an abstract description of the behavior of a reactive system as a series of events occurring in one or more states. A reactive system is a system that constantly responds to external stimuli by changing states or performing actions. Each state diagram represents objects of a single class and the various states of these objects as they move through the system [64]. State diagrams can also depict hierarchy, parallelism, and event broadcasting [143].

In a state diagram, a state is depicted as a rounded rectangle enclosing the state name and an optional list of entry and exit actions and events to be executed upon entry to and exit from the state. The entry and exit actions and events are specified according to the following format:

```
entry/event1;event2;...;eventN;action1;action2;...;
  actionN;
exit/event1;event2;...;eventN;action1;action2;...;
  actionN;
```

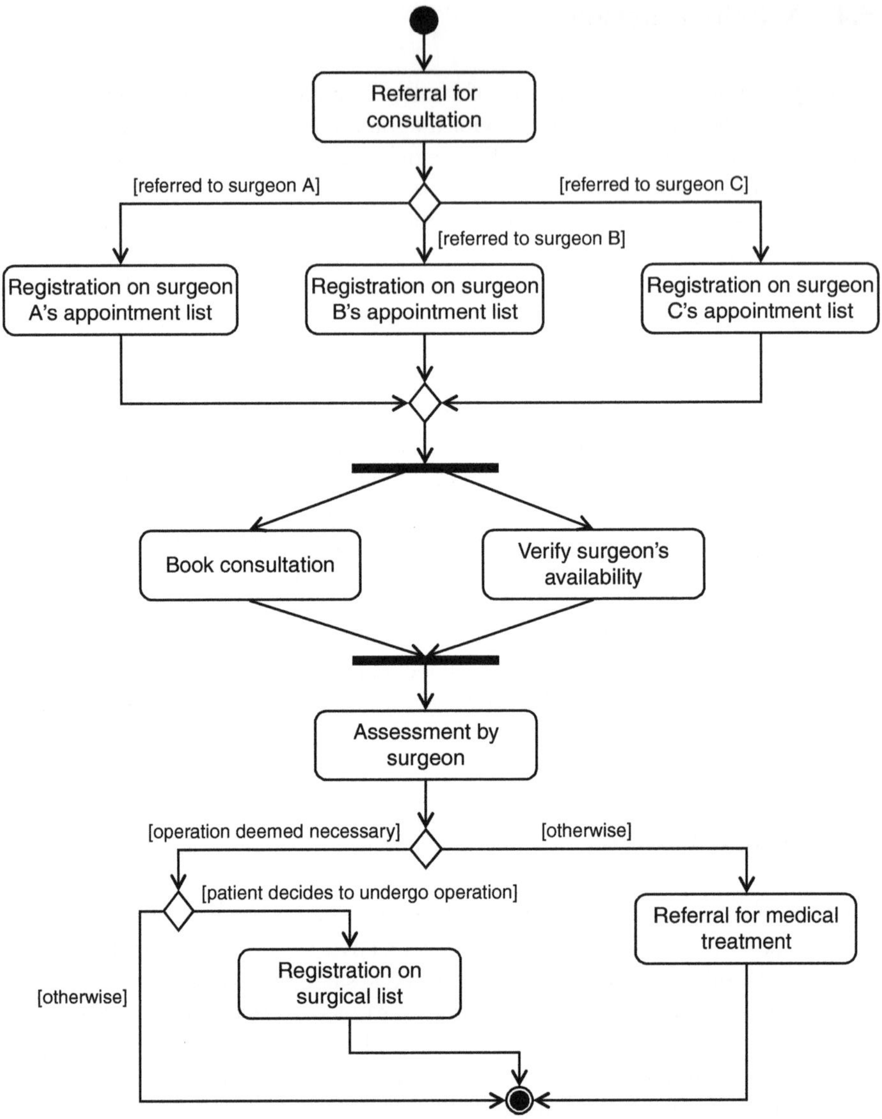

Fig. 5.6 Activity diagram for the process of surgical consultations at an outpatient clinic

The arrow flowing from an initial state to a subsequent state depicts the transition between states. The optional label for a transition arrow lists any events that could trigger the transition, any conditions that must be satisfied for the transition to occur, and any actions associated with the transition.

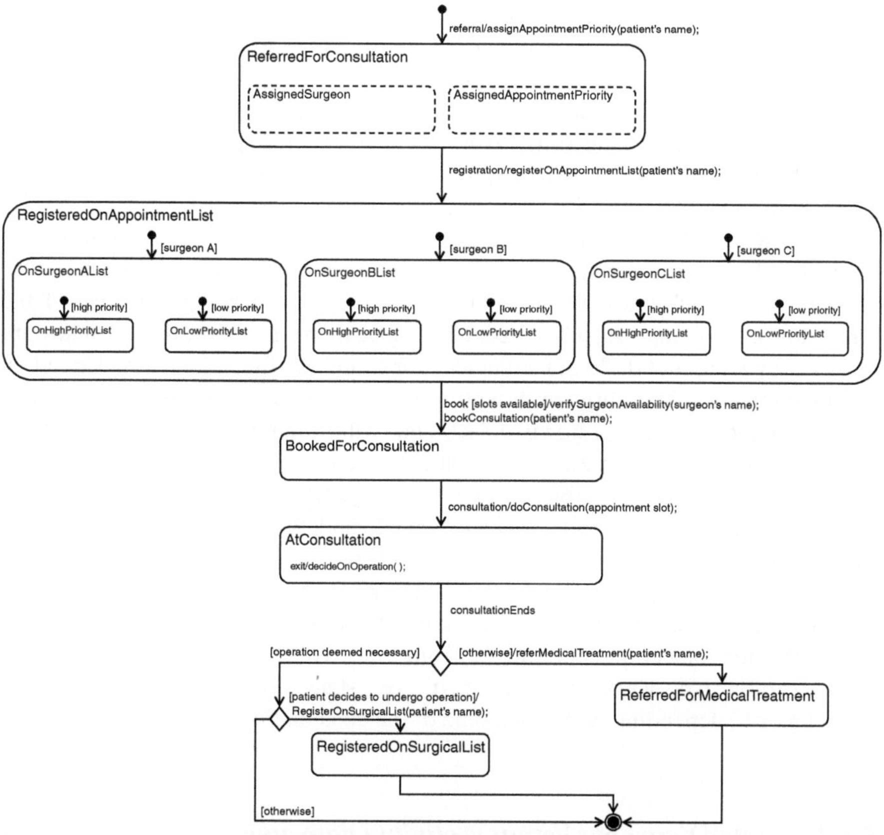

Fig. 5.7 State diagram of a single patient in the process of surgical consultations at an outpatient clinic

The labels use the following format:

```
triggeringEvent[conditionExpression]/event1;
 event2;...;eventN;action1;action2;...;actionN;
```

Diamond-shaped connectors depict decision points where at least one condition must be met for the transition to be completed. The notion of hierarchy (i.e., subordination between states) is represented by placing certain states within other states. The notion of parallelism (i.e., two or more states being active simultaneously) is represented by dashed rectangles. As in activity diagrams, the starting point of a transition is represented by a solid circle, and the end point is represented by a bull's-eye. Every state diagram should have a starting point followed by an initial transition, which should not include a triggering event but which may include associated actions.

The state diagram for a single patient in the process of cardiac surgical consultations at an outpatient clinic is shown in Fig. 5.7. After occurrence of referral event, action assignAppointmentPriority( ) is executed, and the object patient moves to state ReferredForConsultation. This state illustrates the concept of parallelism since its two substates are represented by dashed rectangles, signifying that the object patient can be in both substates at the same time. From there, the object patient moves to state RegisteredOnAppointmentList after event registration occurs and action registerOnAppointmentList( ) is executed.

State RegisteredOnAppointmentList illustrates the concept of hierarchy. This particular state consists of three substates, each of which in turn consists of two substates. Because the object patient can be in only one of the three substates of state RegisteredOnAppointmentList, the substates are enclosed by solid, not dashed, rectangles. For example, if a patient is registered on the appointment list of surgeon A with a low priority, then the object patient can only be in substate OnSurgeonAList and, within that substate, can only be in substate OnLowPriorityList. When book event occurs and only if there are any appointment slots available, actions verifySurgeonAvailability( ) and bookConsultation( ) are executed, and the object patient moves to state BookedForConsultation. From there, after consultation event occurs, the object patient moves to state AtConsultation, and activity decideOnOperation( ) is executed upon exit from this state.

Finally, the object patient moves from state AtConsultation to either state RegisteredOnSurgicalList or state ReferredForMedical Treatment, depending on the outcome of the consultation.

5.5.1 State Diagrams Versus Activity Diagrams

Activity diagrams, described in Sect. 5.4, are elaborate flow charts that often convey behavioral information similar to that conveyed by state diagrams. It is therefore important to clarify the distinction between these two types of diagrammatic representations. State diagrams are concerned with event-driven behavior, whereas flow charts are concerned with transformational behavior [130]. More specifically, a state diagram depicts the states of an object and the actions the object performs in response to explicit triggering events. A state diagram is idle when the object is waiting for an event to occur. Conversely, a flow chart depicts the sequence of activities associated with a process. As such, a flow chart is idle at a node during the execution of activities, and it automatically transitions from node to node upon completion of activities.

In graphic terms, processes (i.e., actions or activities) are associated with transitions and actions in state diagrams, whereas in flow charts, they are associated with the rounded rectangles representing activities. Figure 5.8 shows the processing stages of a state diagram and the corresponding equivalent activities in an activity diagram (flow chart), with alignment of similar points in the process indicated by dotted lines. For example, the transition and action referral/

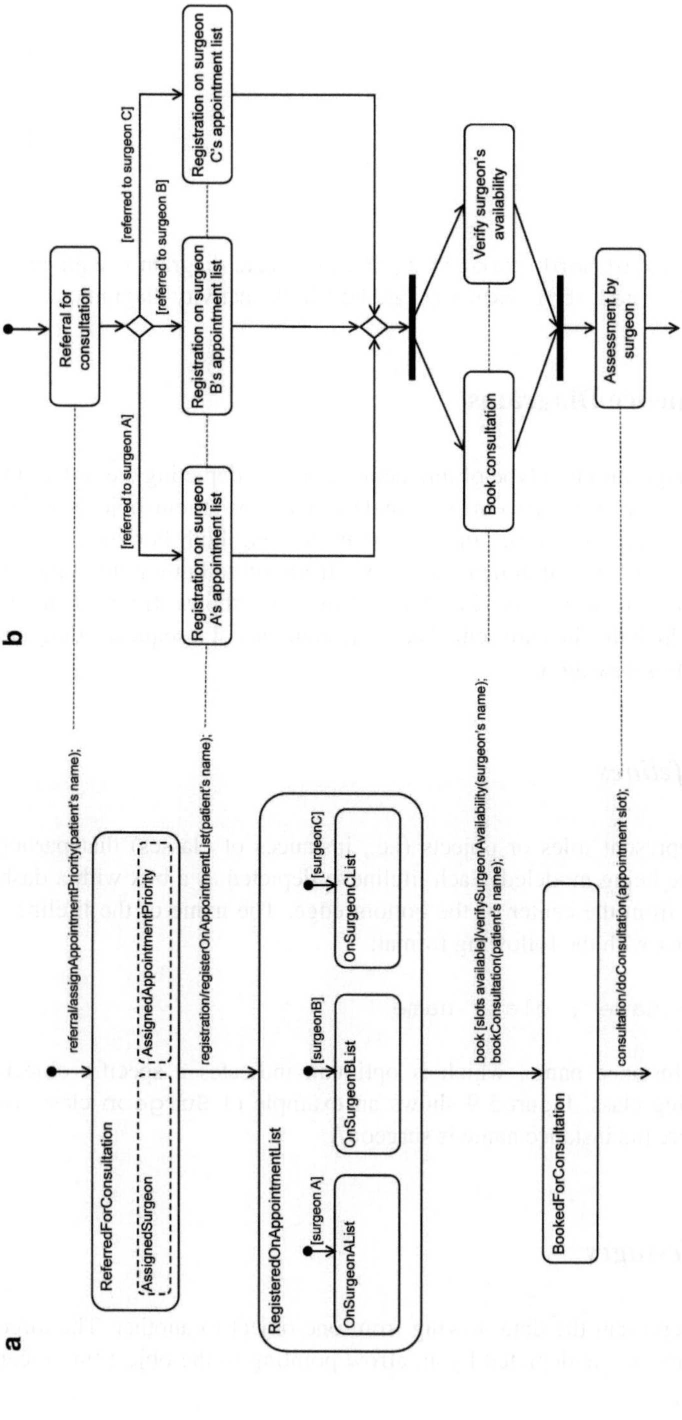

Fig. 5.8 Comparison of a state diagram **(a)** with a flow chart representing an activity diagram **(b)**

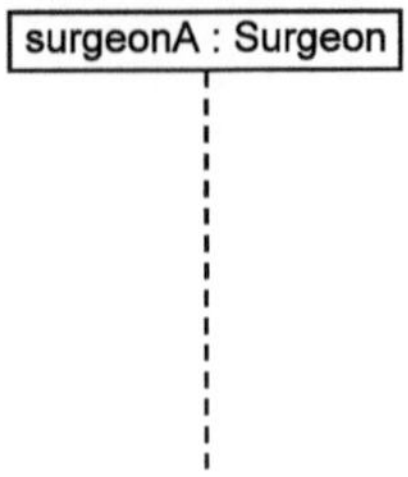

Fig. 5.9 Lifeline diagram with `Surgeon` class, where the instance name is surgeonA (*dashed line* denotes the lifeline)

`assignAppointmentPriority( )` in the state diagram is equivalent to the activity `Referral for consultation` in the activity diagram.

5.6 Sequence Diagrams

Sequence diagrams are a type of interaction diagram depicting the order in which a set of processes within a system occur and the data flow among objects in the system [64]. These diagrams convey this information along both horizontal and vertical dimensions. The vertical dimension shows, from top to bottom, the time sequence of data flow as it occurs; the horizontal dimension shows, from left to right, the objects to which the data are sent. The basic elements of a sequence diagram are its *lifelines* and its *messages*.

5.6.1 Lifelines

Lifelines represent roles or objects (i.e., instances of classes) that participate in the sequence being modeled. Each lifeline is depicted as a box with a dashed line descending from the center of the bottom edge. The name of the lifeline appears inside the box with the following format:

```
instance name : class name
```

where the instance name, which is optional, indicates a specific object of the corresponding class. Figure 5.9 shows an example of `Surgeon` class used in a lifeline where the instance name is surgeonA.

5.6.2 Messages

Messages represent the data flowing from one object to another. The direction of flow of a message is depicted by an arrow pointing to the object that receives the

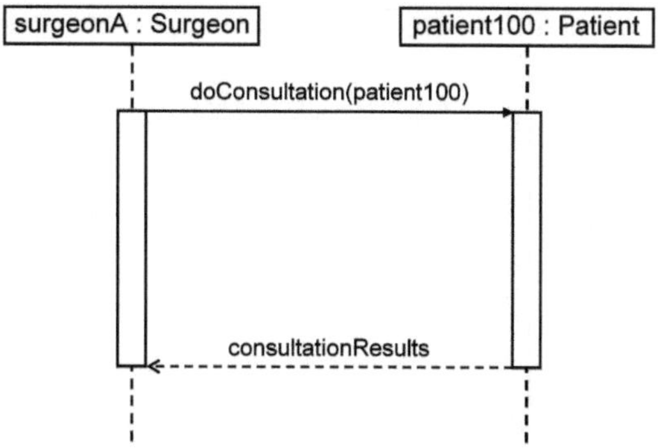

Fig. 5.10 Sequence diagram, showing a message being sent between the object surgeonA and the object patient100

message. The message sent to the receiving object represents an operation to be executed by the class of the receiving object. The message name is placed above the arrow with the following format:

```
[conditionExpression] operation (parameters)
```

where the condition expression and the parameters of the operation are optional. Each message may include a return message. A return message is depicted as a dashed horizontal line with an open arrowhead back to the originating lifeline. The return data from the operation appear as a label above the dashed horizontal line. The time needed for a message to be completed (i.e., from the instant when the message is sent to the instant when a return message is received) is depicted by vertical bars along the lifelines. Figure 5.10 shows the example of a message being sent between the object surgeonA and the object patient100, which is an instance of `Patient` class. In this case, the message is `doConsultation(patient100)` operation, which takes as a parameter the object's name, that is, patient100. The return message is the result of the consultation, that is, `consultationResults`. The time needed for this message to be completed is depicted by the vertical bars along the surgeonA and patient100 lifelines.

Because the vertical dimension of a sequence diagram shows the time sequence of data flow from top to bottom, the message that occurs first is always placed at the top, usually on the left side of the diagram. Subsequent messages (i.e., those occurring at later times) appear below previously occurring messages. The sequence diagram for the process of consultation between a surgeon and a patient is shown in Fig. 5.11. The diagram depicts three lifelines, which correspond to the three objects involved in this particular consultation process: surgeonA, patient100, and clerkA. The first message sent by surgeonA to patient100 is operation `doConsultation(patient100)`, with the patient's name as a parameter. This message appears at the top of the diagram, that is, at the beginning of the time sequence of data flow. During the duration of the first message, a second message, `decideOnOperation( )`, is sent by the object patient100 to itself. For this second message, there is no return

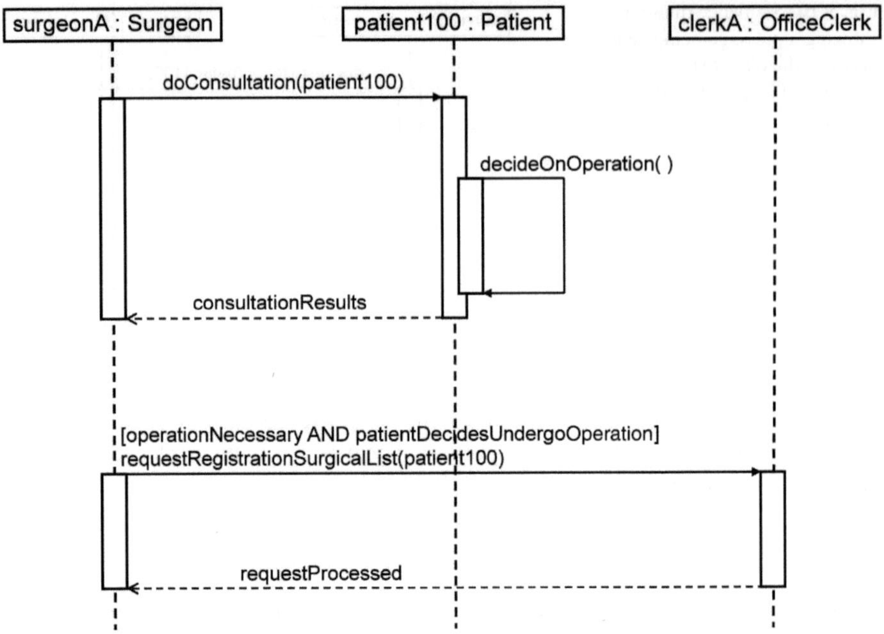

Fig. 5.11 Sequence diagram for the process of surgical consultation, showing interactions between a surgeon and a patient

message. After completion of the second message by the object patient100, a return message (`consultationResults`) is sent to the object surgeonA, and operation `doConsultation(patient100)` is completed. The last message to occur in this process is operation `requestRegistrationSurgicalList (patient100)`, with the patient's name as the parameter. This operation is guarded by two conditions:

```
operationNecessary
patientDecidesUndergoOperation
```

Both conditions must be satisfied for object surgeonA to complete operation `requestRegistrationSurgicalList(patient100)` . The return message for this operation is an acknowledgment of request (`requestProcessed`).

5.7 Timing Diagrams

A timing diagram is a type of interaction diagram that depicts changes of state or value for one or more objects throughout a given period of time [64]. These diagrams can also show interactions between events and the duration constraints that govern

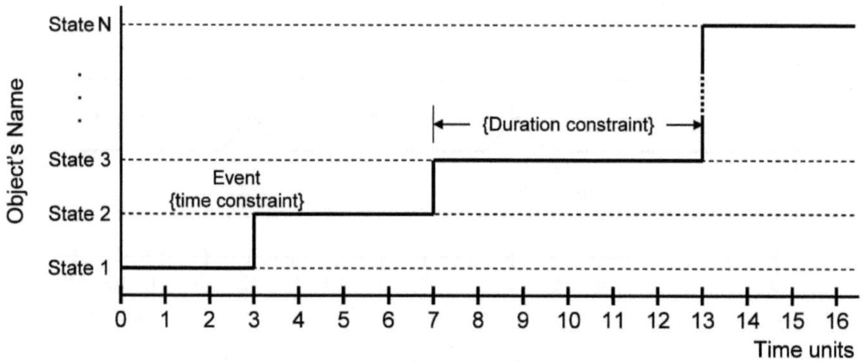

Fig. 5.12 Timing diagram showing structure and nomenclature of a state lifeline

them. The horizontal axis of a timing diagram shows the flow of time from left to right, and the vertical axis shows the state or value of the object. Each object is assigned a horizontal band across the diagram, often called a swim lane. If a swim lane depicts changes of state for an object, it is called a state lifeline; alternatively, if a swim lane depicts changes of value of an object, it is called a value lifeline. Messages, which are depicted as single arrows, can be passed from one lifeline to another.

A state lifeline shows the changes of state of an object over time. The horizontal axis shows time units, whereas the vertical axis lists the object's states. Each state change can have a defined event, a time constraint indicating the instant of time when the event occurs, and a duration constraint indicating the period for which the state is active. The structure and nomenclature of a state lifeline are depicted in Fig. 5.12.

A value lifeline shows the changes in value of an object over time. The horizontal axis shows time units, which should be the same as those for any state lifelines included in the diagram. The value of the object appears between a pair of horizontal lines. These lines cross over at each change in value. Similar to what occurs with state lifelines, each change in value can be related to a defined event, and each can have a time constraint indicating the instant of time when the event occurs and a duration constraint indicating the period for which the value is valid. The structure and nomenclature of a value lifeline are depicted in Fig. 5.13.

A timing diagram for the changes of state and value of a specific patient and a specific appointment slot within the sample process of cardiac surgical consultations at an outpatient clinic is shown in Fig. 5.14. In this case, the diagram comprises three swim lanes. The top swim lane corresponds to the state lifeline of the object patient100 and includes the states `ReferredForConsultation`, `RegisteredOnAppointmentList`, and `BookedForConsultation`. For the purposes of this example, the object patient100 is assumed to start in the `ReferredForConsultation` state. The middle swim lane represents the state lifeline of the object appointmentSlot10 and

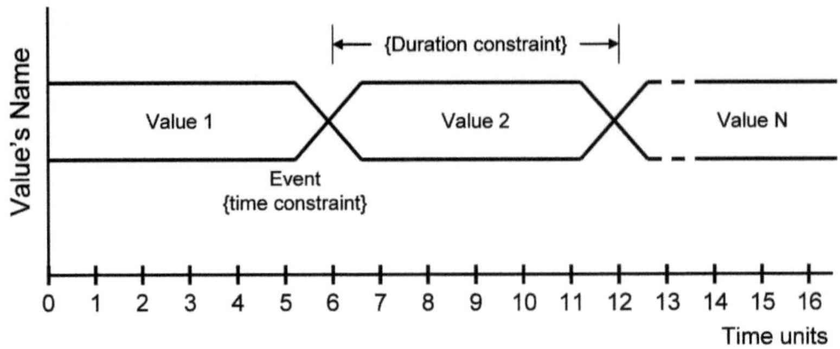

Fig. 5.13 Timing diagram showing structure and nomenclature of a value lifeline

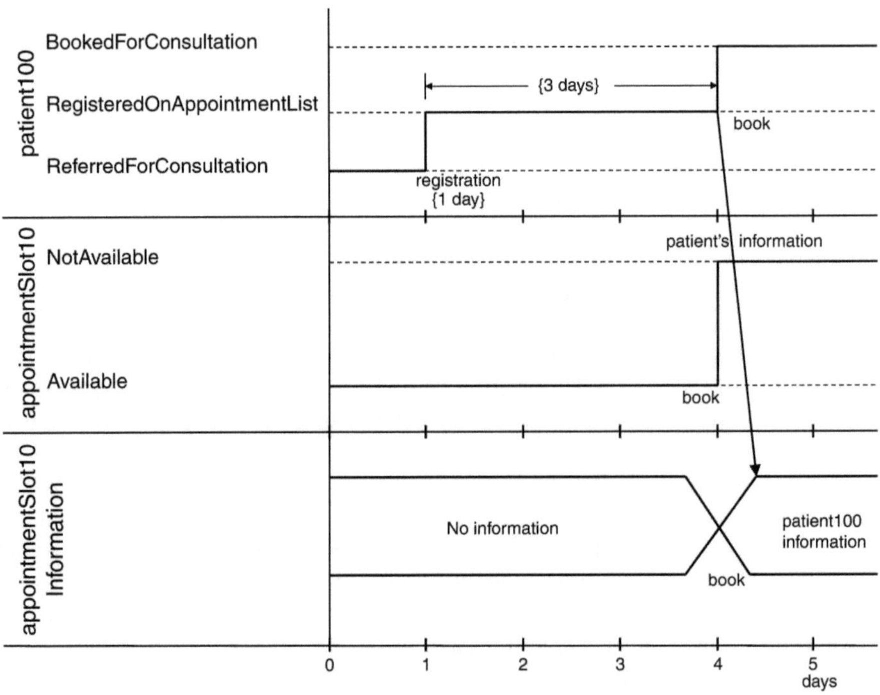

Fig. 5.14 Timing diagram depicting changes of state and value for a patient and an appointment slot within the process of surgical consultations at an outpatient clinic

includes the states `Available` and `NotAvailable`. The bottom swim lane represents the value lifeline of the object appointmentSlot10. The time unit for all swim lanes is one day. In this diagram, the object patient100 is registered on the appointment list one day after being referred for consultation. This time constraint appears as a label (1 day) below the name of the corresponding event (registration). For the purposes of this example, patient100 is kept on the appointment list for three days, after which the patient is booked for the consultation in appointmentSlot10 and appointmentSlot10 moves from state `Available` to state `NotAvailable`. Note that at this point in time a message is sent from the state lifeline of the object patient100 to the value lifeline of the object appointmentSlot10. This message includes the patient's information, which is stored in the object appointmentSlot10.

Chapter 6
Statecharts for Patient Flow

In Chap. 5, we discussed UML state diagrams as a means of describing the process of surgical care. This type of diagram is based on the Statecharts visual formalism developed by computer scientist David Harel. In this chapter, we first review the most important concepts of the formalism. We then focus on simulation of patient flow in surgical care and describe in greater detail the specifications of discrete-event models based on the Statecharts formalism. Discrete-event models are especially effective for simulation of patient flow in health care, as they allow the progression of individual patients through a care process to be described as a series of asynchronous updates in patient records generated in reaction to events produced by parallel states representing concurrent activities. In this regard, the Statecharts formalism is useful for representing patient flow mechanisms in terms of activities, events, states, and transitions between states. This chapter includes examples of Statecharts diagrams for concurrent care activities.

6.1 Visual Formalism

The Statecharts extend the formalism of finite-state machines, which describes states and transitions in a modular fashion, by including notions of hierarchy, parallelism, and event broadcasting [69]. Hierarchy permits subordination between states. Parallelism permits several states to be active concurrently. Broadcasting of events permits one state to detect changes in another state [69, 70, 160]. Graphically, states, which are also called machines, are depicted by rounded rectangles (as described in Sect. 5.5). A transition between states is depicted by an arrow flowing from an initial state to a subsequent state. Diamond-shaped connectors depict decision points, where at least one condition must be met for the transition to be completed. Optional entry and exit actions (to be executed upon entry to and exit from the state, respectively) are listed within the state.

B. Sobolev et al., *Health Care Evaluation Using Computer Simulation: Concepts, Methods, and Applications*, DOI 10.1007/978-1-4614-2233-4_6,

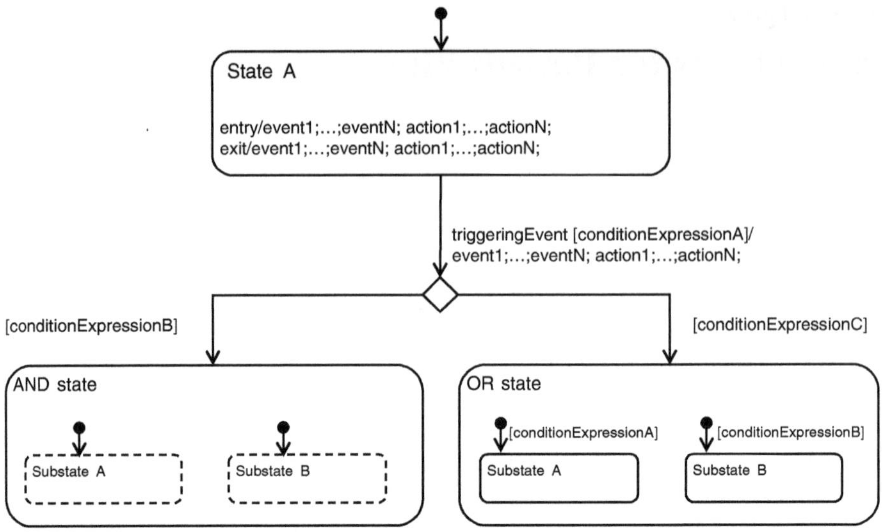

Fig. 6.1 Semantics of the Statecharts visual formalism

A hierarchical relation between states is represented by including substates and internal transitions within a state. States containing substates are called complex states. If the system represented by a Statechart leaves a complex state, then the system also leaves each substate. Parallelism between states is modeled by two types of complex states: AND states and OR states. Residence in an AND state implies that the system represented by the Statechart also resides in all of the direct substates. Substates within an AND state are represented by dashed rectangles. Residence in an OR state implies that the system represented by the Statechart resides in exactly one of the direct substates. Substates within an OR state are represented by solid rectangles. Events can trigger transitions between states, which in turn can generate other events.

The Statecharts formalism defines four kinds of events: those generated by processes in an asynchronous fashion, those generated by an action within a machine, those generated by the change in value of an attribute, and those generated by regular time advances. Transition labels, which specify triggering events and events generated by the transition, consist of a trigger component and an action component. The trigger component consists of the name of the triggering event and an expression for any conditions determining when the transition will occur. The action component specifies the events and actions that will be generated if the transition is executed. Events can be broadcast throughout the Statechart, which means that multiple transitions may be triggered and executed simultaneously [69, 160]. The semantics of the Statecharts visual formalism (as illustrated in Fig. 6.1) is amenable to mathematical analysis [151], and appropriate simulation software can execute the system depicted by the Statecharts formalism, similar to a program code.

6.2 Representing Reactive Systems

Health care systems are reactive, in that they involve patients who are subject to multiple concurrent activities, which are in turn governed by a variety of events and the coordination of the outcomes of these concurrent activities [19]. As an example, booking elective surgery can be described in terms of two activities: planning service-specific staffing and booking the cases of individual surgeons within their assigned blocks of operating time [102]. These two activities, however, may present a complex set of temporal relations with other activities. For instance, the unplanned emergency admission of a patient with a booked procedure may trigger changes in routine activity in the operating room and may lead to cancellations of other procedures and staffing adjustments. In our experience, the Statecharts visual formalism greatly simplifies the description of reactive systems in a way that is amenable to simulation.

To illustrate the capacity of Statecharts in constructing a discrete-event simulation model of patient flow, we consider here the delivery of surgical services, which involves multiple concurrent activities and coordination of their outcomes [19]. Specifically, we focus on the preoperative stage of the process of cardiac surgical care, as described in more detail in Chap. 3. For convenience, we list again in Table 6.1 all of the clinical and managerial activities that take place from the time of a decision to operate until the patient enters the operating room. In the following sections, we analyze the notions of hierarchy, parallelism, and event broadcasting using the activities in Table 6.1 as examples.

6.2.1 Hierarchy

In the context of health care, hierarchy provides the means both to describe steps within activities and to cluster activities. For example, booking inpatient operations involves assigning a date for the operation, confirming the surgeon's availability to operate, booking operating room time and other hospital resources (e.g., a bed in the intensive care unit), booking clinical staff, confirming the anesthesiologist's availability for the in-hospital assessment before the date of the operation, and booking an in-hospital preoperative assessment. For activity `BookingInpatientOperations` and its associated steps (Fig. 6.2), the activity itself is represented by an OR state, whereby the system can be in only one substate at a time. The activities within the OR state are autonomous and thus are executed independently from one another in a sequential order, such that completion of one activity constitutes the start of the next activity.

Table 6.1 Clinical and managerial activities at the preoperative stage of surgical care

Activity	Steps
1 Booking elective surgery	1a Registration of patients on surgical wait list
	1b Booking of patients for operation
2 Processing of inpatient referrals	2a Notification of surgeons about request for inpatient referrals
	2b Surgical consultation with inpatients
3 Booking inpatient referrals for surgery	3a Registration of inpatients on surgical queue
	3b Booking of inpatients for operation
	3c Fast-tracking of patients who live far away
4 Scheduling operating room slots	4a Weekly scheduling of operating time for the coming week by operating room teams
	4b Daily publication of operating room schedule
	4c Changes to the published operating room schedule
5 Canceling scheduled operations	5a Cancellation of scheduled operations by emergency arrivals
	5b Cancellation of scheduled operations by inpatients
	5c Cancellation of scheduled operations for patient-related reasons
	5d Cancellation of scheduled operations for hospital-related reasons
6 Rebooking canceled operations	6a Rebooking of canceled operations
7 Assessing patients preoperatively	7a Preoperative assessment of patients needing elective surgery
	7b In-hospital preoperative assessment of inpatients
	7c Discharge planning before surgery
8 Managing wait lists	8a Audit of wait lists
	8b Management of unplanned emergency admissions
	8c Analysis of patients' queueing behavior

6.2.2 Parallelism

In the context of health care, parallelism provides the means to specify and synchronize concurrent activities. Since parallelism permits multiple states to be active concurrently, it allows representation of components of a health care system that need to be active, or available, simultaneously. For example, multiple beds in an intensive care unit may be available simultaneously for patients recovering from an operation, as illustrated in Fig. 6.3. This figure shows an AND state representing four beds in an intensive care unit. Each bed is represented by a single Statechart comprising two states: `Available` and `Unavailable`. Because the beds are part of an AND state, any bed can be in either the state `Available` or the state `Unavailable`. However, within the Statechart for each bed, only one state can be active; that is, a bed cannot be available and unavailable simultaneously.

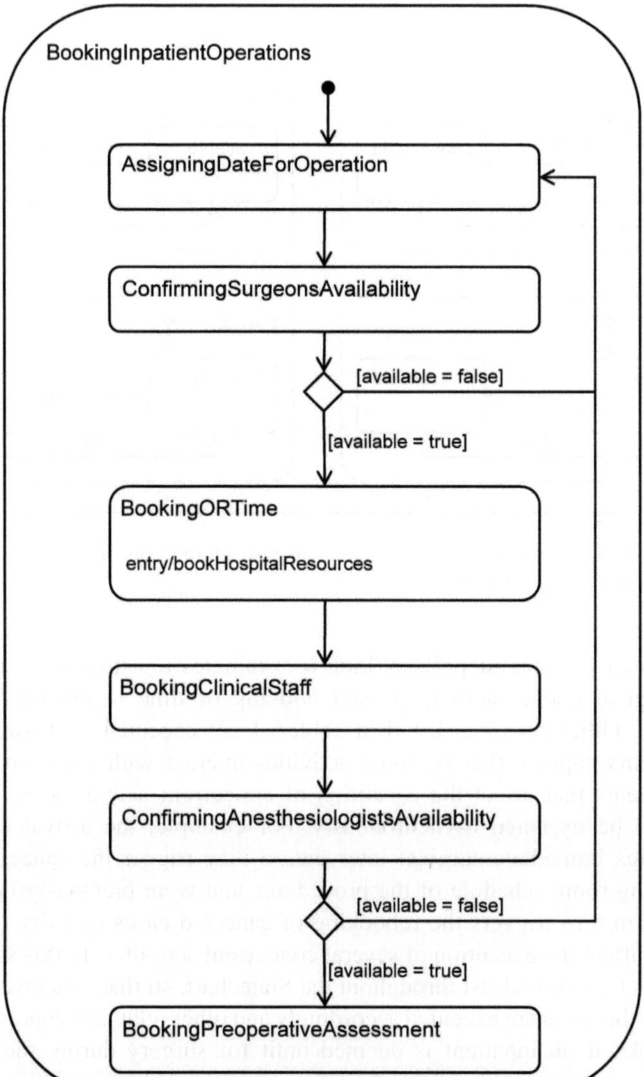

Fig. 6.2 The notion of hierarchy in the Statecharts visual formalism: steps within the activity of booking inpatient operations (OR = operating room)

6.2.3 *Event Broadcasting*

Some of the activities listed in Table 6.1 are executed independently, in sequential order; that is, completion of one activity constitutes the start of the next activity. For example, determining that an inpatient requires surgery after in-hospital assessment

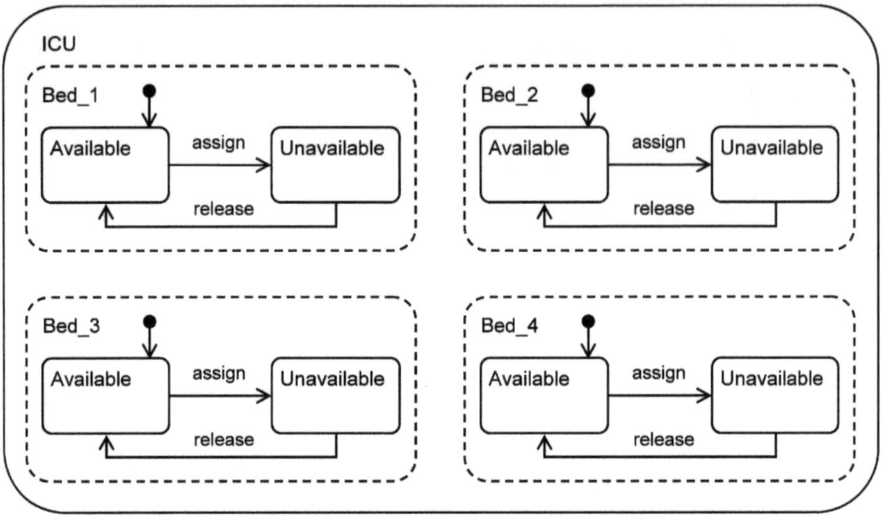

Fig. 6.3 The notion of parallelism in the Statecharts visual formalism: an AND state representing four beds in intensive care unit (ICU)

by the on-call surgeon (step 2b in Table 6.1) initiates registration of the inpatient in the surgical queue (activity 3) and booking of time in the operating room (activity 4). Other activities listed in Table 6.1 are executed or disrupted only if certain events happen; that is, some activities interact with each other and may produce events that affect the execution of concurrent activities. Such activities are said to be executed asynchronously. For example, the arrival of a patient who requires immediate surgical intervention may trigger the cancellation from the operating room schedule of the procedures that were previously booked (step 5a), which in turn triggers the rebooking of canceled cases (activity 6). A single event may affect the execution of several concurrent activities. In this situation, the event needs to be broadcast throughout the Statechart, so that concurrent activities affected by the event are executed accordingly and other related events are triggered. For example, if an inpatient is deemed unfit for surgery during the in-hospital preoperative assessment (because of, say, a pulmonary infection), this event causes the execution of certain concurrent activities: specifically, additional diagnostic tests are ordered, and the operation is rebooked. This event also triggers two simultaneous events: an operating room slot and a bed in the intensive care unit become available for another patient.

An example of event broadcasting (Fig. 6.4) shows three Statecharts: one depicting the states of an inpatient from the time surgery is deemed necessary to the time the inpatient enters the operating room, one depicting the states of a single operating room slot, and one depicting the states of a single bed in the intensive care unit. When the event `booking` in the Statechart for InpatientA is triggered, the inpatient moves to the state `BookedForOperation`.

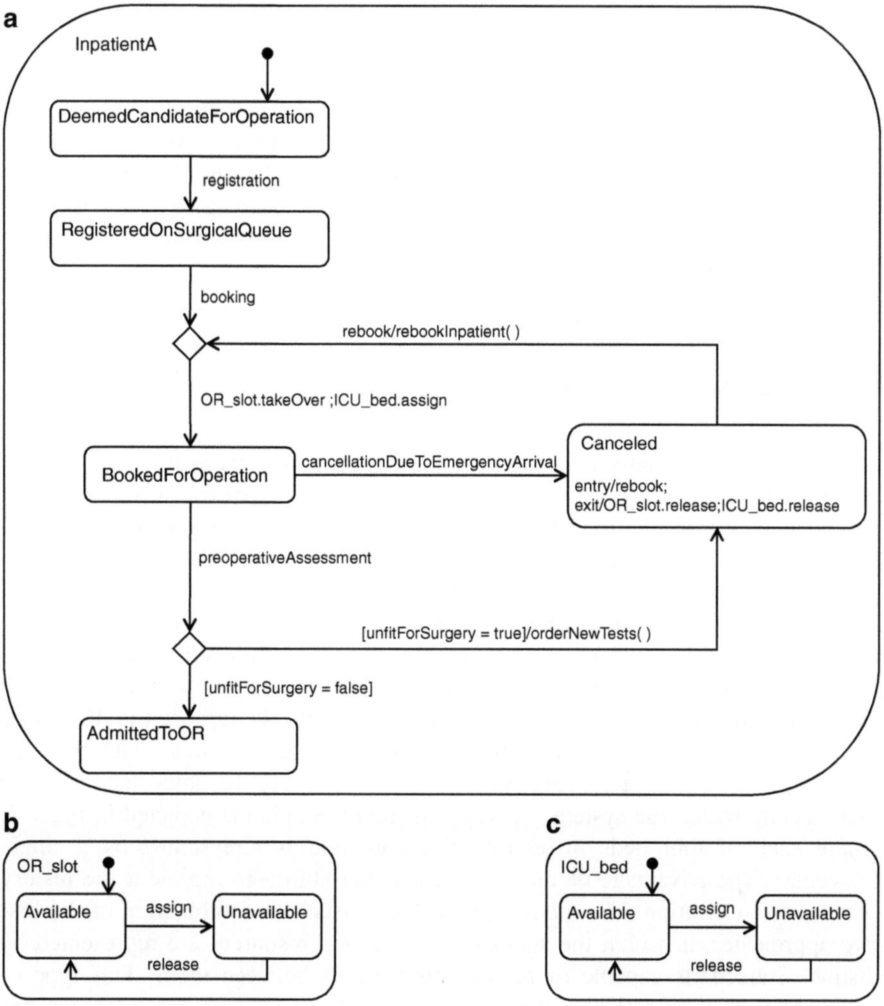

Fig. 6.4 The notion of event broadcasting in the Statecharts visual formalism: (**a**) an inpatient's progression from the time surgery is deemed necessary to the time the inpatient enters the operating room (OR), (**b**) a single OR slot, and (**c**) a single bed in the intensive care unit (ICU)

This event causes the event `assign` to be broadcast to the OR_slot and ICU bed Statecharts, which in turn causes transition from the state `Available` to the state `Unavailable` within each of these two Statecharts. The event `cancellationDueToEmergencyArrival` may disrupt the progression of the inpatient to the operating room, in which case the inpatient moves to the state `Canceled`. Entry into the state `Canceled` triggers the event `rebook`, which causes execution of the activity `rebookInpatient( )` as the inpatient moves from the state `Canceled` back to the state `BookedForOperation`.

If there is no cancellation due to an emergency arrival at this stage, the event `preoperativeAssessment` occurs. However, if the condition `unfitForSurgery` is met after the preoperative assessment, the inpatient again moves to the state `Canceled`. The condition `unfitForSurgery` also causes execution of the activity `orderNewTests( )`. As the patient exits from the state `Canceled`, the event `release` is broadcast to the OR_slot and ICU_bed Statecharts. This event causes transition from the state `Unavailable` to the state `Available` in both of these Statecharts, making both the operating room slot and the intensive care bed available for another patient.

6.3 Representing Patient Flow

The capacity of the Statecharts formalism to represent reactive systems in terms of activities, events, states, and transitions between states gives rise to three distinct approaches to representing a health care system for discrete-event simulation of patient flow: the *patient* approach, the *resource* approach, and the *mixed* approach. The *patient* approach represents a health care system purely in terms of the states that patients may occupy throughout the system. This type of representation is depicted in Fig. 6.4a, where the progression of a single inpatient is described as a number of states from the time surgery is deemed necessary to the time the inpatient enters the operating room. The advantage of this approach is the ability to represent the flow of patients through the health care system. The *resource* approach represents a health care system purely in terms of the states that resources may occupy within the system. This type of representation is depicted in Fig. 6.3, where each of four beds in an intensive care unit is represented by a single Statechart. The advantage of this approach is the ability to represent the history of resource utilization. The *mixed* approach consists of a combination of the first two approaches, in which the states of patients and resources are represented by distinct Statecharts capable of broadcasting events between them. This type of representation is depicted by the three parts of Fig. 6.4. This last approach has the advantage of representing both patient flow and resource utilization in a single conceptual framework.

Conceptually, the progression of individual patients through the simulated health care system may be modeled as a series of updates in patient records in reaction to events generated by the modeled processes of care delivery in an asynchronous fashion. For example, a discrete-event simulation model of patient flow may generate the timing and occurrence of simulation events and store them in dynamic tables that the modeled processes can update and read in reaction to events generated by other processes [71]. The captured data may then be used to generate the histories of simulated individual care paths. To illustrate the simulation of individual care paths, consider the progression of inpatients as illustrated in Fig. 6.4. For this type of patient, five events determine progression through the surgical process: (1) registration in the surgical queue, (2) booking of the operation, (3) preoperative assessment, (4) cancellation of the operation, and (5) admission to the operating room. In a discrete-event simulation, a set of dynamic tables is used to store the timing and occurrence of these five events, as well as information about the simulated inpatients (e.g., patient identification number, sex, and age) (Table 6.2). These data can be used to generate the progression of each individual patient.

The field Event ID is used to record the order of occurrence of events, such that the occurrence of the first event for each patient's progression always has the value 1. For example, patient 1000, a 65-year-old man, was registered in the surgical queue on day 2, was booked for operation on day 5 (with the operation scheduled to occur on day 8), underwent preoperative assessment on day 7, and was admitted to the operating room on day 8, as planned. Patient 1003, a 70-year-old woman, was registered in the surgical queue on day 4, was booked for surgery on day 7 (with the operation scheduled to occur on day 10), and underwent preoperative assessment on day 9, at which time she was found to be unfit for the operation and the surgery was canceled. Also on day 9, this patient was rebooked for surgery (with the operation now scheduled to occur on day 12), and she underwent another preoperative assessment on day 11, after which she was admitted to the operating room (on day 12). Patient 1006, a 75-year-old man, was registered in the surgical queue on day 5, was booked for surgery on day 6 (with the operation scheduled to occur on day 9), and underwent preoperative assessment on day 8, when he was found to be unfit for the operation. The procedure was canceled on day 8, and the patient was rebooked for surgery the same day (with the operation now scheduled to occur on day 11). The patient underwent a second preoperative assessment on day 10, but his operation was canceled on day 11 by the arrival of a more urgent patient. Patient 1006 was rebooked for the operation on day 11 (with the operation scheduled to occur on day 12) and was finally admitted to the operating room on day 12.

In addition to the use of dynamic tables, patient progression can be depicted graphically, as in Fig. 6.5 for patients 1000 and 1003. The x-axis of this patient progression diagram shows the time units that control the flow of time during the simulation (in this case, days), and the y-axis shows the modeled events. The figure clearly shows that the progression of patient 1003 was disrupted on day 9 because of a cancellation.

6.4 Modeling Requirements

As mentioned in Sect. 2.1.2, the use of simulation for evaluating health care policy is based on two premises: first, that simulated individual care paths realistically represent the delivery of health services to a patient population and, second, that simulation produces care paths that are likely under the policy in question. The definition of modeling requirements in discrete-event simulation using the Statecharts formalism leads to models that are based on these two premises and produce more realistic simulated care paths under the policy in question.

Table 6.2 Sample dynamic tables used by a discrete-event simulation model of patient flow to store patient information and the timing and occurrence of events

Table: Patient information

Patient ID	Sex	Age (years)
997	Male	69
1000	Male	65
1003	Female	70
1005	Male	68
1006	Male	75

Table: Registration in surgical queue

Patient ID	Day of event	Event ID
997	1	1
1000	2	1
1003	4	1
1005	2	1
1006	5	1

Table: Booking of operation

Patient ID	Day of event	Event ID	Scheduled day of operation
997	1	2	3
997	3	5	4
1000	5	2	8
1003	7	2	10
1003	9	5	12
1005	4	2	6
1006	6	2	9
1006	8	5	11
1006	11	8	12

Table: Preoperative assessment

Patient ID	Day of event	Event ID
997	2	3
1000	7	3
1003	9	3
1003	11	6
1005	5	3
1006	8	3
1006	10	6

Table: Cancellation

Patient ID	Day of event	Event ID	Reason
997	3	4	Patient arrival
1003	9	4	Unfit for operation
1006	8	4	Unfit for operation
1006	11	7	Patient arrival

Table: Admission to operating room

Patient ID	Day of event	Event ID
997	4	6
1000	8	4
1003	12	7
1005	6	4
1006	12	9

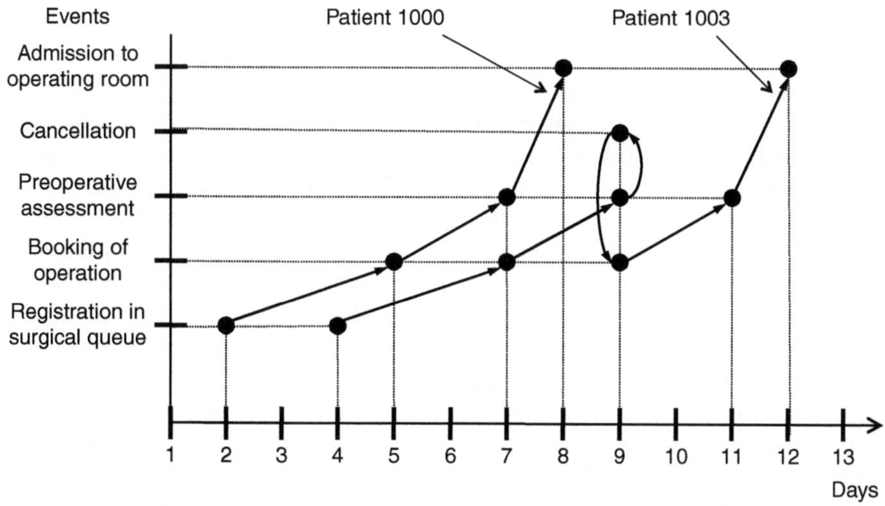

Fig. 6.5 Diagram showing patient progression (see Table 6.2)

In Sect. 3.2, we discussed the taxonomy of a health care process as a tool that can be used in a number of ways: to describe the process within a uniform framework of knowledge, to document possible variation in managing activities across care facilities, to develop a data model for representing patient progression through the process, and to define modeling requirements.

6.5 Modeling Assumptions

Modeling assumptions facilitate the definition of Statecharts representing a health care system without adversely modifying the model's objectives, which could affect results of a simulation experiment. They also help to clarify those aspects of a health care system that can feasibly be simulated. For example, in a discrete-event simulation model of the process of booking patients for an operation, it can be assumed that the clerical staff responsible for booking operations are always available, even though this may not be the case in real life, since staff may be absent because of illness or vacation. Similarly, when modeling the activity of preoperative assessment of patients, it can be assumed, on the basis of historical data, that a certain proportion of patients will be found unfit for the operation; for this assumption, the fitness of each individual patient will be based on a binomial (branching) probability drawn from the distribution of historical data.

6.6 Input Parameters

A simulation experiment involves running the model with inputs that represent policy alternatives and the parameters of organizational arrangements (e.g., frequency, timing, and duration of activities or processes; occupational mixes; distribution probabilities representing historical data) [143]. Other inputs affect system performance without themselves being affected by any change in policy. For example, consider a simulation model of patient flow that requires a different proportion of patients found unfit for surgery after preoperative assessment by an anesthesiologist from run to run. In this case, the binomial probability governing the simulated outcome of the preoperative assessment will be the input parameter for the model. Another example is the modeling requirement to simulate the anesthesiologist's availability to assess patients before the operation only on certain days each week. In this case, the schedule of the anesthesiologist's weekly availability should be the input parameter for the model. The Statecharts formalism is especially suitable for defining the system configurations through the input parameters that realistically represent the delivery of health services to a patient population under the policy in question.

6.7 Output Data

In Chap. 2, we noted that each run generates a group of simulated patients served in a modeled care facility or hospital, with the group size being determined by input parameters, such as arrival and service rates, and by simulation time. The outputs of a discrete-event simulation model usually include variables related to both the simulated health care system and the simulated patients. These variables, which are stored in dynamic tables during the simulation, comprise information about the health care process, the records of individual simulated patients, and the timing and occurrence of simulation events. System-related output data, which consist of all the information about the policy alternative modeled in each simulation run, represent the modeled care facility. Individual patient paths can be re-created by linking the patient-related outputs stored in the dynamic tables, as explained in Sect. 6.3. Study outcomes may then be computed from values taken from fields in the linked data. For example, time from registration in a surgical queue to operation can be computed as the number of days between the registration date and the operation date. Discrete-event models are especially effective for simulation of patient flow, as they simulate individual care paths as a series of asynchronous updates in patient records generated in reaction to events produced by parallel states representing concurrent activities. In this regard, the Statecharts formalism is useful for representing the progression of individual patients through a care process in terms of activities, events, states, and transitions between states.

Part II
Methods

Chapter 7
Design of a Simulation Study

In health services research, an intervention study is a common tool for evaluating policy changes implemented in hospitals, wards, or outpatient services. In Chap. 2, we argued that the methodological rigor of intervention research should be applied in conducting computer simulation studies to evaluate policy changes before they are implemented. In particular, we have proposed that the framework for health care intervention studies be applied to computer simulation experiments. This application is the focus of this chapter. First, we develop the analytical framework of the simulation experiment. Second, we describe how to determine the number of simulation runs and how to allocate the runs in a cluster randomized study design. Finally, we outline a plan for analyzing output data from a simulation experiment.

7.1 Simulation Study as Intervention Research

7.1.1 Computer Simulation

Computer simulation provides a method for evaluating the effects of proposed changes in the delivery of health care before implementation, as discussed in Chap. 2. Evaluative studies using computer simulation involve developing a simulation model of health care processes and conducting simulation experiments to generate data for analysis, as described in Chap. 6. Input parameters of a simulation model represent proposed alternatives, service details, and characteristics of a population of patients and their conditions. Each run of the simulation model generates a group, or cluster, of response pathways for individual patients served in a modeled hospital. During each run, the simulation software records the occurrence and timing of simulated events in the patient population, such as appointments, registrations, and cancellations. In fact, a simulation model can be thought of as a bookkeeping system that records output data generated in response to input data. Output data from simulation experiments can be used to evaluate the performance of

B. Sobolev et al., *Health Care Evaluation Using Computer Simulation: Concepts, Methods, and Applications*, DOI 10.1007/978-1-4614-2233-4_7,

Box 7.1 Drawing inferences from a simulation experiment

Analytical framework
Study hypothesis stating the relation between intervention and its effects
Primary study factor representing intervention
Experimental outcomes representing individual and system responses
Performance measure summarizing the outcome distribution
Change in performance measure between experimental groups representing effect

Experimental design
Unit of randomization specifying entities assigned to experimental groups
Number of simulation runs ensuring high probability of detecting the true effect
Cluster-level factors determining allocation of runs to experimental groups

Plan of analysis
Unit of analysis specifying level of model-based statistical inferences
Testing of statistical hypothesis
Regression methods for estimating the intervention effect
Other factors impeding or enhancing the occurrence of outcomes

the modeled services similar to the use of data that would be obtained from a real-life intervention study of the same question. Therefore, the analytical framework for health care intervention studies can be applied to the analysis of data from simulation experiments.

7.1.2 Three Aspects of Simulation Experiment

Researchers look at three aspects of a simulation experiment: the analytical framework, the experimental design, and the plan of analysis of results, as presented in Box 7.1. The analytical framework operationalizes the study question into a hypothesis by identifying the primary study factor, the experimental outcomes, and the measure of effect size. These three elements correspond to the elements of an intervention study, discussed in detail in Chap. 1. The researcher uses these elements to plan how interventions will be represented in the simulation model and what output data will be used to measure the effectiveness of the intervention. The experimental design, specifies the unit of randomization, determines the number of runs that will be needed, and devises the allocation of runs to experimental groups. The experimental design helps the researcher to plan how the simulations will be run. The plan of analysis identifies the unit of analysis, the hypothesis testing, the regression methods, and the adjustment factors. This information is used in planning how to evaluate the effectiveness of the intervention, for example, in deciding on how to interpret effects.

7.2 Analytical Framework

7.2.1 *Study Hypothesis*

Developing the analytical framework refines the study question into a hypothesis. The study hypothesis states the conjectural nature of the link between study factors and outcome variables in the simulation experiment. In the experiment, the study factors are forced to change their values, and the outcome variables are expected to change their values in response. The purpose of the simulation study is then to test whether a change in the study factors representing the intervention results in a change in the outcome variables (see Chap. 1). As an illustration, consider the study question, *What are the effects of booking elective surgery in advance?* A researcher will first identify the experimental groups, with the control group usually representing the existing method. In this example, the control group consists of patients whose surgery is scheduled by the wait-list method, and intervention group consists of those scheduled by the advance booking method. The researcher will also identify the outcome of interest, which might be surgical wait times. At this point, the study question can be translated into a study hypothesis: *surgical wait times are shorter when elective surgery is booked in advance, relative to booking from wait lists.*

The statistical hypothesis is a more specific statement of the tested relation than the study hypothesis. It includes statements for the null hypothesis (denoted by H_0) and the alternative hypothesis (denoted by H_A). Usually, the null hypothesis states that there is no difference in the performance measure between the experimental groups, and the alternative hypothesis states that there is a difference between the groups.

7.2.2 *Primary Study Factor*

In intervention research, the primary study factor represents the intervention. In designing a simulation experiment, the primary study factors are the input parameters related to the policy being evaluated (see Sect. 2.3). The method of booking surgery is an example of a primary study factor.

7.2.3 *Experimental Outcomes*

In Sect. 2.4, we discussed three types of experimental outcomes: those related to the simulated patients, those related to simulated treatments, and those related to simulated systems of care delivery. Patient-related outcomes represent the effect on

Table 7.1 Examples of experimental outcomes

Outcome	Type	Categories or values
Patient-related		
Time on surgical wait list	Numeric	0 or more weeks
Timing of surgery	Categorical	Within recommended time
		After recommended time
Treatment-related		
Postoperative complication	Categorical	Yes
		No
System-related		
Appointment list census	Numeric	0 or more patients

simulated patients of the delivery of care in the simulated health care system. An example of such an outcome is the number of weeks from registration to removal from the surgical wait list (see Table 7.1). In patient-level simulation models, this outcome is computed from the date of registration on the wait list and the date of removal from the wait list for each simulated patient in the experiment. Treatment-related outcomes represent the effect on a simulated patient's biological or physiological condition of undergoing therapy within the simulated system. An example of such an outcome is whether a patient experiences postoperative complications necessitating admission to the intensive care unit. System-related outcomes represent the effect on the health care system. An example of this outcome is the appointment list census, a count of patients on the appointment list at the end of a specified period. As discussed in Chap. 1, understanding the overall effect of an intervention could require the analysis of multiple outcomes such as these.

Experimental outcomes are computed from the simulated patient records generated by runs of the simulation model with different combinations of input data (see Chap. 6). The output data of a simulation model may directly contain an experimental outcome. For example, simulation models of individual patient trajectories can produce a set of binary responses $\{y_{ijl}\}$ showing whether the surgery of patient $l = 1, \ldots, m_{ij}$ in run $j = 1, \ldots, k$ of experimental group i was canceled on the day of surgery. Alternatively, the experimental outcomes may have to be computed from the output data of the simulation model. For example, consider the outcome of whether a hospital performed the required procedure within the recommended time frame for all patients who had high priority at the time of registration for elective surgery. Determining this response for each simulated hospital would require an assessment of whether each patient underwent surgery on time. The outcome would be a set of binary responses $\{y_{ij}\}$ showing whether all high-priority procedures in run $j = 1, \ldots, k$ of experimental group i were performed within the recommended time frame.

7.2.4 Performance Measures

In intervention studies related to health care, a summary outcome measure represents the distribution of an outcome variable in the patient population. Similarly, in simulation experiments related to health care, a performance measure summarizes the distribution of an experimental outcome in the simulated patient population. In this book, we use the terms *summary measure* and *performance measure* interchangeably because summary measures are used to characterize performance. In most studies, the performance measure combines the observed responses for all patients or hospitals from the simulation experiment into a single number. For example, a simulation experiment might record the timing and occurrence of a clinic appointment for each simulated patient, with the distribution of time to clinic appointment (the experimental outcome) being summarized by the weekly rate of appointments (the performance measure).

Suppose a simulation experiment has been designed to address the question, *Does the method of booking elective surgery affect surgical wait times?* Here, the primary study variable is the method of booking elective surgery, and the outcome variable is time to surgery. Operationalizing the study question involves identifying a performance measure that will provide meaningful information about the effect of the booking method on times to surgery. One available performance measure could be the proportion of patients who undergo surgery within a recommended time frame. Note that this proportion combines into a single quantity multiple, individual wait times of patients undergoing surgery. Another performance measure could be the rate at which patients undergo surgery. This rate combines into a single quantity data about whether the patients undergo surgery and data about how long they wait for the procedure. Performance measures may also involve more than a single number. For example, a surgical access function has multiple numbers, estimating the probabilities of surgery for each week on the wait list. Hospital-level and patient-level performance measures are discussed in more detail in Chap. 8 and Chap. 9, respectively.

7.2.5 Measure of Effect Size

Researchers use observed variation in a performance measure between experimental groups to estimate the effect size of a policy, similar to using variation in a summary measure between study groups in an intervention study (Sect. 1.3). The effect size is usually expressed in terms of absolute or relative differences in performance measures (or related functions) between the experimental groups. As an illustration of an effect-size measure that uses absolute differences, suppose a policy-maker would like to compare clearance times (i.e. the number of weeks it takes to serve all patients currently waiting for an appointment) between two methods of booking appointments (i.e., the experimental groups). A performance measure for this outcome could be the average clearance time, and a corresponding measure of effect size would be the absolute difference in average clearance times between methods of booking appointments. As an illustration of an effect-size measure that uses relative differences, suppose a policy-maker would like to compare the occurrence of a postoperative complication between two methods of booking surgery. A performance measure for this outcome could be the odds of a postoperative complication, and a corresponding measure of effect size would be the odds ratio.

The effect of a policy can be measured at the level of the hospital or at the level of the patient. For example, the absolute difference in average clearance times measures the effect size at the hospital level, whereas the relative difference in the odds of a postoperative complication measures the effect size at the patient level (see previous paragraph). Measures of effect size at the level of the hospital (i.e., cluster) and the patient (i.e., individual) will be discussed further in Chap. 8 and Chap. 9, respectively. In Sect. 7.4, we note that effect sizes can be estimated using regression methods, in which an unknown regression coefficient is linked to an effect-size measure (see also Chap. 11 and Chap. 12).

7.3 Experimental Design

7.3.1 Cluster Randomized Design in Simulation Experiments

As noted in Sect. 7.1, the experimental design is another aspect of a simulation experiment in health care. In Chap. 2, we suggested that the elements of experimental design for simulation experiments be the same as those of an intervention study. Specifically, the experimental design should include the unit of randomization, the number of simulation runs, and the method of allocating individual experimental entities and simulation runs to different experimental groups. For the experimental design of a simulation experiment, we propose applying a cluster randomized design, as discussed in Sect. 1.4, with a simulation run as the randomization unit. For this randomization unit, clusters of patients, rather than individual patients, are assigned to experimental groups. This type of randomization is suitable when the intervention of interest is aimed at a group since each simulation run generates a cluster of patients whose treatment is the same in some respect. For example, all of the patients might be served in the same modeled hospital. Relative to randomization at the level of individual patients, randomization at the level of clusters of patients represents a more complex design, requires more patients to generate equivalent statistical power, and requires more complex analysis [33].

In studies with a cluster randomized design, the number of simulation runs is influenced by characteristics of the cluster, such as the number of individuals in

Table 7.2 Inflation factors calculated as $1 + (m - 1)\rho$ for various cluster sizes m and values of the intracluster correlation coefficient ρ, rounded to one decimal place

	Intracluster correlation coefficient					
Cluster size	0.001	0.01	0.02	0.03	0.04	0.05
10	1.0	1.1	1.2	1.3	1.4	1.4
50	1.0	1.5	2.0	2.5	3.0	3.5
100	1.1	2.0	3.0	4.0	5.0	6.0
200	1.2	3.0	5.0	7.0	9.0	11.0
500	1.5	6.0	11.0	16.0	21.0	26.0
750	1.7	8.5	16.0	23.5	31.0	38.5
1,000	2.0	11.0	21.0	31.0	41.0	51.0

each cluster and the degree of similarity between outcomes within each cluster. If individuals from one cluster are more similar to each other than they are to individuals from other clusters, then more individuals will be needed in a study with a randomized cluster design than in a study where individuals are randomly assigned to experimental groups. The intracluster correlation coefficient quantifies the extent of agreement in the observed outcomes between two individuals from the same cluster or simulation run [59]. More specifically, it is the ratio of the variation between clusters to the total variation [62]. An intracluster correlation coefficient that is greater than zero implies that individuals within the same cluster are similar. The degree of similarity increases with the increasing values of the intracluster correlation coefficient. Another measure of similarity is the coefficient of variation, which is the ratio of the between-cluster variation and the event rate.

The inflation factor, also known as the design effect, is a multiplicative factor indicating how many more individuals are needed to detect an effect in a study with randomization of clusters, rather than randomization of simulated individuals. This inflation factor is a function of both the number of individuals per cluster and a measure of the degree of similarity between individuals. When the performance measure is an individual-level mean or proportion, the inflation factor is equal to $1 + (m - 1)\rho$, where m is the cluster size and ρ is the intracluster correlation coefficient [49]. For a small cluster size of 50 and a low intracluster correlation coefficient of 0.001, the inflation factor is 1.05, and the number of individuals to be simulated is therefore about 5% higher with randomization at the level of clusters rather than individuals. For a large cluster size of 750 and a high intracluster correlation coefficient of 0.04, the inflation factor is 31, and it would therefore be necessary to simulate about 31 times as many individuals in a cluster randomized design. The inflation factor is directly related to both the cluster size and the intracluster correlation coefficient (Table 7.2). As cluster size increases, the inflation factor increases for a given intracluster correlation coefficient. Similarly, as the intracluster correlation coefficient increases, the inflation factor increases if cluster size is held constant.

7.3.2 *Unit of Randomization*

The design of a simulation experiment has at its core the unit of randomization, the entity that will be randomly assigned to one of the experimental groups. This might range from a basic entity, such as a simulated patient, to a more complex entity, such as a network of simulated hospitals. In situations where the health care intervention of interest is directed at a group of individuals, such as all patients in a particular hospital, the group, rather than the individual patient, is the natural unit of randomization. Considering that each simulation run will generate a group (or cluster) of patients served in a modeled hospital, we suggest that the simulation experiment should have a cluster randomized design, with the unit of randomization being the simulation run [153]. As shown in [51], the cluster randomized design provides methodological advantages when the intervention requires policy changes at the organizational level and when the expected effect is to be evaluated at both the organizational and the individual level.

7.3.3 *Number of Simulation Runs*

The number of factors involved in health care interventions is usually substantial. Even seemingly straightforward management alternatives may have underlying complexities related to, for example, interactions between the managerial and clinical activities of surgical care. If this complexity is adequately captured in the model's specifications, it will produce substantial variability in the experimental outcomes. Therefore, the design of a simulation experiment should ensure a sufficient number of simulation runs for detecting, with high probability, the anticipated effect of the controlled variation in multiple study factors in the statistical analysis of experimental data. For example, hospital-level interventions may result in similar outcomes for patients from the same simulation run because of hospital-level factors. The number of runs are estimated using formulas that adjust for similarity of individuals' outcomes within runs, using a measure such as the intracluster correlation coefficient.

In general, three factors determine the number of simulation runs needed to compare individual-related or cluster-related outcomes across experimental groups: the anticipated effect size, the statistical power desired, and the significance level. The effect size here represents the smallest anticipated difference between experimental groups. The number of runs should be set so that if such a difference exists, then it is very likely that a statistically significant result will be obtained. The choice of the measure of effect size depends on the performance measure. The statistical power will be the probability that the null hypothesis is correctly rejected. It is usually thought of as the complement of the probability of missing a real effect. Therefore, higher power means a lower chance of missing the effect. The significance level is a cutoff point for the p value, below which the null hypothesis

Table 7.3 Example of design points representing combinations of values for experimental factors, a full factorial design

	Experimental factor		
Design point	Booking surgical consultations	Booking elective surgery	Allocating operating room slots
1	Individual lists	Wait-list booking	Weekly split
2	Individual lists	Wait-list booking	Daily split
3	Individual lists	Advance booking	Weekly split
4	Individual lists	Advance booking	Daily split
5	Pooled list	Wait-list booking	Weekly split
6	Pooled list	Wait-list booking	Daily split
7	Pooled list	Advance booking	Weekly split
8	Pooled list	Advance booking	Daily split

is rejected. The p value is the probability of obtaining the effect size observed in the experiment if the null hypothesis of no difference is actually true. If the p value for the test is less than the significance level, the researcher concludes that it would be improbable to have observed the data obtained in the experiment if there was actually no effect. By extension, the researcher then concludes that there is evidence of an effect. The steps for determining the number of simulation runs are presented in Appendix B.

7.3.4 Allocation of Runs Across Experimental Groups

In simulation experiments with a cluster randomized design, the unit of randomization is the simulation run, each with different values for the various experimental factors. Each run generates a group of simulated patients (the individual experimental entities) served in a modeled hospital (the cluster). In a stratified cluster randomized design, the simulation runs are grouped initially into homogeneous strata according to a combination of characteristics of the run and are then randomly assigned, within each stratum, to either the intervention or the control group.

A full factorial cluster randomized design would have one simulation run for every possible combination of the values of the cluster-level experimental factors, with the term *design point* being used to refer to each such combination of values. For example, in a simulation experiment with three factors (e.g., method of booking surgical consultation appointment, method of booking elective surgery, and allocation of operating room slots) each having two categories, a full factorial design would have eight design points (= $2 \times 2 \times 2$) (Table 7.3). Combinations of values for each simulation run are assigned using a design matrix. Such a matrix could be represented by coding values of the cluster-level experimental factors as indicator variables. For example, the method of booking appointment could be coded as 0 for the individual-lists method and 1 for the pooled-list method, the method of booking

Table 7.4 Example of allocating runs in a full factorial design

Run	Variable I_1	Variable I_2	Variable I_3
1	0	0	0
2	0	0	1
3	0	1	0
4	0	1	1
5	1	0	0
6	1	0	1
7	1	1	0
8	1	1	1

Abbreviations: I_1 = indicator variable for method of booking consultation, I_2 = indicator variable for method of booking surgery, I_3 = indicator variable for method of allocating operating room slots

surgery could be coded as 0 for wait-list booking and 1 for advance booking, and allocation of operating room slots could be coded as 0 for the weekly-split method and 1 for the daily-split method (as in Table 7.4).

The coding with indicator variables in Table 7.4 helps to explain how a design matrix is constructed. In a design matrix, these indicator variables are represented by columns, and a simulation run is represented by a row. The corresponding design matrix $\boldsymbol{X}$ for the full factorial design shown in Table 7.4 is as follows:

$$\boldsymbol{X} = \begin{pmatrix} 0\ 0\ 0 \\ 0\ 0\ 1 \\ 0\ 1\ 0 \\ 0\ 1\ 1 \\ 1\ 0\ 0 \\ 1\ 0\ 1 \\ 1\ 1\ 0 \\ 1\ 1\ 1 \end{pmatrix}.$$

The first row of this design matrix (i.e., [0 0 0]) indicates that the simulation run will use the individual-lists method of booking surgical consultation appointment, the wait-list method of booking elective surgery, and the weekly-split method of allocating operating room slots.

The researcher may encounter situations where the number of design points does not equal the number of simulation runs needed to detect an effect. If there is a large number of environmental factors or if the environmental factors have many possible values, the number of runs in a full factorial design may greatly exceed the number of runs needed to detect an effect. In these circumstances, the researcher may opt to use a subset of the design points. Conversely, the number of runs needed to detect an effect may exceed the number of design points. In these circumstances, the researcher needs to know which design points to use multiple times.

In situations where the researcher wants to ensure an optimal distribution of experimental factors across the runs, the Fedorov algorithm can be used [55].

With this algorithm, the initial design is based on a random selection of design points (i.e., combinations of the values of the cluster-level experimental factors) from the full factorial design. The Fedorov algorithm then switches pairs of design points from the initial design, and the remainder of the design points to maximize the determinant of the information matrix for the design output [6]. The information matrix is related to the inverse of the variance–covariance matrix; therefore, maximizing the determinant of the information matrix is equivalent to minimizing the determinant of the variance–covariance matrix. The resulting set of design points determines the combinations of values of the environmental factors to be assigned to each run. A group of individuals randomly generated in a run with these combinations of values is then allocated to an experimental group.

For example, suppose a researcher needs 10 simulation runs per experimental group for a simulation experiment comparing two methods of booking surgical consultation appointment. Also, suppose the method of booking surgery (two categories) and the allocation of operating room slots (two categories) may have an influence on the outcome of interest. The transposed design matrix of an optimal design that was obtained by the Fedorov algorithm is as follows:

$$X = \begin{pmatrix} 0\,0\,0\,0\,0\,0\,0\,0\,0\,0\,1\,1\,1\,1\,1\,1\,1\,1\,1\,1 \\ 0\,0\,0\,0\,0\,1\,1\,1\,1\,1\,0\,0\,0\,0\,0\,1\,1\,1\,1\,1 \\ 0\,0\,1\,1\,1\,0\,0\,0\,1\,1\,0\,0\,0\,1\,1\,0\,0\,1\,1\,1 \end{pmatrix}^{\mathrm{T}}.$$

In this optimal design matrix, the 11th simulation run would be assigned the pooled-list method of booking the surgical consultation appointment, the wait-list method of booking surgery, and the weekly-split method of allocating operating room slots. The matrix shows that more than one simulation run is assigned to each design point. For example, two simulation runs will be assigned to design point 1 and three simulation runs will be assigned to design point 2.

Ensuring a balanced distribution of individuals' (i.e., patients') attributes across the runs is an important aspect of the experimental design. Each simulated patient is randomly assigned values for attributes, such as age and sex. The value of each attribute is obtained by sampling from the distribution of a random variable, which has parameter values derived from historical data. For example, if historical data show that 80% of the population are male, then the simulation model could use a binary random variable with a probability parameter of 0.80 to assign the sex of a simulated patient. In this example, a value of 1 would represent a male simulated patient, and a value of 0 would represent a female simulated patient. Each run of the simulation model will generate a group of simulated patients whose distribution of attributes is similar to that from the historical data. A balanced distribution of both environmental factors and the attributes across runs will allow the researcher to attribute any observed differences in the experimental outcome to differences in the primary study factor (i.e., the intervention).

7.4 Plan of Analysis

The plan for analysis of data from a simulation experiment will guide the assessment of performance of the intervention. The analysis of the experimental output involves statistical comparison of outcomes across experimental groups, such that a difference between groups will be interpreted as the effect of the intervention. In Chap. 1, we discussed how the unit or units of analysis, the regression methods, and other explanatory factors relate to statistical inferences in intervention studies. The same elements are also used by researchers when planning analyses for a simulation experiment.

7.4.1 Unit of Analysis

The unit of analysis is the entity upon which statistical inferences will be based, for example, a hospital, a ward, a clinic, or a patient. The unit of analysis contrasts with the unit of randomization, the entity that is randomly assigned to an experimental group, and the unit of observation, the entity for which data are collected. In some cases, the same entity serves as the unit of randomization, observation, and analysis. In a cluster randomized study, the unit of randomization is the cluster, and the unit of observation could be the individual, the cluster, or both. The unit of analysis represents the level at which the researcher wants to make generalizations about the simulated population, as described below.

If the researcher is interested in how the intervention will affect an individual simulated patient, then the unit of analysis will be the individual patient. On the other hand, if the researcher is interested in how the intervention will affect a collection of simulated patients, then the unit of analysis would be the cluster of patients (i.e., the hospital). To illustrate, consider the study question, *does the method of booking appointments at the preadmission clinic affect the proportion of hospitals with less than 10% of procedures canceled for patient-related reasons?* This study question focuses on performance at the level of the hospital (frequency of cancellations), so the hospital is the unit of analysis. Similarly, the intervention (the method of booking appointments at the preadmission clinic) is applied at the hospital level, so the hospital is the natural unit of randomization in a cluster randomized design. Conversely, the outcome of interest (whether a hospital had less than 10% of procedures canceled for patient-related reasons) requires data from each patient in the hospital, so the unit of observation will be the patient. However, because data on hospital characteristics are also required for this analysis, there is a second unit of observation, the hospital.

7.4.2 Hypothesis Testing

The data generated from a simulation experiment are used to test the statistical hypothesis and determine if there is evidence to reject the null hypothesis. Testing of a statistical hypothesis could be two-sided or one-sided. With two-sided testing, the null hypothesis states that there is no difference in the performance measure between the intervention group and the control group, and the alternative hypothesis states that a difference may exist, without specifying the direction of the difference. In other words, the alternative hypothesis states that the intervention group performs either better or worse than the control group. With one-sided testing, the alternative hypothesis does specify a direction, stating either that the intervention group performs better than the control group or that the control group performs better than the intervention group. Two-sided tests should be used unless there is a specific reason to test the effect in one direction [22]. An expectation that the difference will be in a particular direction is not sufficient justification for performing a one-sided test. In the context of health care, interventions may be complex, and the results of simulation experiments could be surprising. Therefore, if the true effect is in the opposite direction from the expected effect, specification of a one-sided test would prevent detection of the true result [22].

To illustrate two-sided and one-sided hypothesis testing, suppose a policy-maker wants to compare surgical wait times between two methods of booking surgery: wait-list booking and advance booking. In these examples, the performance measure of interest could be the rate of surgery, defined as the average number of elective surgeries per week. The rate characterizes the distribution of the surgical wait times by summarizing how many patients undergo surgery per time unit. With the two-sided hypothesis, the researcher investigates whether the surgery rates differ between the two methods of booking, regardless of which performs better. Therefore, a two-sided statistical hypothesis would be formulated as follows:

H_0: There is no difference in the surgery rate between the wait-list booking and advance booking methods.

H_A: There is a difference in the surgery rate between the wait-list booking and advance booking methods.

In contrast, with a one-sided hypothesis, the researcher investigates whether the surgery rate is higher in hospitals that use advance booking. This one-sided statistical hypothesis would be formulated as follows:

H_0: The surgery rate among patients treated in hospitals that use advance booking is lower than among patients treated in hospitals that book procedures from wait lists.

H_A: The surgery rate among patients treated in hospitals that use advance booking is higher than among patients treated in hospitals that book procedures from wait lists.

If in fact the surgery rate is higher in hospitals that book procedures from wait lists, the analysis would not be able to detect the difference with the one-sided hypothesis.

Two types of errors may occur in hypothesis testing. A type I error is defined as the null hypothesis being mistakenly rejected (i.e., there is evidence of a difference in the performance measure between experimental groups when such a difference does not exist). For example, in the two-sided hypothesis comparing two methods of booking surgery, a type I error would be made if the rates of surgery were the same for the two booking methods, but the statistical results led the researcher to conclude that the rates were different. In contrast, a type II error is defined as the null hypothesis being mistakenly accepted (i.e., there is no evidence for a difference in the performance measure between experimental groups when such a difference exists). To illustrate, a type II error would be made if the rates differed between the two booking methods, but the statistical results led the researcher to claim that the rates were the same. In reality, researchers never know whether their conclusions accurately reflect the true situation or whether an error has occurred, but they can limit the chances of such errors through the design of the simulation experiment, as described in Sect. 7.3. The probability of a type I error, denoted by α, is related to the significance level (i.e., the probability that a result is due to chance). The probability of a type II error, denoted by β, is the complement of statistical power. Both the significance level and statistical power influence the number of runs required in a simulation experiment (see Appendix B).

7.4.3 Regression Methods

Quantifying the effects of an intervention (i.e., estimating the effect size) requires statistical comparison of outcomes between experimental groups using regression methods. Different regression methods are applied according to the type of experimental outcomes, which may be measured at different levels, may take different forms, or may be captured with different frequencies over the course of the simulation experiment (Table 7.5). For example, linear regression measures effect size in terms of a difference between means for comparisons of continuous outcomes. Logistic regression measures effect size in terms of an odds ratio for comparisons of a binary outcome between groups. Discrete-time survival regression measures effect size in terms of a rate ratio for comparisons of outcomes related to the occurrence and timing of an event. Furthermore, controlling for other cluster-level or individual-level factors that may influence the outcome of interest necessitates adjustment by multivariable regression methods. Also, similarities between simulated individuals in each cluster necessitate adjustment of the chosen regression method for within-cluster correlation. Here, we briefly describe two regression methods with some examples of experimental outcomes for each approach.

First, as noted briefly above, experimental outcomes that measure a binary response for each cluster are analyzed with logistic regression models. Examples of such binary outcomes include whether or not a hospital had no cancellations

Table 7.5 Link between the elements of analytical framework and regression analysis

Element	Linear regression	Logistic regression	Discrete-time survival regression
Experimental outcome	Continuous	Binary	Time to event
Performance measure	Average	Odds	Event rate
Measure of the effect	Difference in averages	Ratio of odds	Ratio of rates, ratio of odds
Regression coefficient	Difference in averages	Difference in log odds	Difference in log odds
Effect-size estimate	Regression estimate	Exponential of regression estimate	Exponential of regression estimate

of high-priority procedures and whether or not a hospital had delays of the anesthesiology consultation for fewer than half of all patients. With this type of analysis, the experimental outcome is modeled as a function of the primary study variable, with adjustments for cluster-level factors. The exponential of the regression coefficient of the primary study variable yields the odds ratio for measuring the effect of the intervention at the cluster (i.e., hospital) level.

Second, experimental outcomes that measure the occurrence and timing of an event for each simulated individual (i.e., patient) are analyzed with discrete-time survival models. Examples of these types of outcomes include the number of weeks from a referral to a consultation with the surgeon and the number of weeks from registration on a wait list for surgery to unplanned emergency admission. With this type of analysis, the experimental outcome is again modeled as a function of the primary study variable, but this time with adjustments for both cluster-level and individual-level factors. The exponential of the regression coefficient of the primary study variable yields the weekly odds ratio for measuring the effect of the intervention at the individual level. To account for correlation between individuals, generalized estimating equations are used to determine the standard error of the regression estimates more accurately (i.e., by using the robust estimator for the covariance matrix) [94]. Regression methods for the analysis of cluster-level outcomes and individual outcomes are described in more detail in Chaps. 11 and 12, respectively.

During the regression analysis itself, the primary study variable and other explanatory variables are entered into multivariable regressions. Each categorical variable is included in the regression model as a set of indicator variables. The number of indicator variables in each set is one fewer than the number of categories, and the reference group is represented by a value of 0 for each indicator variable. For example, consider the primary study variable representing three experimental groups: reference, intervention 1, and intervention 2. For this variable, a set of two indicator variables (I_1 and I_2) are created to represent the three groups. The reference group takes a value of 0 for both indicator variables, and the two other groups (intervention 1 and intervention 2) represent the comparison categories (Table 7.6).

Table 7.6 Coding for two indicator variables representing three groups

Group	Variable I_1	Variable I_2
Reference	0	0
Intervention 1	1	0
Intervention 2	0	1

In a linear regression model, the regression coefficient for variable I_1 would estimate the difference in the averages of the experimental outcome between intervention group 1 and the reference group. Likewise, in this linear regression model, the regression coefficient for variable I_2 would estimate the effect of intervention 2 as compared with the reference group by the difference in the averages of the experimental outcome between intervention group 2 and the reference group. In contrast, in a logistic regression model, the regression coefficient for variable I_1 would estimate the difference in the log odds of an event in intervention group 1 compared to the reference group. The regression coefficient for variable I_2 would estimate the difference in the log odds of an event in intervention group 2 compared with the reference group.

7.4.4 Other Explanatory Factors

In Sect. 2.3, we introduced three types of experimental factors that investigators purposely vary to determine their influence on the performance measure: primary study factors, environmental factors, and attributes of experimental units. Primary study factors represent the intervention of interest. The environmental factors and attributes of experimental units may impede or promote the response of interest. Identifying environmental factors and attributes of experimental units allows the statistician to use regression methods to adjust for any differences in distributions between experimental groups.

Environmental factors are input parameters that contain information external to the individual simulated entity. An example of an environmental factor could be the method the hospital uses to allocate operating room slots (Table 7.7). It is possible that a particular primary study factor in one simulation experiment could be an environmental factor in another experiment. For example, the method of booking surgery is the primary study factor if the study question is *Does the method of booking elective surgery affect surgical wait times?* If the study question were instead, *Does the allocation of operating room slots affect surgical wait times?* the primary study factor would be the allocation of operating room slots, and the method of booking surgery would become an environmental factor. Attributes of individual simulated entities are output data containing information about the characteristics of the simulated patients, such as sex or number of coexisting medical conditions. These attributes may also be referred to as patient attributes.

Table 7.7 Examples of experimental factors

Factor	Type	Categories or values
Primary study factor		
Method of booking surgery	Categorical	Advance booking
		Wait-list booking
Environmental factors		
No. of surgeons	Numeric	≥1
Allocation of operating room slots between elective and urgent procedures	Categorical	Weekly split
		Daily split
Patient attributes		
Sex	Categorical	Female
		Male
Age group (years)	Categorical	<50
		50–59
		60–69
		70–79
		≥80

In designing a simulation experiment, the researcher determines the experimental factors to be varied in the experiment, the levels to be used for categorical variables, and whether any of the quantitative variables should be categorized, whereby a categorical variable would be used to represent a quantitative variable. For example, as shown in Table 7.7, age may be input as a categorical variable, with data categorized into age groups. Alternatively, age may be input as a numeric variable with data values in years. In designing a simulation model, the researcher determines the input parameters that represent the distribution of these attributes in the population (e.g., the probability that a simulated patient will be female).

Chapter 8
Planning a Study at the Cluster Level

In health care simulation studies involving patient care paths, each simulation run generates a cluster of outcomes. Such outcomes might come from a group of simulated patients served in a modeled hospital or surgical service. In Chap. 1, we introduced the notion of intervention studies employing a cluster randomized design, in which hospitals, physicians' practices, or surgical services, rather than individual patients, are randomly assigned to study groups. Similar to the situation for intervention studies, in simulation experiments with a cluster randomized design, it is simulation runs, rather than individual experimental units, that are randomized across experimental groups. Then, in Chap. 2, we observed that the outputs of simulation experiments could be used to evaluate the performance of the modeled services, similar to data that would be obtained from a real-life intervention study of the same question. Therefore, we suggested employing the analytical framework of intervention studies to the analysis of data from simulation experiments.

In Chap. 7, we drew a parallel between summary measures and performance measures, arguing that a summary measure represents the outcome distribution observed in real life and a performance measure summarizes the distribution of an experimental outcome. With guidance from the study question, experimental outcomes can be evaluated at the level of the individual or the cluster. In cluster-level analysis, the cluster of simulated individuals is considered as the unit of inference, and performance measures are computed across cluster-level outcomes. In this chapter, we present two performance measures suitable for assessing the effect of an intervention at the cluster level: proportions and averages. We relate these performance measures to the study hypothesis, the experimental outcome, and the corresponding measures of effect for comparisons across experimental groups. We also present formulas for determining the number of runs for an experiment that would be sufficient to detect the effect of an intervention on the basis of cluster-level performance measures.

B. Sobolev et al., *Health Care Evaluation Using Computer Simulation: Concepts, Methods, and Applications*, DOI 10.1007/978-1-4614-2233-4_8,

8.1 Cluster-Level Proportions

Cluster-level proportions summarize system performance by measuring the fraction of clusters that satisfy a specified criterion. Whether the cluster-level proportion is suitable for assessing the effect of an intervention is related to the study hypothesis, the experimental outcome, and the corresponding measures of effect for comparisons across experimental groups. The outcome for a cluster-level indicator variable is often calculated from the outcomes of the individual entities (e.g., simulated patients) within each cluster. There are many scenarios for which evaluation using cluster-level proportions might be suitable.

8.1.1 A Scenario Involving Cluster-Level Proportions

In this chapter, we use the following scenario to illustrate the evaluation of system performance by using cluster-level proportions. We will refer to this hypothetical situation as Scenario 8.1: A health services researcher is studying alternative methods of booking patients for consultation appointments in a surgical clinic. Most hospitals have a separate wait list for each surgeon, and patients are seen by the surgeon named in the referral on a first-come, first-served basis (i.e., the individual wait-lists method). Some hospitals have started to use a single, pooled wait list, whereby patients are seen on a first-come, first-served basis, but each appointment is made with the first available surgeon (i.e., the pooled wait-list method). The researcher is curious to know if the method of booking these consultation appointments affects whether any high-priority elective procedures will be performed after the recommended time frame. He formulates the following study question: *Does the method of booking surgical consultation appointments affect whether any of the hospital's high-priority elective procedures experience surgical delay?*

8.1.2 Type of Study Hypothesis

In the context of health care simulations, cluster-level proportions summarize the performance of a system when the study hypothesis involves the chance of a cluster meeting a performance criterion. For such hypotheses, the cluster might be a group of simulated patients in a hospital or a ward. The performance criterion might be whether the hospital has any canceled procedures.

On the basis of the study question, researchers determine if the cluster-level proportion is an appropriate performance measure for formulating the statistical hypothesis. Two features of the study question are used to make this determination. The first feature is whether the question is formulated at the level of the cluster. As such, the unit of analysis is the cluster. For example, in Scenario 8.1, the hospital (rather than the patient) is the entity of interest; in other words, the researcher is interested in outcomes at the level of the hospital. The second feature is whether the question has an experimental outcome that takes one of two possible values (i.e., meeting or not meeting the criterion). As such, the experimental outcome is binary. In Scenario 8.1, the outcome is whether or not surgery is delayed for any of the hospital's high-priority elective procedures.

Provided the unit of analysis is the cluster and the experimental outcome is binary, the study question can be operationalized into a statistical hypothesis for cluster-level proportions (see Sect. 7.2). Such statistical hypotheses identify the primary study factor, the experimental outcome, and the performance measure. These hypotheses also consist of statements about whether the proportions differ between experimental groups. In Scenario 8.1, the primary study factor is the method for booking surgical consultation appointments. For this scenario, the following two-sided statistical hypothesis would apply, where H_0 is the null hypothesis and H_A is the alternative hypothesis:

H_0: There is no difference in the proportion of hospitals with surgical delay for high-priority elective procedures between hospitals using the individual-lists method for booking surgical consultation appointments and those using the pooled-list method.

H_A: There is a difference in the proportion of hospitals with surgical delay for high-priority elective procedures between hospitals using the individual-lists method for booking surgical consultation appointments and those using the pooled-list method.

8.1.3 Type of Experimental Outcome

Cluster-level proportions are estimated from experimental outcomes that are binary and that are observed for each cluster. In a health care intervention study, this type of experimental outcome generally indicates whether or not a hospital meets the performance criterion. For example, in Scenario 8.1, the experimental outcome is whether or not the hospital has any surgical delays for high-priority elective procedures.

Data generated by simulation experiments that would be suitable for estimating cluster-level proportions for Scenario 8.1 have two properties. First, each observed value of the experimental outcome corresponds to one hospital, with the hospital being the unit of analysis. Second, the variable corresponding to the experimental outcome can take on one of two values: 0 if the hospital does not have delay of surgery for any high-priority elective procedures and 1 if the hospital does have such delays. As such, this variable is what is known as an indicator variable. Indicator variables are coded as 1 if the event of interest occurs and as 0 otherwise. To determine the observed value for the indicator variable representing the cluster-level outcome, the researcher will require data at the individual level. In particular, he will require information about each patient's priority for elective surgery, the recommended time frame for the surgery, and how long the patient waited for surgery. If any patient undergoes surgery after the recommended time frame in a given hospital, the value of the indicator variable for that hospital is set to 1; otherwise, it is set to 0.

8.2 Measuring Performance with Proportions

8.2.1 Definition

Cluster-level proportions define the fraction of clusters that satisfy a specified criterion. In the context of health services research, the proportion of hospitals meeting a criterion, which is a common performance measure, would be a cluster-level proportion. For example, researchers might want to determine the proportion of hospitals with cancellations of high-priority elective procedures, the proportion of hospitals in which fewer than half of initial surgical consultations are delayed, or the proportion of hospitals in which the operating room is not fully booked more than 10% of the time [138, 144].

A performance measure that is related to the cluster-level proportion is the cluster-level odds. The cluster-level odds can be expressed as the ratio of the probability of a cluster meeting the performance criterion to the probability of the cluster not meeting the performance criterion (i.e., its complement). These odds are equivalent to the ratio of the expected number of times the cluster will meet a specified criterion to the expected number of times the cluster will not meet the criterion. Proportions have a lower limit of 0 and an upper limit of 1. Odds have a lower limit of 0 and no upper limit.

8.2.2 Estimation

The cluster-level proportion, p^{c}, is estimated as the ratio of the observed number of clusters meeting the performance criterion to the total number of clusters:

$$\hat{p}^{\mathrm{c}} = \frac{\text{no. of clusters meeting criterion}}{\text{total no. of clusters}}. \tag{8.1}$$

The hat symbol $\hat{}$ denotes a quantity that is estimated from the observed data in a simulation experiment. Therefore, $\hat{p}^{\mathrm{c}}$ is an estimated value for the cluster-level proportion.

Consider Scenario 8.1, where the researcher is interested in monitoring procedures delayed after the recommended time frame. The estimated cluster-level performance measure, the proportion of hospitals with surgical delay for any high-priority elective procedures, is expressed as follows:

$$\hat{p}^{c} = \frac{\text{no. of hospitals with delay}}{\text{total no. of hospitals}}.$$

Suppose that the researcher in this scenario assigns 50 groups of simulated patients to each method of booking surgical consultation appointments. A group of simulated patients has been served in one modeled hospital; therefore, we may say that 50 hospitals have been assigned to each booking method. Suppose further that the researcher observes that overall 84 of the 100 hospitals in the study have delays for high-priority elective procedures. The estimated cluster-level proportion would therefore be $84/100 = 0.84$.

The cluster-level proportion in (8.1) can be expressed in terms of the experimental outcome for each cluster. Suppose y_j is the binary response for whether run $j = 1, \ldots, k$ meets the performance criterion (i.e., the experimental outcome). The cluster-level proportion can then be calculated as follows:

$$\hat{p}^{c} = \frac{\sum_{j=1}^{k} y_j}{k}, \tag{8.2}$$

where the numerator, $\sum_{j=1}^{k} y_j$, counts the number of clusters that meet the performance criterion.

A confidence interval specifies a range of values that quantify the uncertainty of an estimate. For example, a 95% confidence interval will contain the true parameter value 95 times out of 100. The lower and upper boundaries of the confidence interval are called confidence limits. For a large number of clusters, the normal approximation to the binomial distribution can be used to obtain approximate $100(1-\alpha)\%$ lower and upper confidence limits for the cluster-level proportion:

$$\begin{aligned} \text{LCL} &= \hat{p}^{c} - z_{\alpha/2}\sqrt{\text{Var}(\hat{p}^{c})}, \\ \text{UCL} &= \hat{p}^{c} + z_{\alpha/2}\sqrt{\text{Var}(\hat{p}^{c})}, \end{aligned} \tag{8.3}$$

where $z_{\alpha/2}$ is the $100(1-\alpha/2)$th quantile of the standard normal distribution and $\text{Var}(\hat{p}^{c}) = \hat{p}^{c}(1-\hat{p}^{c})/k$ is the variance for the estimated proportion [37]. For 95% confidence limits, $\alpha = 0.05$ and $z_{0.025} = 1.96$.

For Scenario 8.1, the approximate 95% confidence limits for the proportion of hospitals with delay of surgery for high-priority elective procedures are calculated using (8.3) as follows:

$$\begin{aligned} \text{LCL} &= 0.84 - 1.96\sqrt{(0.84)(1-0.84)/100} \approx 0.77, \\ \text{UCL} &= 0.84 + 1.96\sqrt{(0.84)(1-0.84)/100} \approx 0.91. \end{aligned}$$

Equation (8.3) estimates confidence limits using the normal approximation to the binomial distribution. The approximate lower or upper confidence limit calculated with this equation may lie below 0 or above 1, respectively. If the number of clusters is small, then an exact confidence interval may be derived from the binomial distribution [37]. A continuity correction is used if either the number of clusters meeting the performance criterion (i.e., $k\hat{p}^{\mathrm{c}}$) or the number of clusters not meeting the performance criterion (i.e., $k[1-\hat{p}^{\mathrm{c}}]$) is not above 5.

The cluster-level odds are estimated as the ratio of the cluster-level proportion to its complement:

$$\text{odds} = \frac{\hat{p}^{\mathrm{c}}}{1-\hat{p}^{\mathrm{c}}}. \tag{8.4}$$

For example, if the proportion of hospitals allowing delays for high-priority elective procedures is 0.84, then the odds of a hospital having delay are estimated as follows:

$$\text{odds} = \frac{0.84}{1-0.84} \approx 5.3.$$

8.2.3 *Interpretation*

The cluster-level proportion represents the fraction of simulated clusters (e.g., hospitals) meeting a specified criterion. The percentage of clusters meeting the criterion is estimated by multiplying this proportion by 100. This quantity can be interpreted as the number of clusters, out of every 100, expected to meet the performance criterion. For example, given a proportion of 0.84 for hospitals with delay of high-priority elective procedures, the researcher would expect about 84 out of every 100 hospitals to have surgical delays for this category of patients.

The cluster-level odds is a ratio expressing the expected number of times the cluster will meet a specified criterion in relation to the expected number of times it will not meet the criterion. Odds of exactly 1 imply that the likelihood of the cluster meeting the performance criterion is the same as the likelihood that it will not meet the criterion. Odds greater than 1 imply that the cluster is more likely than not to meet the criterion, whereas odds less than 1 imply that the cluster is more likely to *not* meet the criterion. For example, the odds of 5.3 that a hospital will have delays of high-priority elective procedures mean that the probability that a hospital will have delays is 5 times the probability that it will not have delays.

8.3 Comparing Proportions

8.3.1 *Definition*

Comparing cluster-level proportions and quantifying their differences between experimental groups necessitate a measure of effect size. The cluster-level odds ratio is a measure of differences in cluster-level proportions between two experimental groups. The odds ratio expresses the relative difference in odds between group 1 and group 2:

$$\text{odds ratio} = \frac{\text{odds for group 2}}{\text{odds for group 1}}. \tag{8.5}$$

In this measure, the odds for the reference group (i.e., group 1) is presented in the denominator, and the odds for the comparison group (i.e., group 2) is presented in the numerator.

8.3.2 *Crude Estimate*

A crude estimate of the odds ratio can be produced using simulated data from two experimental groups. Suppose y_{ij} is the binary response for run $j = 1, \ldots, k$ of group $i = 1, 2$ meeting the performance criterion. The cluster-level proportion for group i can be calculated as follows:

$$\hat{p}_i^{\mathrm{c}} = \frac{\sum_{j=1}^{k} y_{ij}}{k}. \tag{8.6}$$

In a cluster-level analysis, the crude odds ratio is estimated as the ratio of the observed odds for the comparison group to the observed odds for the reference group:

$$\text{crude odds ratio} = \frac{\hat{p}_2^{\mathrm{c}}/(1-\hat{p}_2^{\mathrm{c}})}{\hat{p}_1^{\mathrm{c}}/(1-\hat{p}_1^{\mathrm{c}})}, \tag{8.7}$$

where $\hat{p}_1^{\mathrm{c}}$ is the estimated cluster-level proportion for the reference group and $\hat{p}_2^{\mathrm{c}}$ is the estimated cluster-level proportion for the comparison group.

Consider Scenario 8.1, where the researcher assigned 50 hospitals to each experimental group and observed a total of 84 out of 100 hospitals with delays for high-priority elective procedures. Suppose that 45 of the 84 hospitals with surgical delays are from the experimental group using the individual-lists method of booking surgical consultations and the remaining 39 hospitals are from the group using the pooled-list method. If the hospitals using the individual-lists method are deemed to form the reference group, and the hospitals using the pooled-list method are deemed to form the comparison group, the estimated odds ratio of hospitals with delays for high-priority elective procedures is calculated as follows (see (8.7)):

$$\begin{aligned} \text{crude odds ratio} &= \frac{(39/50)/(1-39/50)}{(45/50)/(1-45/50)} \\ &= \frac{0.78/(1-0.78)}{0.90/(1-0.90)} \approx 0.39. \end{aligned}$$

8.3.3 *Interpretation*

Cluster-level odds ratios compare the odds (or proportions) between experimental groups. An odds ratio of 1 implies that the odds of a cluster meeting the performance criterion are equal for the comparison and reference groups. An odds ratio greater than 1 implies that the odds of a cluster meeting the criterion are higher in the comparison group than in the reference group. Conversely, an odds ratio less than 1 implies that the odds of a cluster meeting the criterion are lower in the comparison group than in the reference group.

The percent difference in the odds of a cluster in the comparison group meeting the criterion relative to the odds of a cluster in the reference group meeting the criterion is calculated by subtracting 1 from the odds ratio and then multiplying the value by 100 [2]. For example, the odds ratio of 0.39 for Scenario 8.1, calculated above, means that the odds of delay for high-priority elective procedures are about 61% lower (i.e., $[0.39-1]\times 100\% = -61\%$) among hospitals using pooled lists for booking surgical consultation appointments than among hospitals using individual lists.

8.4 Number of Runs for Comparing Proportions

When planning a simulation experiment, the number of simulation runs should be large enough to allow the researcher to detect the anticipated effect of the intervention with high probability. In Appendix B, we outline the steps for estimating the number of simulation runs, a process that depends on the performance measure of interest. Here, we describe how to determine the number of simulation runs when the cluster-level proportion is used as the performance measure. In addition to the performance measure, the number of runs depends on the significance level, the statistical power, and the anticipated difference between experimental groups in the proportions of clusters meeting a performance criterion.

Suppose a researcher wants to test the null hypothesis that the cluster-level proportions for two groups are equal against a two-sided alternative. Calculating the number of simulation runs requires knowledge of the cluster-level proportion for the reference group, p_1^c, and the smallest anticipated difference between the cluster-level proportions for the comparison and reference groups, δ. Given p_1^c and δ, the proportion for the comparison group, p_2^c, is calculated as $\delta + p_1^c$.

To compare proportions at the cluster level, k runs are randomized to each experimental group [58]:

$$k = \left[\frac{z_{\alpha/2}\sqrt{2\bar{p}^c(1-\bar{p}^c)} + z_{\beta}\sqrt{p_1^c(1-p_1^c)+p_2^c(1-p_2^c)}}{\delta} \right]^2, \tag{8.8}$$

where $z_{\alpha/2}$ is the $100(1-\alpha/2)$th quantile of the standard normal distribution, z_β is the $100(1-\beta)$th quantile of the standard normal distribution, and $\bar{p}^c = (p_1^c + p_2^c)/2$ is the average proportion for two groups with an equal number of runs [58]. In these expressions, α represents the significance level and β represents the type II error (or the complement of the statistical power) (see Appendix B).

Statistical software can be used to obtain the needed quantiles of the standard normal distribution (i.e., $z_{\alpha/2}$ and z_β). For example, a significance level of 0.05 corresponds to the 97.5th quantile of the standard normal distribution, which has a value of 1.96 (i.e., $z_{0.025} = 1.96$), and a statistical power of 90% corresponds to a type II error rate of 0.10 and the 90th quantile of the standard normal distribution, which has a value of 1.28 (i.e., $z_{0.10} = 1.28$). For a one-sided alternative, $z_{\alpha/2}$ is replaced with z_α in (8.8). This formula is derived by assuming asymptotic normality.

In Scenario 8.1, the researcher wants to evaluate the effect of the method of booking surgical consultation appointments—either individual lists or a pooled list—on the proportion of hospitals with delays for high-priority elective procedures. Suppose that provisional runs of the simulation model indicate that, among hospitals using the individual-lists method, the hypothesized proportion of hospitals with delay is 0.90 (i.e., $p_1^c = 0.90$). The number of runs needed to detect a reduction in this proportion from 0.90 to 0.80 (i.e., $\delta = -0.10$) is estimated with a two-tailed probability of 0.05 (i.e., $\alpha = 0.05$) and 90% statistical power (i.e., $\beta = 0.10$). Using (8.8),

$$k = \left[\frac{1.96 \times \sqrt{2 \times 0.85 \times 0.15} + 1.28 \times \sqrt{(0.90 \times 0.10) + (0.80 \times 0.20)}}{-0.10}\right]^2$$
$$\approx 265.6.$$

Therefore, the estimated number of simulation runs per method is 266 to ensure 90% statistical power to detect the 0.10 difference at the significance level of 0.05.

The significance level, statistical power, and effect size all affect the number of simulation runs. When estimating the number of runs, the values of these factors may be unknown, so it is advisable to use a range of values for the calculations. Estimating the number of runs using a range of values serves two purposes. First, if the value of an element is unknown, the researcher is not forced to choose a random value, which might unduly influence planning of the experiment. Second, it allows the researcher to understand how widely the number of runs will vary with variations in certain determining factors.

As an illustration, we calculated the number of runs for Scenario 8.1, varying the significance level between 0.01 and 0.05, the statistical power between 80% and 90%, and the difference between the cluster-level proportions from −0.50 to −0.10, as depicted in Fig. 8.1. In the figure, the horizontal axis shows the magnitude and direction of the smallest anticipated difference in the proportion of hospitals with surgical delays between groups, and the vertical axis represents the number of simulation runs needed per group. For these calculations, the proportion for the reference group, p_1^c, was fixed at 0.90. Therefore, a value of −0.10 on the

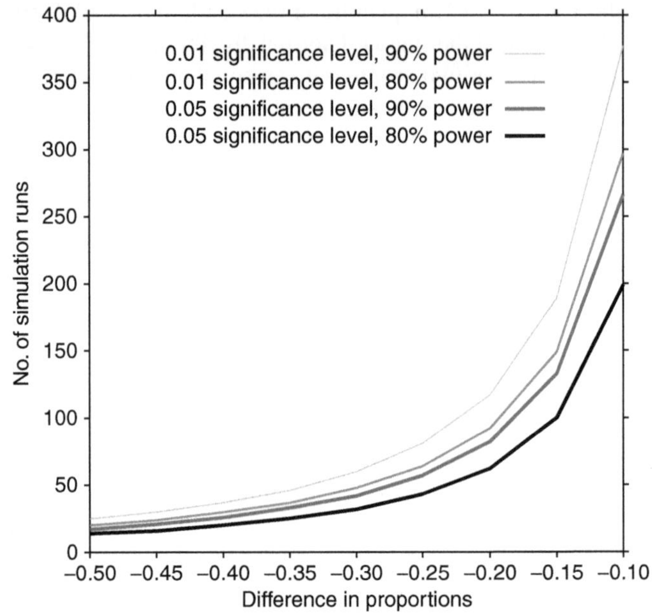

Fig. 8.1 Number of simulation runs for comparing cluster-level proportions in Scenario 8.1 in relation to significance level, statistical power, and difference in proportions ($p_2^c - p_1^c$, where p_1^c is the proportion for the reference group and p_2^c is the proportion for the comparison group)

horizontal axis corresponds to values of 0.90 and 0.80 for the proportions of hospitals with surgical delays in the reference group, p_1^c, and the comparison group, p_2^c, respectively.

Figure 8.1 shows that as the significance level decreases, the number of simulation runs increases, for fixed values of statistical power and difference in proportions. For example, the number of simulation runs increases from 266 to 377 when the significance level decreases from 0.05 to 0.01, for 90% statistical power and a 0.10 decrease in proportions. This makes sense intuitively since a researcher who wants to lower the chances of incorrectly claiming that the method of booking appointments affects the frequency of surgical delay will require more data. The number of simulation runs also increases as statistical power increases, with the significance level and difference in proportions held constant. For example, the number of simulation runs increases from 199 to 266 as the statistical power increases from 80% to 90%, for a significance level of 0.05 and a 0.10 decrease in proportions. Again, more data are required if the researcher wants to increase the chances of correctly claiming that the method of booking appointments affects the frequency of surgical delays.

Finally, the number of simulation runs increases as the magnitude of the effect size decreases, for a given significance level and statistical power. For example, the number of simulation runs increases from 82 to 266 as the difference between proportions decreases from 0.20 to 0.10, for a significance level of 0.05 and with 90% statistical power. This makes sense intuitively, since it is more difficult to detect smaller differences, so more data are required to detect such differences.

8.5 Cluster-Level Averages

Cluster-level averages are suitable for questions formulated at the level of the cluster, where the cluster (e.g., a hospital) is the unit of analysis, and for questions for which the outcome measure is continuous. The average is used to estimate the expected value of the distribution of an outcome variable. Whether the cluster-level average is suitable for assessing the effect of an intervention depends on the study hypothesis, the experimental outcome, and the corresponding measures of effect for comparisons across experimental groups. There are many scenarios for which evaluation using cluster-level averages might be suitable.

8.5.1 A Scenario Involving Cluster-level Averages

In this chapter, we use the following scenario to illustrate the evaluation of system performance using cluster-level averages. We will refer to this hypothetical situation as Scenario 8.2: A health services researcher is studying alternative methods of booking surgical consultation appointments. Most hospitals have a separate wait list for each surgeon, and patients are seen by the surgeon named in the referral on a first-come, first-served basis (i.e., the individual-lists method). Some hospitals have started to use a single, pooled wait list, whereby patients are seen on a first-come, first-served basis, but each appointment is made with the first available surgeon (i.e., the pooled-list method). The researcher is curious to know if the method of booking these consultation appointments affects the clearance time for an appointment list (i.e., the ratio of the existing demand to clinic capacity) [39]. Her question of interest is *Does the method of booking surgical consultation appointments affect clearance times for appointment lists?*

8.5.2 Type of Study Hypothesis

The cluster-level average is an appropriate performance measure when the expected value of observations from clusters is of interest. In these situations, the cluster is the unit of analysis, and the experimental outcome is a continuous or discrete measure. For such hypotheses, the cluster might be a group of simulated patients in a hospital or ward. The continuous measure might be the number of weeks required to serve all patients currently waiting for an appointment.

The study question in Scenario 8.2 can be operationalized into a statistical hypothesis, where the intervention is the method of booking surgical consultation appointments, the experimental outcome is the clearance time for the appointment lists, and the performance measure is the cluster-level average. The following two-sided statistical hypothesis would be of interest:

H_0: There is no difference in the average clearance time for appointment lists between hospitals using the individual-lists method of booking consultation appointments and those using the pooled-list method.

H_A: There is a difference in the average clearance time for appointment lists between hospitals using the individual-lists method of booking consultation appointments and those using the pooled-list method.

8.5.3 Type of Experimental Outcome

Cluster-level averages are estimated from experimental outcomes that are continuous or discrete and observed for each cluster. Examples of such outcomes include the number of weeks required to clear the list of patients waiting for a surgical consultation appointment (as in Scenario 8.2), the time by which 90% of patients will have undergone surgery, and the number of patients waiting on surgical wait lists [39, 145].

Data generated by simulation experiments that would be suitable for estimating cluster-level averages for Scenario 8.2 should have two properties. First, each observed value of the experimental outcome corresponds to one hospital, with the hospital being the unit of analysis. Second, the variable corresponding to the experimental outcome is a continuous or discrete variable, measuring the number of weeks required to serve all patients currently waiting for an appointment. It refers to the moving average clearance time for appointment lists and is estimated as the average of observed clearance times over 18 weeks for each hospital.

8.6 Measuring Performance with Averages

8.6.1 Definition

The average is often used to estimate the expected value of a distribution of one outcome variable. Examples of cluster-level averages include the average number of weeks required to clear the list of patients who are waiting for an appointment and the average number of patients currently waiting on a hospital's surgical wait lists [39, 145]. If the distribution is symmetric, then the population mean equals the population median, where the median is the point at which half of the values lie above and half of the values lie below.

8.6.2 Estimation

The cluster-level average, μ^c, is estimated as the sum of the observed values of the experimental outcome divided by the total number of clusters:

$$\hat{\mu}^c = \frac{\text{sum of observed values of outcome}}{\text{total no. of clusters}}. \tag{8.9}$$

The hat symbol ^ denotes a quantity that is estimated from the observed data in a simulation experiment. Therefore, $\hat{\mu}^c$ is an estimated value for the cluster-level average μ^c.

As an illustration, consider Scenario 8.2, where the researcher is interested in clearance times. The estimated cluster-level average clearance time for appointment lists is expressed as follows:

$$\hat{\mu}^c = \frac{\text{sum of observed hospital clearance times}}{\text{total no. of hospitals}}.$$

Suppose the researcher in Scenario 8.2 assigns 30 groups of simulated patients to each method of booking surgical consultation appointments. Again, a group of simulated patients is conceptualized as all those served in one modeled hospital; therefore, we may say that 30 hospitals have been assigned to each booking method. Suppose further that the researcher sums the observed clearance times for all 60 hospitals and obtains a total of 265 weeks. From (8.9), the cluster-level average is estimated as follows:

$$\hat{\mu}^c = \frac{265}{60} \approx 4.4 \text{ weeks}.$$

The cluster-level average in (8.9) can be expressed in terms of the observed outcomes from a simulation experiment. Suppose y_j is the continuous or discrete response for run $j = 1, \ldots, k$. The cluster-level average can then be calculated as follows:

$$\hat{\mu}^c = \frac{\sum_{j=1}^{k} y_j}{k}. \tag{8.10}$$

For a large number of clusters, the normal approximation to the t distribution can be used to obtain approximate $100(1 - \alpha)\%$ lower and upper confidence limits for the cluster-level average:

$$\begin{aligned} \text{LCL} &= \hat{\mu}^c - z_{\alpha/2}\sqrt{\text{Var}(\hat{\mu}^c)}, \\ \text{UCL} &= \hat{\mu}^c + z_{\alpha/2}\sqrt{\text{Var}(\hat{\mu}^c)}, \end{aligned} \tag{8.11}$$

where $z_{\alpha/2}$ is the $100(1-\alpha/2)$th quantile of the standard normal distribution, $\text{Var}(\hat{\mu}^c) = \hat{\sigma}^2/k$ is the variance of the estimated average, and $\hat{\sigma}^2 = \sum_{j=1}^{k}(y_j - \hat{\mu}^c)^2/(k-1)$ is the variance of the observed outcomes [37]. For 95% confidence limits, $\alpha = 0.05$ and $z_{0.025} = 1.96$. If the number of clusters in the simulation experiment is small, then the t distribution will be used in (8.11), instead of the normal distribution.

In Scenario 8.2, suppose the researcher calculates that the variance of the observed clearance times is 0.9. Then, using (8.11), the approximate 95% confidence limits for the average clearance time in weeks are calculated as follows:

$$\text{LCL} = 4.4 - 1.96\sqrt{0.9/60} \approx 4.2,$$

$$\text{UCL} = 4.4 + 1.96\sqrt{0.9/60} \approx 4.6.$$

8.6.3 Interpretation

Cluster-level averages quantify the expected value of the distribution of an outcome variable. As such, they are estimates of cluster-level population means. In Scenario 8.2, the clearance time for all hospitals is, on average, about 4.4 weeks (95% confidence interval 4.2–4.6). In this example, the point estimate of the cluster-level population mean is 4.4 weeks, and there is a 95% chance that the interval from 4.2 to 4.6 weeks captures the true value of this mean.

8.7 Comparing Averages

8.7.1 Definition

Comparing averages between experimental groups necessitates a measure of effect size. The difference compares averages in two groups by subtracting the average for group 1 from the average for group 2:

$$\text{difference} = \text{average for group 2} - \text{average for group 1}, \qquad (8.12)$$

In this measure, the average for the reference group (i.e., group 1) is subtracted from the average for the comparison group (i.e., group 2).

8.7.2 *Crude Estimate*

A crude estimate of the difference in cluster-level averages can be produced using simulated data from two experimental groups. Suppose y_{ij} is the continuous or discrete response for run $j = 1, \ldots, k$ in group $i = 1, 2$. The cluster-level average for group i can be calculated as follows:

$$\hat{\mu}_i^{c} = \frac{\sum_{j=1}^{k} y_{ij}}{k}. \tag{8.13}$$

In a cluster-level analysis, the crude difference is estimated as the difference in averages between the comparison group and the reference group:

$$\text{crude difference} = \hat{\mu}_2^{c} - \hat{\mu}_1^{c}, \tag{8.14}$$

where $\hat{\mu}_1^{c}$ is the estimated cluster-level average for the reference group and $\hat{\mu}_2^{c}$ is the estimated cluster-level average for the comparison group.

Consider Scenario 8.2, where the researcher is interested in comparing average clearance times for hospitals using one of two methods of booking consultation appointments: the individual-lists method (the reference group) and the pooled-list method (the comparison group). Suppose the average clearance time in the reference group is 5.2 weeks and the average clearance time in the comparison group is 3.6 weeks. Then, using (8.14), the crude difference between the cluster-level average clearance times can be estimated as follows:

$$\text{crude difference} = 3.6 - 5.2 \approx -1.6.$$

8.7.3 *Interpretation*

The crude difference is a measure of the effect size for comparing averages between experimental groups. If the crude difference is 0, then the averages for the reference group and the comparison group are the same. If the crude difference is greater than 0, the average is greater in the comparison group than in the reference group. Conversely, if the crude difference is less than 0, the average is less in the comparison group than in the reference group. For example, the calculated crude difference of -1.6 weeks in Scenario 8.2 means that the the clearance time for appointment lists is almost 2 weeks shorter among hospitals using the pooled-list method for booking surgical consultation appointments than among those using the individual-lists method.

8.8 Number of Runs for Comparing Averages

Similar to calculations for cluster-level proportions, when the performance measure of interest is a cluster-level average, the number of simulation runs depends upon the significance level, the statistical power, and the smallest anticipated difference in averages between experimental groups.

Suppose a researcher wants to test the null hypothesis that the cluster-level averages for two groups are equal against a two-sided alternative. Calculating the number of simulation runs requires knowledge of the difference in averages between groups, δ, and the common standard deviation, σ. To compare averages at the cluster level, the number of runs to be randomized to each group, k, is given by the following formula [127]:

$$k = \frac{2\sigma^2(z_{\alpha/2} + z_\beta)^2}{\delta^2}, \tag{8.15}$$

where $z_{\alpha/2}$ is the $100(1 - \alpha/2)$th quantile of the standard normal distribution, and z_β is the $100(1 - \beta)$th quantile of the standard normal distribution. In these expressions, α represents the significance level and β represents the type II error (or the complement of the statistical power) (see Appendix B). At a significance level of 0.05, $z_{\alpha/2}$ corresponds to the 97.5th quantile of the standard normal distribution, which has a value of 1.96 (i.e., $z_{0.025} = 1.96$), and a statistical power of 90% corresponds to a type II error rate of 0.10 and the 90th quantile of the standard normal distribution, which has a value of 1.28 (i.e., $z_{0.10} = 1.28$).

In Scenario 8.2, the researcher wants to evaluate the effect of the method of booking consultation appointments on the average clearance time for the appointment list. Suppose that provisional runs of the simulation model indicate that the common standard deviation is about 2 weeks. The number of simulation runs needed to detect a difference of 1 week in the average clearance time can be estimated using (8.15) with a significance level of 0.05 and 90% statistical power:

$$k = \frac{2(2)^2(1.96 + 1.28)^2}{(-1)^2} \approx 84.0.$$

Therefore, the estimated number of simulation runs per method is 84 to ensure 90% statistical power to detect a difference of 1 week at a significance level of 0.05.

The formula for the number of simulation runs in (8.15) assumes a large number of clusters available for observation. If the number of clusters is small, it is recommended that the number of runs be determined on the basis of the t distribution. Because the degrees of freedom for the t distribution depend on the number of runs, there is no closed-form formula in this case. Instead, statistical software using iterative methods is employed to determine the number of simulation runs.

To demonstrate the variation in the number of runs required to detect a range of effect sizes for different significance levels and different values of statistical power,

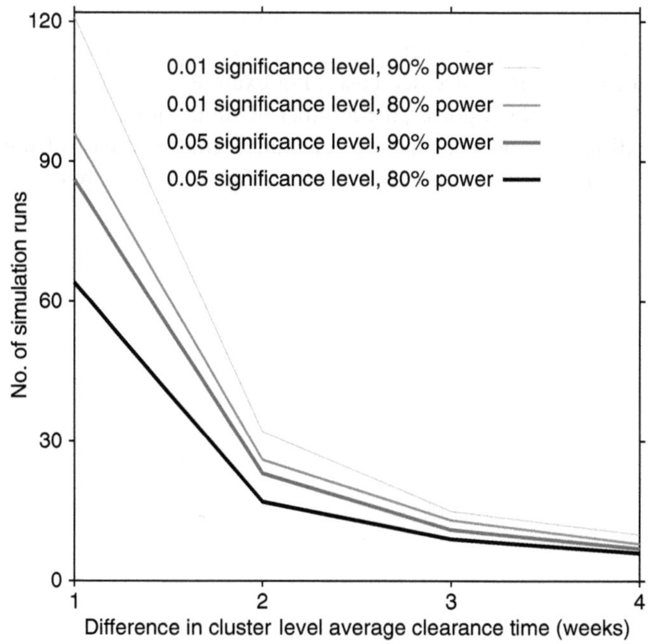

Fig. 8.2 Number of simulation runs for comparing cluster-level averages in Scenario 8.2 in relation to significance level, statistical power, and difference in averages ($\mu_2^c - \mu_1^c$, where μ_1^c is the average clearance time for the reference group and μ_2^c is the average clearance time for the comparison group)

we used the `power.t.test` function of R statistical software to compute the number of runs for Scenario 8.2 on the basis of the t distribution (Fig. 8.2). In the figure, the horizontal axis shows the magnitude and direction of the anticipated difference in the average clearance time between the comparison group and the reference group, and the vertical axis represents the number of simulation runs needed per group. A value of 1 on the horizontal axis corresponds to a difference of 1 week in the average clearance time between the two groups.

Figure 8.2 shows that as the significance level decreases, the number of simulation runs increases, for fixed values of statistical power and difference in averages. For example, the number of simulation runs increases from 86 to 121 when the significance level decreases from 0.05 to 0.01, for 90% statistical power and a 1-week difference in clearance times. This makes sense intuitively, since a researcher who wants to lower the chances of incorrectly claiming that the booking method affects the average clearance time will require more data. The number of simulation runs also increases as statistical power increases, with the significance level and difference in averages held constant. For example, the number of simulation runs increases from 64 to 86 as statistical power increases from 80% to 90%, for a significance level of 0.05 and a decrease of 1 week in cluster-level averages. Again, more data are required if the researcher wants to increase the chances of correctly claiming that the booking method affects the clearance time. Finally, for a given significance level and statistical power, the number of simulation runs increases as the magnitude of the effect size decreases. For example, with a significance level of 0.05 and at 90% statistical power, the number of simulation runs increases from 23 to 86 as the difference between average clearance times decreases from 2 weeks to 1 week. Again, this corresponds to our intuition that more data are required to detect smaller differences.

Chapter 9
Planning a Study at the Individual Level

In Chap. 8, we introduced two performance measures suitable for evaluating the effect of an intervention when the cluster of simulated individuals is the unit of inference. In this chapter, the simulated individual, which in health care is usually the patient, is the unit of inference. We present performance measures for evaluating the effect of an intervention on outcomes measured for each individual. In particular, we discuss individual-level proportions and rates in relation to the study hypothesis, the experimental outcome, and the corresponding measures of effect. When planning a simulation experiment, researchers decide upon the performance measures and determine the number of simulation runs using the chosen measures. Methods for estimating the number of runs on the basis of individual-level performance measures are presented in this chapter.

9.1 Individual-Level Proportions

In the context of health care evaluation, individual-level proportions quantify the fraction of individuals experiencing an event of interest. This type of performance measure contrasts with cluster-level proportions, which define the fraction of clusters or groups of patients that meet a specific criterion (as described in Sect. 8.2). For example, the study hypothesis of a health services researcher who is investigating the likelihood that a patient's elective surgery is canceled will differ from the hypothesis of another researcher who is interested in whether a hospital cancels fewer than 10% of its elective procedures. The first of these two researchers would use an individual-level proportion to draw a conclusion, whereas the second would use a cluster-level proportion. When estimating individual-level proportions, the individual patient is the unit of analysis, and the experimental outcome takes one of two possible values (i.e., whether or not the patient has experienced the event of interest).

B. Sobolev et al., *Health Care Evaluation Using Computer Simulation: Concepts, Methods, and Applications*, DOI 10.1007/978-1-4614-2233-4_9,

9.1.1 A Scenario Involving Individual-Level Proportions

In this chapter, we use the following scenario to illustrate the evaluation of system performance using individual-level proportions. We will refer to this hypothetical situation as Scenario 9.1: A surgeon approaches a simulation researcher expressing concern that a large number of his elective procedures are being canceled from the final operating room list. The surgeon has admitting rights at a hospital that has been using the wait-list booking method to schedule elective surgeries. He suspects that the advance booking method would reduce the chances of a patient's surgery being canceled. On the basis of the information provided by the surgeon, the researcher formulates the following study question: *Does the method of booking elective surgery affect the probability of cancellation of an elective procedure from the final operating room list?*

9.1.2 Type of Study Hypothesis

In the previous chapter, we noted that the suitability of a proportion for assessing the effect of an intervention is related to the study hypothesis, the experimental outcome, and the corresponding measures of effect for comparisons across experimental groups. The performance of a system can be summarized using proportions when the study hypothesis involves the probability of an individual experiencing an event of interest. For studies with this type of hypothesis, the individual is the unit of analysis, and the experimental outcome takes one of two possible values (i.e., whether or not the individual has experienced the event of interest).

From Scenario 9.1, researchers obtain information about the experimental groups, the experimental outcome, and the performance measure, which can be used to operationalize the study question into a statistical hypothesis. The experimental groups in this scenario will represent the two methods of booking elective surgery: wait-list booking and advance booking. The experimental outcome, which will be recorded for each patient scheduled for elective surgery, is whether or not the patient's procedure is canceled from the final operating room list. The individual-level (i.e., patient-level) proportion is an appropriate performance measure because the study hypothesis is formulated at the level of the patient and the outcome is binary. The study question can be operationalized into the following statistical hypothesis:

H_0: There is no difference in the proportion of patients whose elective surgery is canceled from the final operating room list between patients treated in hospitals using the wait-list method of booking surgery and those treated in hospitals using the advance booking method.

H_A: There is a difference in the proportion of patients whose elective surgery is canceled from the final operating room list between patients treated in hospitals using the wait-list method of booking surgery and those treated in hospitals using the advance booking method.

9.1.3 Type of Experimental Outcome

Individual-level proportions are estimated from experimental outcomes that take one of two values and that are observed for each individual. In a health care intervention study, this type of experimental outcome generally indicates whether or not an individual patient has experienced the event of interest. For example, in Scenario 9.1, the event of interest is cancellation from the final operating room list, and the experimental outcome records whether or not the patient's surgery has been canceled.

Data generated by simulation experiments that would be suitable for estimating cluster-level proportions for Scenario 9.1 should have two properties. First, each observed value of the experimental outcome corresponds to a single patient, with the patient being the unit of analysis. Second, the variable corresponding to the experimental outcome is binary and can take one of two values: 0 if the patient's procedure is not canceled from the final operating room list and 1 if the patient's procedure is canceled. As such, this variable is an indicator variable.

9.2 Measuring Performance with Proportions

9.2.1 Definition

In the context of health care simulations, individual-level proportions quantify the fraction of simulated individuals experiencing an event of interest. For instance, this type of performance measure can be used to summarize the proportion of simulated patients whose procedures are canceled from the final operating room list, the proportion of simulated patients whose surgical consultation appointments are delayed, or the proportion of surgeries performed on days when the operating room is less than fully booked.

Related to the individual-level proportion, the individual-level odds show the ratio of the probability of an individual experiencing the event of interest to the probability of the individual not experiencing the event (i.e., its complement). These odds are equivalent to the ratio of the expected number of times the event will occur to the expected number of times it will not occur [2].

9.2.2 Estimation

The individual-level proportion, p, is estimated as the ratio of the observed number of individuals experiencing the event of interest to the total number of individuals:

$$\hat{p} = \frac{\text{no. of individuals experiencing event}}{\text{total no. of individuals}}. \tag{9.1}$$

The hat symbol ^ denotes a quantity that is estimated from the observed data in a simulation experiment. Therefore, $\hat{p}$ is the estimated value for the proportion p.

To illustrate, consider Scenario 9.1, where the surgeon is interested in cancellations of elective procedures from the final operating room list. The individual-level performance measure, the proportion of patients with cancellation of elective surgery, is estimated as follows:

$$\hat{p} = \frac{\text{no. of patients with cancellation}}{\text{total no. of patients}}.$$

Suppose that in Scenario 9.1, the researcher observes that 7,179 out of 43,004 patients in the simulation study experience cancellation of their procedures from the final operating room list. The estimated proportion would therefore be 7,179/43,004 ≈ 0.17.

The individual-level proportion in (9.1) can be expressed in terms of the observed outcomes from a simulation experiment. Suppose there are k runs with m_j individuals in run $j = 1, \ldots, k$. Suppose also that y_{jl} is the binary response for an event for individual $l = 1, \ldots, m_j$ in run j. This outcome variable takes the value 1 if the individual experiences the event and 0 otherwise. The proportion of individuals experiencing the event is estimated as follows:

$$\hat{p} = \frac{\sum_{j=1}^{k} \sum_{l=1}^{m_j} y_{jl}}{\sum_{j=1}^{k} m_j}, \tag{9.2}$$

where the numerator, $\sum_{j=1}^{k} \sum_{l=1}^{m_j} y_{jl}$, counts the number of individuals that experienced the event of interest.

Confidence limits for an individual-level proportion are computed from the variance of this estimated proportion. In contrast to the variance of a cluster-level proportion (Sect. 8.2), the variance of an individual-level proportion requires statistical techniques that account for correlation between individual outcomes in each run. The ratio estimator is appropriate for estimating the variance of $\hat{p}$ [35,49]:

$$\text{Var}(\hat{p}) = \frac{k}{(k-1)(\sum_{j=1}^{k} m_j)^2} \sum_{j=1}^{k} \left(\sum_{l=1}^{m_j} y_{jl} - m_j \hat{p} \right)^2. \tag{9.3}$$

The approximate $100(1-\alpha)\%$ lower and upper confidence limits for the individual-level proportion can be calculated as

$$\begin{aligned} \text{LCL} &= \hat{p} - z_{\alpha/2}\sqrt{\text{Var}(\hat{p})}, \\ \text{UCL} &= \hat{p} + z_{\alpha/2}\sqrt{\text{Var}(\hat{p})}, \end{aligned} \tag{9.4}$$

where $z_{\alpha/2}$ is the $100(1-\alpha/2)$th quantile of the standard normal distribution. For 95% confidence limits, $\alpha = 0.05$ and $z_{0.025} = 1.96$.

For Scenario 9.1, the approximate 95% confidence limits for the proportion of patients with cancellation of their procedure from the final operation room list are calculated using (9.4) and estimates of $\hat{p} = 0.17$ and $\mathrm{Var}(\hat{p}) = 0.0052$:

$$\mathrm{LCL} = 0.17 - 1.96\sqrt{0.0052} \approx 0.03,$$
$$\mathrm{UCL} = 0.17 + 1.96\sqrt{0.0052} \approx 0.31.$$

The individual-level odds are estimated as the ratio of the observed individual-level proportion to its complement:

$$\text{odds} = \frac{\hat{p}}{1-\hat{p}}. \qquad (9.5)$$

Using (9.5), the odds that a patient's surgery will be canceled from the final operating room list are estimated as follows:

$$\text{odds} = \frac{0.17}{1-0.17} \approx 0.20.$$

9.2.3 Interpretation

The individual-level proportion represents the fraction of simulated individuals (e.g., patients) who experience an event of interest. The percentage of individuals experiencing the event is estimated by multiplying this proportion by 100. This quantity can be interpreted as the number of individuals, out of every 100, expected to experience the event. For example, given a proportion of 0.17 for patients whose procedures are canceled from the final operating room list, the surgeon can expect that surgery will be canceled for about 17 out of every 100 patients.

The individual-level odds is a ratio expressing the expected number of times an individual will experience the event of interest in relation to the expected number of times the individual will not experience the event. Odds of exactly 1 imply that the likelihood of the individual will experience the event is the same as the likelihood that the individual will not experience the event. Odds greater than 1 imply that the individual is more likely than not to experience the event, whereas odds less than 1 imply that the individual is more likely to *not* experience the event. For example, the odds of 0.20 that a patient's surgery will be canceled from the final operating room list mean that the probability of cancellation is one-fifth of the probability of no cancellation.

Individual-level proportions can be combined to provide additional information. For example, the cumulative proportion of individuals experiencing an event within a certain time frame can be used to generate an access curve [139]. Access curves, which show the estimated cumulative probability of an event on the vertical axis and time along the horizontal axis, allow researchers to estimate the probability

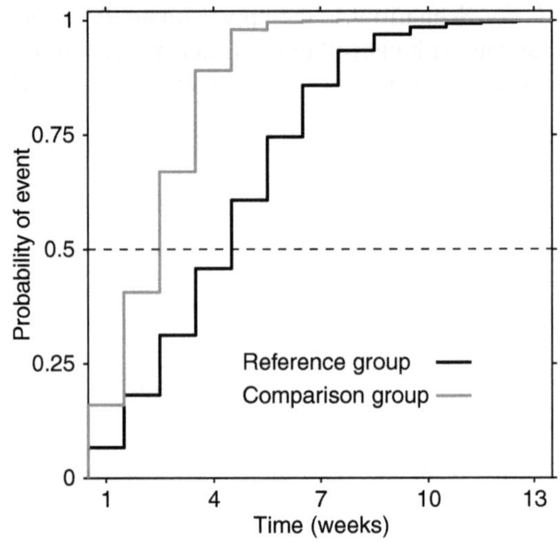

Fig. 9.1 Probability of an event within a certain time, by experimental group

that an individual will experience the event within a given time period. In Fig. 9.1, the estimated probability of event within 4 weeks is 0.46 for the reference group and 0.89 for the comparison group. Conversely, for a given probability, the access curve allows estimation of the time within which a certain proportion of individuals will experience the event. These times are estimated by the first time a step in the access curve is equal to or greater than the specified proportion. In Fig. 9.1, 50% of individuals experienced the event within 5 weeks for the reference group and within 3 weeks for the comparison group.

9.3 Comparing Proportions

9.3.1 Definition

In Chap. 8, we presented the odds ratio as a measure of differences in the odds of an event between two experimental groups. The odds ratio expresses the relative difference in the odds between group 1 and 2:

$$\text{odds ratio} = \frac{\text{odds for group 2}}{\text{odds for group 1}}. \tag{9.6}$$

In this measure, the odds for the reference group (i.e., group 1) is presented in the denominator and the odds for the comparison group (i.e., group 2) is presented in the numerator.

9.3.2 Crude Estimate

A crude estimate of the individual-level odds ratio can be produced using simulated data from two experimental groups. Suppose there are k runs per experimental group, with m_{ij} individuals in run $j = 1, \ldots, k$ of group $i = 1, 2$. Suppose also that y_{ijl} is the binary response for an event for individual $l = 1, \ldots, m_{ij}$ in run j of group i. The individual-level proportion for group i can be calculated as follows:

$$\hat{p}_i = \frac{\sum_{j=1}^{k} \sum_{l=1}^{m_{ij}} y_{ijl}}{\sum_{j=1}^{k} m_{ij}}. \tag{9.7}$$

In individual-level analysis, the crude odds ratio is estimated as the ratio of the observed individual-level odds for the comparison group to the observed odds for the reference group:

$$\text{crude odds ratio} = \frac{\hat{p}_2/(1-\hat{p}_2)}{\hat{p}_1/(1-\hat{p}_1)}, \tag{9.8}$$

where $\hat{p}_1$ is the estimated individual-level proportion for the reference group and $\hat{p}_2$ is the estimated proportion for the comparison group.

Consider Scenario 9.1 where the researcher assigns 30 hospitals to each experimental group and observes that elective procedures for 7,179 of 43,004 simulated patients are canceled from the final operating room list. Further suppose that 3,552 of the cancellations occur among the 21,430 patients in the wait-list booking group and the remaining 3,627 cancellations occur among the 21,574 patients in the advance booking group. If the patients whose surgery is booked by the wait-list booking method are deemed to form the reference group, and the patients whose surgery is booked by the advance booking method are deemed to form the comparison group, the estimated odds ratio of cancellation from the final operating room list is calculated as follows (see (9.8)):

$$\begin{aligned}
\text{crude odds ratio} &= \frac{(3{,}552/21{,}430)/(1 - 3{,}552/21{,}430)}{(3{,}627/21{,}574)/(1 - 3{,}627/21{,}574)} \\
&\approx \frac{0.1657/(1-0.1657)}{0.1681/(1-0.1681)} \approx 0.98.
\end{aligned}$$

9.3.3 Interpretation

Individual-level odds ratios are used to compare the odds (or proportions) between experimental groups. An odds ratio of 1 implies that the odds of an individual experiencing the event of interest are equal for the comparison and reference groups.

An odds ratio greater than 1 implies that the odds of an individual experiencing the event are higher for the comparison group than for the reference group. Conversely, an odds ratio less than 1 implies that the odds of an individual experiencing the event are lower for the comparison group than for the reference group. The percent difference in the odds of an event between the comparison and reference groups is calculated by subtracting 1 from the odds ratio and then multiplying the value by 100 [2]. For example, the odds ratio of 0.98 calculated above for Scenario 9.1, means that the odds that a patient will be canceled from the final operating room list are about 2% lower (i.e., $[0.98 - 1] \times 100\% = -2\%$) in hospitals using the advance booking method than in hospitals using the wait-list method.

9.4 Number of Runs for Comparing Proportions

In Appendix B, we outline the steps for estimating the number of simulation runs, a process ensuring that the anticipated effect of an intervention will be detected with high probability. Here, we describe how to determine the number of simulation runs when the proportion is used as the performance measure in individual-level analysis. In addition to the performance measure of interest, the number of runs depends on the significance level, the statistical power, the intracluster correlation coefficient, and the anticipated difference between experimental groups in the proportions of individuals experiencing the event of interest.

Suppose a researcher wants to test the hypothesis that the individual-level proportions for two groups are equal against a two-sided alternative. Calculating the number of simulation runs requires knowledge of the proportion for the reference group, p_1, and the anticipated difference between the proportions for the comparison and reference groups, δ. Given p_1 and δ, the proportion for the comparison group, p_2, is calculated as $\delta + p_1$. In a cluster randomized experiment, such as that in Scenario 9.1, the number of individuals per cluster, m, and the intracluster correlation coefficient, ρ, are also needed. The intracluster correlation coefficient is the ratio of between-cluster variation to total variation:

$$\hat{\rho} = \frac{\text{MSB} - \text{MSW}}{\text{MSB} + (m_0 - 1)\text{MSW}}, \tag{9.9}$$

where MSB and MSW are the pooled mean square errors between and within runs, respectively. Researchers use preliminary simulation runs to estimate the intracluster correlation coefficient. In particular, for two groups,

$$\text{MSB} = (K-2)^{-1} \sum_{i=1}^{2} \sum_{j=1}^{k_i} m_{ij} (\hat{p}_{ij} - \hat{p}_i)^2 , \tag{9.10}$$

$$\text{MSW} = (M - K)^{-1} \sum_{i=1}^{2} \sum_{j=1}^{k_i} m_{ij} \hat{p}_{ij} (1 - \hat{p}_{ij}) \,, \tag{9.11}$$

$$m_0 = (K - 2)^{-1} \left(M - \sum_{i=1}^{2} \sum_{j=1}^{k_i} m_{ij}^2 / M_i \right) \,, \tag{9.12}$$

where K is the total number of simulation runs, k_i is the number of simulation runs in group i, m_{ij} is the number of individuals in run j of group i, M_i is the number of individuals in group i, M is the total number of individuals simulated, $\hat{p}_{ij}$ is the individual-level proportion for run j in group i, and $\hat{p}_i$ is the proportion in group i [49].

To compare proportions at the individual level, the number of runs, each with m subjects, to be randomized to each experimental group is given by the following formula:

$$k = \frac{(z_{\alpha/2} + z_\beta)^2 [p_1(1 - p_1) + p_2(1 - p_2)]}{m(p_2 - p_1)^2} \text{IF}, \tag{9.13}$$

where the inflation factor,

$$\text{IF} = 1 + (m - 1)\rho, \tag{9.14}$$

shows the increase in the number of simulation runs required to achieve the same statistical power as in a design with randomization at the level of simulated individuals [49]. In (9.13), $z_{\alpha/2}$ is the $100(1-\alpha/2)$th quantile of the standard normal distribution, and z_β is the $100(1-\beta)$th quantile of the standard normal distribution. In these expressions, α represents the significance level and β represents the type II error (or the complement of the statistical power) (see Appendix B).

Consider again the researcher who wants to evaluate the effect of two methods of booking surgery on the proportion of patients with cancellation of their procedures from the final operating room list. Among hospitals using wait-list booking, preliminary simulation runs indicate that the hypothesized percentage of cancellations is 17% (i.e., $p_1 = 0.17$), and MSB ≈ 0.1765, MSW ≈ 0.1390, and $\hat{m}_0 \approx 716.702$. Therefore, the intracluster correlation coefficient is estimated as

$$\hat{\rho} = \frac{0.1765 - 0.1390}{0.1765 + (716.702 - 1) \times (0.1390)} \approx 0.000376 \,.$$

If advance booking decreases the proportion of cancellations by at least 1.5% (i.e., $\delta = 0.015$ and $p_2 = 0.17 - 0.015 = 0.155$), the researcher would like to correctly detect this difference, when it exists, with 90% certainty (i.e., $\beta = 1 - 0.90 = 0.10$) and would like to restrict to 5% the chance of mistakenly claiming there is a difference when none is present (i.e., $\alpha = 0.05$). In the preliminary runs, an average of 717 patients are served in each hospital. Using (9.14), the inflation factor,

$$\mathrm{IF} = 1 + (717 - 1) \times 0.000376 \approx 1.27,$$

indicates that the cluster randomized design requires 27% more patients than a design with randomization of individual simulated patients. Using (9.13), the estimated number of simulation runs per method is

$$k = \frac{(1.96 + 1.28)^2 \times [(0.17 \times 0.83) + (0.155 \times 0.845)]}{717 \times (0.015)^2} \times 1.27 \approx 22.5.$$

Hence, 23 hospitals per experimental group would suffice to test this hypothesis.

The significance level, statistical power, and effect size, as well as the intracluster correlation coefficient and the number of individuals per cluster, all affect the number of simulation runs. When estimating the number of runs, the values of these factors may be unknown, so it is advisable to use a range of values for the calculations. Estimating the number of runs using a range of values serves two purposes. First, if the value of a factor is unknown, the researcher is not forced to choose a random value, which might unduly influence planning of the experiment. Second, it allows the researcher to understand how widely the number of runs will vary with variations in certain determining factors.

As an illustration, we calculated the number of runs for Scenario 9.1, varying the significance level between 0.01 and 0.05, the statistical power between 80% and 90%, and the difference between the patient-level proportions from -0.10 to 0.10 (Fig. 9.2). In the figure, the horizontal axis shows the magnitude and direction of the smallest anticipated difference in the proportion of patients with cancellation of elective surgery in the advance booking and wait-list booking groups, and the vertical axis represents the number of simulation runs needed per group. In this example, the proportion for the wait-list booking group (the reference group) was fixed at 0.17. Therefore, a value of -0.10 on the horizontal axis corresponds to values of 0.17 and 0.07 for the proportions of patients with cancellation of procedures in the reference group, p_1, and the comparison group, p_2, respectively.

The number of simulation runs increases when the significance level decreases, with other factors affecting the number of runs held constant (Fig. 9.2). There is also an inverse relation between the number of runs and the statistical power. With all other elements fixed, the number of simulation runs increases with increasing statistical power. As the absolute value of the difference in proportions decreases from 0.10, the number of simulation runs gradually increases, for fixed values of significance level and statistical power, to a difference of about 0.02. For absolute differences less than 0.02, the number of runs tends rapidly toward infinity as the difference approaches 0.

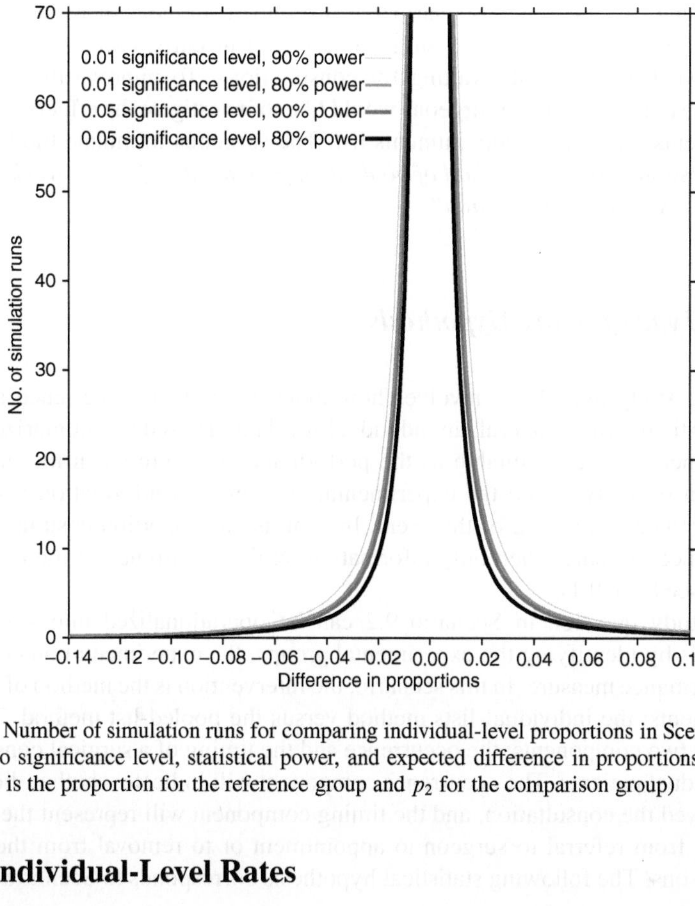

Fig. 9.2 Number of simulation runs for comparing individual-level proportions in Scenario 9.1 in relation to significance level, statistical power, and expected difference in proportions ($p_2 - p_1$, where p_1 is the proportion for the reference group and p_2 for the comparison group)

9.5 Individual-Level Rates

In health care evaluation, the event rate is a measure of how often the event of interest, such as adverse event, hospitalization, or death at discharge from hospital, occurs in the experiment during the period of observation. Data on both the occurrence and timing of an event that are recorded at the level of the individual can be used to estimate the rate of an event. Unlike proportions, rates have a lower limit of 0 and no upper limit. The study hypothesis and the type of experimental outcome determine whether the individual-level rate is suitable for evaluating the effect of an intervention.

9.5.1 A Scenario Involving Individual-Level Rates

In this chapter, we use the following scenario to illustrate the evaluation of system performance using individual-level rates as a performance measure. We will refer to this hypothetical situation as Scenario 9.2: A group of surgeons shares consultation, operation, and office duties in a surgical service. Currently, each surgeon has his or her own list of patients waiting for consultations. To improve their patients' access to a consultation, the surgeons would like to investigate the effects of pooling their patients on a single appointments list. The surgeons formulate the following study question: *Does the method of booking appointments affect the weekly rate of receiving a surgical consultation?*

9.5.2 Type of Study Hypothesis

When the study hypothesis involves how many individuals experience an event over a particular time interval, an individual-level rate is used to summarize system performance. A rate is suitable as the performance measure when the individual is the unit of analysis and the experimental outcome has information about both the occurrence and timing of the event. In contrast, a proportion is suitable as the performance measure when only information on the occurrence of the event is of interest (see Sect. 9.1).

The study question in Scenario 9.2 can be operationalized into a statistical hypothesis by identifying the experimental groups, the experimental outcome, and the performance measure. In this scenario, the intervention is the method of booking appointments: the individual-lists method versus the pooled-list method. The outcome has two components: the occurrence and the timing of a surgical consultation for individual patients. The occurrence component will indicate whether the patient has received the consultation, and the timing component will represent the number of weeks from referral to surgeon to appointment or to removal from the list for other reasons. The following statistical hypothesis corresponds to Scenario 9.2:

H_0: There is no difference in the rate of surgical consultation between hospitals using the individual-lists method and those using the pooled-list method.
H_A: There is a difference in the rate of surgical consultation between hospitals using the individual-lists method and those using the pooled-list method.

9.5.3 Type of Experimental Outcome

An experimental outcome that is recorded at the level of the individual and that has data about both the occurrence and timing of an event can be used to estimate an event rate. In this situation, the experimental outcome is represented by two variables. One variable indicates whether an individual has experienced the event of interest, and the other variable records the time to the event, if it occurred, or the time the individual was last observed, if the event did not occur.

Data generated by simulation experiments that would be suitable for estimating individual-level rates for Scenario 9.2 should have two properties. First, each observed value of the experimental outcome corresponds to a single patient, with the patient being the unit of analysis. Second, the variables corresponding to the experimental outcome is composed of one variable indicating whether the patient received a surgical consultation and another variable indicating the number of weeks from referral to consultation or last observation.

9.6 Measuring Performance with Rates

9.6.1 Definition

In general, event rates quantify the number of occurrences of an event over a specified time interval. In the context of simulation studies, individual-level rates quantify the number of simulated individuals who experience one event over a time interval. For example, a response to changes in the management of consultation clinics could be summarized by changes in the weekly rate of surgical consultation appointments or the weekly rate of elective surgery.

9.6.2 Estimation

The individual-level rate, λ, is estimated as the observed number of individuals experiencing the event of interest divided by the total person-time at risk:

$$\hat{\lambda} = \frac{\text{no. of individuals experiencing event}}{\text{total time at risk}}. \tag{9.15}$$

The hat symbol $\hat{}$ denotes a quantity that is estimated from the observed data in a simulation experiment. Therefore, $\hat{\lambda}$ is the estimated value of the rate. In (9.15), total time at risk is a measure combining times at risk contributed by all studied individuals. The time at risk is the period in which an individual may experience the event. The total person-time is the sum of the observed time to the event of interest, loss to follow-up, or end of the simulation study, whichever occurs first, for all individuals in a study.

In Scenario 9.2, the rate of consultation appointments is defined as follows:

$$\lambda = \frac{\text{no. of patients receiving appointment}}{\text{sum of weeks spent waiting for appointment}}.$$

Suppose that the researcher in Scenario 9.2 observes a total of 42,992 appointments among the 45,307 patients over a total of 175,827 weeks of waiting, then the estimated rate of appointment would be 42,992/175,827 $\approx$ 0.24 appointments per patient-week of waiting.

The individual-level rate in (9.15) can be expressed in terms of the observed outcomes from a simulation experiment. Suppose there are k runs with m_j individuals in run $j = 1, \ldots, k$ with a total follow-up time of t_j. The binary response y_{jl} is an indicator of the occurrence of the event for individual l in run j. The rate of individuals experiencing the event of interest can be estimated by

$$\hat{\lambda} = \frac{\sum_{j=1}^{k} \sum_{l=1}^{m_j} y_{jl}}{\sum_{j=1}^{k} t_j}, \tag{9.16}$$

where the numerator, $\sum_{j=1}^{k} \sum_{l=1}^{m_j} y_{jl}$, counts the number of individuals that experienced the event of interest, and the denominator, $\sum_{j=1}^{k} t_j$, represents the total time that individuals were at risk of experiencing the event.

Confidence limits for an individual-level rate are computed from the variance of this estimated rate. With simulation runs (i.e., clusters) being the unit of randomization, statistical techniques that account for correlation between individual outcomes in each run are needed. The ratio estimator is appropriate for estimating the variance of $\hat{\lambda}$ [49]:

$$\mathrm{Var}(\hat{\lambda}) = \frac{k}{k-1} \sum_{j=1}^{k} \left[\frac{(\hat{\lambda}_j - \hat{\lambda}) t_j}{\sum_{j'=1}^{k} t_{j'}} \right]^2, \tag{9.17}$$

where $\hat{\lambda}_j = \sum_{l=1}^{m_j} y_{jl}/t_j$ is the estimated event rate in run j. Therefore, the approximate $100(1-\alpha)\%$ lower and upper confidence limits for the individual-level event rate are estimated by

$$\begin{aligned} \mathrm{LCL} &= \hat{\lambda} - z_{\alpha/2}\sqrt{\mathrm{Var}(\hat{\lambda})}, \\ \mathrm{UCL} &= \hat{\lambda} + z_{\alpha/2}\sqrt{\mathrm{Var}(\hat{\lambda})}, \end{aligned} \tag{9.18}$$

where $z_{\alpha/2}$ is the $100(1 - \alpha/2)$th quantile of the standard normal distribution.

For Scenario 9.2, the approximate 95% confidence limits for the weekly rate of consultation appointments are calculated using (9.18) and estimates of $\hat{\lambda} = 0.24$ and $\mathrm{Var}(\hat{\lambda}) = 0.0035$:

$$\begin{aligned} \mathrm{LCL} &= 0.24 - 1.96\sqrt{0.0035} \approx 0.12\,, \\ \mathrm{UCL} &= 0.24 + 1.96\sqrt{0.0035} \approx 0.36\,. \end{aligned}$$

9.6.3 *Interpretation*

Individual-level rates quantify the expected number of individuals who will experience an event over a specified time interval. Generally, it is convenient to scale the rates so as to present the expected number of events over a certain standardized number of person-time units. For example, the rate of 0.24 appointments per patient-week can also be expressed as 24 appointments per 100 patient-weeks.

9.7 Comparing Rates

9.7.1 *Definition*

Comparing cluster-level proportions and quantifying their differences between experimental groups necessitate a measure of effect size. The rate ratio expresses the relative difference in the rates between two experimental groups. The rate ratio expresses the relative difference in rates between group 1 and group 2:

$$\text{rate ratio} = \frac{\text{rate for group 2}}{\text{rate for group 1}}. \tag{9.19}$$

In this measure, the rate for the reference group (i.e., group 1) is presented in the denominator and the rate for the comparison group (i.e., group 2) is presented in the numerator.

9.7.2 *Crude Estimate*

A crude estimate of the individual-level rate ratio can be produced using simulated data from two experimental groups. Suppose there are k runs per experimental group, with m_{ij} individuals in run $j = 1, \ldots, k$ of group $i = 1, 2$, with a total follow-up time of t_{ij}. The binary response y_{ijl} is an indicator of the occurrence of the event for individual l in run j of group i. The rate of individuals in group i experiencing the event of interest can be estimated by

$$\hat{\lambda}_i = \frac{\sum_{j=1}^{k} \sum_{l=1}^{m_{ij}} y_{ijl}}{\sum_{j=1}^{k} t_{ij}}. \tag{9.20}$$

The crude rate ratio is estimated as the ratio of the observed rate for group 2 to the observed rate for group 1:

$$\text{crude rate ratio} = \frac{\hat{\lambda}_2}{\hat{\lambda}_1}, \tag{9.21}$$

where $\hat{\lambda}_1$ is the estimated rate for the reference group and $\hat{\lambda}_2$ is the estimated rate for the comparison group.

To illustrate the estimation of a rate ratio, consider Scenario 9.2, where the researcher observes 42,992 appointments over 175,827 patient-weeks. Of the 42,992 appointments, about half occur in hospitals that use the individual-lists method and about half in hospitals that use the pooled-list method (21,251 and 21,741 appointments, respectively). Although the numbers of appointments are roughly equally distributed, the total patient-weeks are lower with the pooled-list method (66,318 patient-weeks) than with the individual-lists method (109,509 patient-weeks). Using (9.21) and the individual-lists method as the reference group, the estimated rate ratio of appointments is

$$\text{crude rate ratio} = \frac{(21{,}741/66{,}318)}{(21{,}251/109{,}509)} \approx \frac{0.328}{0.194} \approx 1.69.$$

That is, the appointment rate in the comparison group was about 1.7 times of that in the reference group.

9.7.3 Interpretation

Health services researchers use rate ratios to compare rates between groups. A rate ratio of 1 indicates that the event rates are equal in the comparison and reference groups. A rate ratio greater than 1 indicates that the event rate is higher in the comparison group than in the reference group. Conversely, a rate ratio less than 1 indicates that the event rate is lower in the comparison group than in the reference group. The percent difference in the rate at which individuals experience an event in the comparison and reference groups is calculated by subtracting 1 from the rate ratio and multiplying it by 100. For example, the rate ratio of 1.69 for Scenario 9.2, calculated above, means that the appointment rate is about 69% higher ($= [1.69 - 1] \times 100\%$) for patients treated in hospitals using the pooled-list method than in hospitals using the individual-lists method for booking appointments.

9.8 Number of Runs for Comparing Rates

In Appendix B, we outline the steps for estimating the number of simulation runs to ensure that the anticipated effect of an intervention will be detected with high probability. Here, we describe how to determine the number of simulation runs when the performance measure of interest is a rate. In cluster randomized studies, the number of simulation runs depends upon the specification of the hypothesis, as well as characteristics of the cluster. In addition, the number of runs depends upon the significance level, the statistical power, the coefficient of variation, and the anticipated relative difference in rates between the two experimental groups.

Suppose that the group of clinicians in Scenario 9.2 wants to test the null hypothesis that the appointment rates for the two groups of patients are equal against a two-sided alternative. Calculating the number of simulation runs requires knowledge of the population rate in the reference group, λ_1, and the difference that the clinicians want to be able to detect, measured as the ratio of the rate for the comparison group to the rate for the reference group (i.e., $\delta = \lambda_2/\lambda_1$). For example, if the rate for the comparison group is expected to be 10% higher relative to the reference group, then $\delta = 1.1$. In designing a cluster randomized experiment, the total exposure time per cluster, t, is also required, along with the coefficient of variation for rates, cv, which is the ratio of the between-cluster variation to the rate. It is assumed that the coefficient of variation is constant across groups.

To compare the event rate between two experimental groups, the number of runs to be randomized for each group is calculated as follows:

$$k = \frac{(z_{\alpha/2} + z_\beta)^2(\lambda_1 + \lambda_2)}{t(\lambda_1 - \lambda_2)^2}\mathrm{IF}, \tag{9.22}$$

where the inflation factor,

$$\mathrm{IF} = 1 + \frac{cv^2(\lambda_1^2 + \lambda_2^2)t}{\lambda_1 + \lambda_2}, \tag{9.23}$$

shows the increase in the number of simulation runs required to achieve the same statistical power as in a design with randomization at the level of individual simulated patients [49]. When cv is 0, (9.22) reduces to the sample-size formula for independent observations. In (9.22), α represents the significance level and β represents the type II error (or the complement of the statistical power) (see Appendix B).

The number of simulation runs estimated by (9.22) assumes that the clusters have equal total time at risk for simulated individuals and also assumes that the coefficient of variation is common across both experimental groups. If these assumptions are not valid, then the number of runs can be estimated by the Hayes method [74]:

$$k = 1 + \frac{(z_{\alpha/2} + z_\beta)^2}{(\lambda_1 - \lambda_2)^2} \times \left(\frac{\lambda_1}{t_1} + \frac{\lambda_2}{t_2} + \sigma_1^2 + \sigma_2^2\right), \tag{9.24}$$

where $z_{\alpha/2}$ is the $100(1-\alpha/2)$th quantile of the standard normal distribution, z_β is the $100(1-\beta)$th quantile of the standard normal distribution, λ_i is the rate in experimental group i, t_i is the harmonic mean of the exposure times in group i, and σ_i^2 is the variance of the distribution of rates in group i. This variance can be estimated as the difference between the variance of the observed rates in cluster j of group i and the ratio of λ_i and the total time at risk per cluster in group i. When the number of clusters is small, one simulation run is added to the estimate in (9.24) to account for use of the t distribution instead of the normal distribution [137].

Suppose researchers want to compare the appointment rate between hospitals using the two methods of booking appointments and would like to be able to detect a 10% higher appointment rate when pooling patients on a single list compared with having individual wait lists (i.e., $\delta = 1.1$). They would also like to have a 90% chance of correctly claiming a difference between the two booking methods, if one exists, and to limit to 5% the chance of incorrectly detecting a difference, if none is present. The null hypothesis, that there is no difference in the appointment rates, will be tested against a two-sided alternative hypothesis, since the clinicians are interested in whether the rates differ in the anticipated direction or the reverse direction [58].

From a pilot study, the appointment rate after referral is observed to be 20 per 100 patient-weeks in hospitals using the individual-lists method. Provisional runs yield a total of about 2,931 patient-weeks that are spent waiting, over the simulation period, by patients in a hospital. The estimated coefficient of variation is 0.071. Using (9.23), the inflation factor is calculated as follows:

$$\text{IF} = 1 + \frac{(0.071)^2 \times [0.20^2 + (0.20 \times 1.1)^2] \times 2{,}931}{0.20 + (0.20 \times 1.1)} \approx 4.1.$$

Using (9.22),

$$k = \frac{(1.96 + 1.28)^2 \times [0.20 + (0.20 \times 1.1)]}{2{,}931 \times [0.20 - (0.20 \times 1.1)]^2} \times 4.1 \approx 15.4,$$

so the estimated number of simulation runs per method is 16. Increasing the coefficient of variation to 0.10 increases the inflation factor to 7.1, which corresponds to about 27 simulation runs per method. As described in Sect. 9.4, the significance level, statistical power, and effect size, as well as the coefficient of variation and time at risk, all affect the number of simulation runs. Researchers may find that the values of these factors are unknown, as might be the case for the total time at risk per cluster. Appendix B provides guidance on how to determine values for factors influencing the number of runs. For example, preliminary runs of the simulation model will help to estimate an appropriate value for time at risk in each cluster.

As an illustration, we calculated the number of runs for Scenario 9.2, varying the significance level between 0.01 and 0.05, the statistical power between 80% and 90%, and the relative difference between the rates between 0.80 and 1.6 (Fig. 9.3). In the figure, the horizontal axis shows the smallest anticipated relative difference in the weekly rate of appointment between patients served in hospitals using the pooled-list method and patients served in hospital using individual-lists method, and the vertical axis represents the number of simulation runs needed per group. In this example, the weekly rate in the individual-lists group (the reference group) was fixed at 20 appointments per 100 patient-weeks. Therefore, a value of 1.2 on

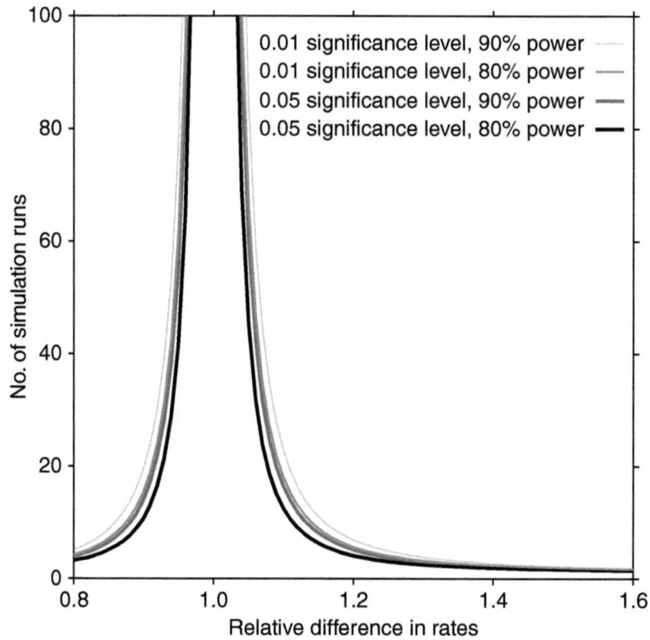

Fig. 9.3 Number of simulation runs for comparing individual-level rates in Scenario 9.2 in relation to significance level, statistical power, and difference in rates (λ_2/λ_1, where λ_1 is the rate for the reference group and λ_2 is the rate for the comparison group)

the horizontal axis corresponds to a value of 0.20 appointments per patient-week for the reference group (λ_1) and a value of 0.24 appointments per patient-week ($= 0.20 \times 1.2$) for the comparison group (λ_2).

As the significance level decreases, the number of simulation runs increases with other factors affecting the number of runs held constant (Fig. 9.3). There is also an inverse relation between the number of runs and the statistical power. With all other elements fixed, the number of simulation runs increases with increasing statistical power. As the relative difference in rates tends away from 1, the required number of simulation runs decreases. For small relative differences, the number of runs tends rapidly toward infinity.

Chapter 10
Reporting on a Simulation Study

In Chap. 2, we argued that clear, transparent, and complete reporting of a simulation study helps the reader to understand and interpret the study, as well as to evaluate the quality of its findings. In this chapter, we outline the information that should be reported from a simulation study in the area of health care evaluation. In particular, we describe the elements to be reported in relation to the study question, the methods, and the results of the simulation itself.

10.1 CONSORT Guidelines

Researchers use peer-reviewed articles, commissioned reports, and other publications to communicate evidence generated by simulation studies. Policy-makers use the reported evidence to understand the potential effect of different management or service alternatives on the delivery of health care. Unfortunately, it is often difficult to assess the validity of evidence from a particular study because of poor reporting. Conversely, clear, transparent, and complete reporting allows the reader to understand how the simulation study was designed, performed, analyzed, and interpreted.

We mentioned in Sect. 2.5 that the CONSORT Group developed and disseminated recommendations to improve the quality of reporting of medical trials. The first version of the CONSORT statement for the reporting of randomized controlled trials was published in 1996. It recommended reporting 22 items corresponding to the sections of an article (i.e., Title, Abstract, Introduction, Methods, Results, and Discussion), as well as a flow diagram to show the progression of participants through the study [13]. The CONSORT statement for reporting randomized controlled trials was revised in 2001 and again, most recently, in 2010 [108, 109, 132]. In 2004, an extension of the statement was created to cover the reporting of cluster randomized trials [33]. This extension recommended additional reporting elements: the rationale for adopting a cluster randomized design, the methods of accounting

B. Sobolev et al., *Health Care Evaluation Using Computer Simulation: Concepts, Methods, and Applications*, DOI 10.1007/978-1-4614-2233-4_10,

for clustering in sample-size calculations and in the statistical analysis, and the flow of clusters and participants through the study. In 2010, the statement for reporting randomized controlled trials was updated with minor changes [109, 132]. In the following sections, we describe our adaptation of the most recent version of the recommendations for reporting cluster randomized trials to the reporting of simulation studies.

In our view, the same rigor that is suggested for reporting real-world studies should be applied to reporting simulation studies. Researchers already recognize the need to include sufficient information in their reports to allow the reader to understand the design of a simulation study [32]. We propose that the CONSORT statement for cluster randomized trials be applied to the reporting of simulation studies in health care evaluation that randomize groups of simulated patients to interventions. In addition, we propose that this statement be further expanded to include items needed for reporting simulation models (see Table 10.1). If the reporting standards for simulation studies are raised in this way, policy-makers will have a better understanding of the resulting evidence and will therefore be able to make better-informed decisions.

The reporting recommendations for cluster randomized trials refer to study elements that overlap with the elements of the analytical framework for simulation studies described in Chap. 7. The hypothesis, the main element (see Sect. 7.2), provides a link between the primary study factor and the experimental outcome, which correspond to items 4 (experimental groups) and 6 (experimental outcomes) of the CONSORT statement, respectively. The performance measure and the measure of effect size tell the reader how the system's performance will be quantified and compared and are covered by item 12 (statistical methods) of the statement. The experimental design (see Sect. 7.3) deals with runs of the simulation model, which include the unit of randomization, the method of allocation, and the total number of runs, that is, the items covered by items 2 (background), 1 (study design), and 7 (number of simulation runs), respectively, of the statement. The plan of analysis in our simulation framework (see Sect. 7.4) guides the reader in assessing the performance of the intervention. Respectively, the unit of analysis is covered by item 5 (objectives) of the statement, and regression methods are covered by item 12 (statistical methods), along with other explanatory factors that might influence the experimental outcome.

On the other hand, some of the items to be included in the report of a simulation study differ from those recommended for cluster randomized trials. First, we suggest expanding item 3 to include details of the simulation model, which will help the reader to understand the intervention and the potential care paths for participants. Second, in our view, the items on allocation concealment (item 9), implementation (item 10), and blinding (item 11) may not be applicable to a simulation study and so might reasonably be omitted. Specifically, with the reference to item 9, the computer algorithms allocate the simulation runs to the experimental groups, so there is no risk of a researcher or other person influencing the outcome of the experiment through knowledge of the allocation of runs. With the reference to item 10, the computer, not a specific person, generates the random allocation sequence and assigns clusters to

Table 10.1 Checklist of items to include when reporting on simulation experiments with a cluster randomized design in the area of health care evaluation

Section of article and topic	Item	Description
Title and abstract:		
Study design	1	How simulated patients and simulation runs were allocated to experimental groups, specifying that allocation was based on simulation runs (i.e., clusters)
Introduction:		
Background	2	Scientific background and explanation of rationale for evaluating interventions using a simulation experiment with a cluster design
Methods:		
Participants	3	Description of the simulated patient population, health services setting, and management and policy alternatives
Simulation model		
Simulation approach	3a	Type of computer simulation model
Modeled activities	3b	Information about the activities included in the simulation model
Modeling requirements	3c	Set of statements that identifies the features of the model
Modeling assumptions	3d	Set of assumptions that facilitate development of the model without adversely affecting the model's objective or results
Configurations of the model	3e	Description of the configurations of the model that define various policy alternatives
Input parameters	3f	Set of parameters and data used by the model to simulate various scenarios
Output data	3g	Set of data generated by the model, representing the simulated scenarios
Experimental groups	4	Precise details of the interventions intended for each experimental group and whether they pertain to the cluster (hospital) level, the individual (patient) level, or both
Objectives	5	Specific objectives and hypotheses and whether they pertain to the cluster (hospital) level, the individual (patient) level, or both
Experimental outcomes	6	Clearly defined primary and secondary experimental outcomes related to the unit of analysis, and whether they pertain to the cluster (hospital) level, the individual (patient) level, or both
Number of simulation runs	7	How the total number of simulation runs was determined (including method of calculation, number of simulation runs, cluster size, a coefficient of intracluster correlation, and an indication of the coefficient's uncertainty)

(continued)

Table 10.1 (continued)

Section of article and topic	Item	Description
Randomization		
Sequence generation	8	Method used to generate the random allocation sequence, including details of any restrictions (e.g., blocking, stratification, matching)
Allocation concealment	9	Not applicable
Implementation	10	Not applicable
Blinding (masking)	11	Not applicable
Statistical methods	12	Statistical methods used to compare groups in terms of primary outcome(s), indicating how clustering was taken into account and methods for additional analyses, such as subgroup analyses and adjusted analyses
Results:		
Participant flow	13	Flow of simulation runs and simulated participants through each stage (a diagram being strongly recommended), with reporting (for each experimental group) of the numbers of runs and participants randomly assigned and analyzed for the primary outcome
Recruitment and follow-up periods	14	Simulated dates defining the periods of recruitment and follow-up
Baseline data	15	Baseline information for each group at the cluster (hospital) and the individual (patient) levels, as applicable
Numbers analyzed	16	Numbers of simulation runs and simulated individuals for each experimental group included in the analysis
Outcomes and estimation	17	For each primary and secondary outcome, a summary of results for each group, at the cluster (hospital) or individual (patient) level as applicable; for each primary and secondary outcome, the estimated effect size and its precision (e.g., 95% confidence interval); and for each primary outcome, an intracluster correlation coefficient
Ancillary analyses	18	Method used to address multiplicity, ideally by reporting any other analyses performed, including subgroup analyses and adjusted analyses, indicating those that were prespecified and those that were exploratory
Adverse events	19	All important adverse events or side effects in each experimental group
Discussion:		
Limitations	20	Trial limitations, addressing any sources of potential bias or imprecision, and, if relevant, risks associated with multiplicity of analyses
Generalizability	21	Generalizability of the trial's findings to other clusters or other simulated patients (as relevant)
Overall evidence	22	General interpretation of the results in the context of current evidence

experimental groups, which eliminates the risk of bias. Finally, with the reference to item 11, it is not necessary to blind simulated patients or simulated care providers, because sharing of information among simulated entities is impossible.

In the remainder of this chapter, we discuss the individual items to be reported for a simulation study, numbered as in Table 10.1 but grouped according to the three main aspects of the simulation framework, as described in preceding paragraphs in this section (i.e., the items do not appear in numeric order). For each item, we provide a brief explanation of its importance, along with one or two examples of appropriate reporting, quoted from previously published studies by our research group. The examples also specify the section of the publication from which they are quoted. These sections usually correspond to the item's recommended article section in Table 10.1, but on occasion may depart from these recommendations.

10.2 Reporting the Study Question

In this section, we describe five items to be reported from a simulation experiment with a cluster randomized design that will help the reader to understand the study question.

10.2.1 Study Design

Similar to the original CONSORT statement, we recommend specifying the study design.

Item 1: How simulated patients and simulation runs were allocated to experimental groups, specifying that allocation was based on simulation runs (i.e., clusters).

Explanation

We suggest that the simulation design be mentioned in the article title. This allows readers to understand from the outset the context of the results (e.g., why it was feasible to have a large number of study participants). Specifying the particular design of the simulation experiment will help the reader to assess the appropriateness of the statistical analyses. More specifically, an experiment with a cluster randomized design requires statistical methods to account for correlations between patients when inferences are made at the level of the patient. This item is also used to report the method of allocation used in designing a simulation experiment (see Sect. 7.3).

Examples

The following two examples show how the study design can be reported in the title or in the "Methods" section of an article.

Title–"Evaluation of methods for scheduling clinic appointments in surgical service: a Statecharts-based simulation study" [145].

Methods–"... we used a cluster randomized design, according to which the simulation runs, rather than the simulated patient entities, were randomly assigned to the three study groups according to appointment system ..." [145].

10.2.2 Background

Similar to the CONSORT extension statement, we suggest describing the background and rationale for using a simulation experiment with a cluster design.

Item 2: Scientific background and explanation of rationale for evaluating interventions using a simulation experiment with a cluster design.

Explanation

A substantial amount of time and effort on the part of many experts is required to develop a simulation model representing the delivery of care for use in a simulation experiment. Therefore, the reasons for conducting the experiment (e.g., limited feasibility of real-world experiments or desire to improve understanding of the issue before real-world implementation of a policy alternative) should be clearly stated to justify the costs incurred. Notably, a cluster randomized design requires more complex statistical methods to account for correlations between simulated patients. To justify the need for these methods, the rationale for using a cluster design should also be reported. Through this justification, this item also provides information about the unit of randomization (see Sect. 7.3).

Examples

The following two sentences are examples of reporting the background and rationale for a simulation experiment using a cluster design in the "Introduction" section of an article.

Introduction–"Patient flow simulation provides an alternative to evaluating proposed changes when hospital intervention studies are not feasible due to ethical, safety, economical or other reasons" [156].

Introduction–"Because booking surgery involves complex decision-making at the level of the hospital, we applied a cluster randomized design in which the unit of randomization was the hospital and the units of analysis were both the hospital and the individual patient" [144].

10.2.3 Objectives

We recommend reporting the cluster-level and individual-level objectives and hypotheses, which conforms with the CONSORT guidelines.

Item 5: Specific objectives and hypotheses and whether they pertain to the cluster (hospital) level, the individual (patient) level, or both.

Explanation

For simulation studies, as for any other research study, a clear statement of specific objectives and hypotheses is recommended. The statement of objective should identify the primary study factor, the experimental outcomes of interest, and whether the hypothesis relates to the cluster (e.g., hospital, clinic, or service), the individual (e.g., patient), or both (see Sect. 7.2). In addition, a statement about the level of inference will help the reader to assess the appropriateness of the statistical methods used and will also help the reader to interpret the results. This item also provides information about the unit of analysis (see Sect. 7.4).

Example

In the following paragraph, the study objectives are described at both the cluster level and individual level.

Introduction–"In this analysis, we compared pre-booking and booking from wait lists in terms of cancellations originating with the hospital and time to surgery in the context of cardiac surgical care ... At the hospital level, the outcome was cancellation of one or more elective procedures with high priority from the final operating room schedule. At the patient level, the outcome was time between registration on a wait list and the operation" [144].

10.2.4 Experimental Groups

As in the CONSORT statement, we suggest reporting the interventions modeled in the simulation experiment.

Item 4: Precise details of the interventions intended for each experimental group and whether they pertain to the cluster (hospital) level, the individual (patient) level, or both.

Explanation

A description of the interventions modeled in the simulation study allows the reader to compare them with current practice and to make decisions about their feasibility in the real world. Reporting should also clearly indicate whether the interventions were applied to the cluster or to individuals. This item corresponds to the primary study factor in the analytical framework of a simulation experiment (see Sect. 7.2).

Example

The following example describes the interventions that were modeled and compared in a simulation study.

Methods–"In our model, patients referred for consultation with a surgeon were kept on the appointment list with a designated priority (high or low) until an opening for a clinic appointment became available. In the case of individual appointment lists, consultations were scheduled with the surgeon named in the referral. This method ensured that the surgeon chosen by the referring physician assessed each patient. In the case of pooled appointment lists, consultations were scheduled with the first available surgeon. In the case of the shortest appointment list, patients were placed on the appointment list of the surgeon with the fewest patients waiting. This method maintains an even distribution of patients among surgeons, while giving each surgeon an individual list of specific patients" [145].

10.2.5 Experimental Outcomes

Similar to the CONSORT extension statement, we suggest that cluster-level and individual-level experimental outcomes be defined and reported.

Item 6: Clearly defined primary and secondary experimental outcomes related to the unit of analysis and whether they pertain to the cluster (hospital) level, the individual (patient) level, or both.

Explanation

In studies with a cluster randomized design, inferences can be made at the level of the cluster or the individual. A statement about the level of the experimental outcomes will help the reader to assess the appropriateness of the statistical methods. Similarly, reporting the level of the outcome will help the reader to interpret the results. This item corresponds to the experimental outcome in the analytical framework for a simulation experiment (see Sect. 7.2).

Example

In the following example, the experimental outcomes of interest at both the cluster level and individual level are described.

Methods–"... the simulation records contained the following patient-level experimental responses: time on the appointment list, time on the surgical wait list, priority of registration for operation, and size of the surgical wait list at registration. The experimental response at the hospital level was the number of patients on the appointment list" [145].

10.3 Reporting the Study Methods

In this section, we describe 12 items that will help the reader to understand the methods used in a simulation study. These items cover descriptions of the simulation model, the design of the simulation experiment, and the statistical tools used for analysis.

10.3.1 Participants

As in the CONSORT statement, we recommend that the simulated population and setting be described.

Item 3: Description of the simulated patient population, health services setting, and management and policy alternatives.

Explanation

A description of the simulated patient population will help the reader to understand the people represented by the simulated population. A description of the health services setting will help the reader to understand the situations in which the results of the simulation might be applied. Finally, a description of the policy alternatives will help the reader to understand the interventions being studied.

Examples

The following examples describe the simulated patient population and health care setting for a simulation study.

Methods–"We modeled three care paths following angiography that patients with established coronary artery disease are likely to experience according to initial presentation and subsequent decisions leading to surgery: elective, inpatient and emergency, as reported elsewhere" [144].

Introduction–"We studied a setting in which weekly availability of surgeons for operations depended on their schedules for consultations, planned operations, on-call duties and vacations" [144].

10.3.2 Simulation Approach

As an addition to the CONSORT extension statement suitable for simulation studies, we suggest reporting the type of computer simulation model.

Item 3a: Type of computer simulation model.

Explanation

Specifying the simulation approach, in terms of the type of computer simulation model used, will help the reader to assess the capability of the model to simulate various scenarios and to understand both the input data required by the model and the output data generated by the simulation.

Example

The following excerpt shows how the type of computer simulation model might be reported.

Methods–"We simulated the delivery of surgical care using a discrete-event model. Using the Statecharts language, we described the progress of individual patients through surgical care as a series of asynchronous updates in patient records. The updates were produced in response to events generated by parallel finite state machines representing concurrent clinical and managerial activities" [145].

10.3.3 Modeled Activities

As a second addition to the CONSORT extension statement, the processes and activities that were implemented in the simulation model should be reported.

Item 3b: Information about the activities included in the simulation model.

Explanation

We suggest that all care processes (e.g., perioperative activities) included within the simulation model be reported, including a brief description of their functionality. This information will help the reader to understand the capability of the model to simulate various scenarios. Information about the modeled activities may be reported in the form of a diagram, a list, or a table.

Example

The following example describes the modeled activities in a simulation experiment.

Methods–"In this study, the modeled processes encompassed the continuum of clinical and managerial activities in cardiac surgical care. The diagram ... shows activities at preoperative, operative, and postoperative stages included in the simulation model. Table 10.1 provides further explanation of the modeled activities" [145].

10.3.4 Modeling Requirements

Another addition to the CONSORT extension statement should be the reporting of the features of the model in terms of the modeling requirements.

Item 3c: Set of statements that identifies the features of the model.

Explanation

A description of the modeling requirements will help the reader to understand the required functioning of the model. The modeling requirements consist of a detailed description of what the model must do (e.g. a detailed description of the perioperative activities, as they are to be implemented in the simulation model) (see Sect. 6.4).

Example

The modeling requirements of a simulation model could be described in the following manner.

Methods–"In our model, patients referred for consultation with a surgeon were kept on the appointment list with a designated priority (high or low) until an opening for a clinic appointment became available. After the consultation, the office of the consulting surgeon registered on his or her wait list patients who required coronary revascularization, designating the required procedure as high, medium, or low priority according to the affected coronary anatomy and the patient's symptoms. The hospital's booking office assigned patients to the operating room slots that had been allocated to the consulting surgeon according to their priority and date of registration on the wait list" [145].

10.3.5 Modeling Assumptions

A further addition to the CONSORT extension statement would be reporting the modeling assumptions.

Item 3d: Set of assumptions that facilitate development of the model without adversely affecting the model's objective or results.

Explanation

Statements describing the modeling assumptions will help the reader to identify those aspects of the process that, if ignored, simplified, or not varied during the simulation, do not adversely affect the objective or results of the study. Information about the modeling assumptions will also help the reader to understand the capability of the model to simulate various scenarios. This type of information may be reported in the form of a list or a table (see Sect. 6.5).

Example

The following excerpt is an example of how assumptions of a simulation model could be described.

Appendix–"In constructing the simulation model, we made the following simplifying assumptions.

1. For each simulation week, the random numbers of referrals for consultations, of emergency patients, and of inpatients were drawn from Poisson distributions, to allow for fluctuations in demand for service.
2. Referred patients could have high or low priority for surgical consultation: patients with high priority were scheduled before those with low priority, and patients with the same priority were scheduled by their respective referral times.
3. Sixteen consultation appointments were available each week, and all patients attended their appointments.
4. Seven operating room slots for elective surgery and eight for urgent procedures were available each week.
5. Two methods for allocating operating room slots over weekdays were studied: weekly or daily split between elective and urgent procedures" [145].

10.3.6 Configurations of the Model

We also suggest reporting the configuration of the model, which represents a fifth addition to the CONSORT extension statement.

Item 3e: Description of the configurations of the model that define various policy alternatives.

Explanation

When the intervention of interest is complex, a description of the various model configurations will help the reader to understand how the alternative policies were modeled.

Example

In the following paragraph, the configurations of a model defining different interventions are reported.

Methods–"We developed four configurations of the discrete-event simulation model to implement the two methods of booking appointments and the two methods of booking elective operations ... In configurations A and B, which used the individual-lists method of booking surgical consultation appointments, there were three priority lists, with surgeon-specific referral rates represented by three internal queues. During each simulated week, the model booked patients waiting on the appointment list of the surgeon who was available for the clinic that week. In configurations C and D, which used the pooled-list method, there was a single priority list for appointments, with an aggregated referral rate represented by a single internal queue. During each simulated week, the model booked patients waiting on the pooled list for an appointment with the surgeon who was available for the clinic that week" (see Sect. 14.2).

10.3.7 Input Parameters

A sixth addition to the CONSORT extension statement would be the input parameters for a simulation model.

Item 3f: Set of parameters and data used by the model to simulate various scenarios.

Explanation

We suggest that all input parameters used by the simulation model be explicitly reported (see Sect. 6.6). This information, which may be presented in the form of a list or table, will help the reader to understand the various scenarios being simulated. It will also help the reader to understand the capability of the model to simulate different scenarios.

Example

The following sentence provides an example of reporting the input parameters for a simulation model.

Appendix–"Table A.1 shows the values of the model input parameters that were used in all simulation runs, including the number of priority groups, arrival rates, branching probabilities, and surgical capacities" [145].

10.3.8 Output Data

As a complement to reporting the input parameters, we also suggest reporting the output data generated by the simulation model (see Sect. 6.7). This represents another addition to the CONSORT extension statement specific to simulation studies.

Item 3g: Set of data generated by the model, representing the simulated scenarios.

Explanation

We suggest that the output data generated by the simulation model be fully reported. This information will help the reader to understand the capability of the model to generate suitable data for comparing performance measures of interest.

Example

The output data generated by a simulation model could be reported as in the following example.

Methods–"The outcomes of the simulation model were the total number of patients waiting for appointments during the weeks with no appointments available, and the individual times from referral to appointment and from appointment to surgery" [156].

10.3.9 Number of Simulation Runs

As recommended in the CONSORT guideline, we suggest reporting the derivation of the number of simulation runs.

Item 7: How the total number of simulation runs was determined (including method of calculation, number of simulation runs, cluster size, a coefficient of intracluster correlation, and an indication of the coefficient's uncertainty).

Explanation

Reporting the details of how the number of runs was calculated will allow the reader to understand how large an effect the study was designed to detect (see Sect. 7.3).

Example

The following paragraph describes how the total number of simulation runs was determined.

Methods–"We estimated that 256 runs would have 90% power to detect a 15% difference in the weekly operation rate between groups of patients in a two-sided 5% significance test ... In calculating the sample size for inferences at the patient level, we estimated an average of 1,730 patient-weeks per simulation run and assumed a coefficient of variation for rates to be 0.25" [144].

10.3.10 Randomization: Sequence Generation

We recommend reporting the method of randomization used to assign interventions to simulation runs. This corresponds to a reporting requirement included in the original CONSORT statement.

Item 8: Method used to generate the random allocation sequence, including details of any restrictions (e.g., blocking, stratification, matching).

Explanation

We suggest reporting how the interventions were randomly assigned to simulation runs. Reporting the method of randomization allows the reader to assess whether the cluster characteristics were distributed similarly across experimental groups.

Example

The following excerpt describes the method of randomization used to assign interventions to simulation runs.

Methods–"... we used the Fedorov algorithm to ensure an optimal distribution of the experimental factors across the runs" [145].

10.3.11 Statistical Methods

Another reporting recommendation for the study methods relates to the statistical methods used to evaluate the results of a simulation experiment, which corresponds to a CONSORT recommendation.

Item 12: Statistical methods used to compare groups in terms of primary outcome(s), indicating how clustering was taken into account and methods for additional analyses, such as subgroup analyses and adjusted analyses.

Explanation

In a cluster randomized design, inferences can be made at the level of the cluster or the individual. Reporting the statistical methods allows the reader to understand how clustering was taken into account in the individual-level analysis. Reporting regression methods involves reporting the performance measure and the measure of effect size. This item corresponds to the measure of effect size and regression methods in the analytical framework for a simulation experiment (see Sects. 7.2 and 7.4).

Example

The following sentence describes the statistical methods used to compare two interventions in a simulation study.

Methods–"The odds ratios derived from discrete-time survival regressions measured the effects of using the individual list and shortest list methods on the weekly proportion of patients on the appointment lists who received their appointments and who underwent the operation, relative to what occurred with the pooled list method" [145].

10.3.12 Ancillary Analyses

Finally, we suggest reporting any ancillary analysis that was performed, in accordance with the original CONSORT statement.

Item 18: Method used to address multiplicity, ideally by reporting any other analyses performed, including subgroup and adjusted analysis, indicating those that were prespecified and those that were exploratory.

Explanation

We suggest that multiple analyses of the same data be reported so that the reader can assess the risk of false-positive results.

Example

The following paragraph describes ancillary analyses that were performed in a simulation study.

Methods–"Several statistical instruments were employed to compare the outcomes of the simulation experiments. We used a two-sample *t*-test to compare the mean number of patients waiting for appointments ... We analysed waiting times as prospective observations from referral to appointment, surgery or removal from the waiting list ..." [156].

10.4 Reporting the Results

In this section, we describe nine items that will help the reader to understand the results of a simulation study.

10.4.1 Recruitment and Follow-Up Periods

As in the CONSORT statement, we recommend reporting the simulated periods of recruitment and follow-up.

Item 14: Simulated dates defining the periods of recruitment and follow-up.

Explanation

A statement about the periods of recruitment and follow-up will inform the reader of the duration of the simulation runs. This information will help the reader to assess if the number of simulated patients and observed events of interest were realistic for the simulated duration. Information on the individual follow-up times will allow the reader to assess if simulated patients were observed for variable lengths of time.

Examples

The following examples of reporting the recruitment and follow-up periods from a simulation study.

Methods–"Each run was 108 weeks long, representing six 18-week cycles of clinic and theater slot allocation to surgeons" [156].

Methods–"We analysed waiting times as prospective observations from referral to appointment, surgery or removal from the waiting list. We treated records with no appointment or surgery time (due to the end of the simulation run, removal from the surgical waiting list, or cancellation of a scheduled operation by an emergency patient) as censored observations, with the assumption that the waiting time would otherwise have been longer" [156].

10.4.2 Participant Flow

We also suggest reporting the number of runs (i.e., simulated clusters) and the number of simulated individuals in experimental groups at various stages of a simulation study. This conforms with a recommendation in the CONSORT extension statement.

Item 13: Flow of simulation runs and simulated participants through each stage (a diagram being strongly recommended), with reporting (for each experimental

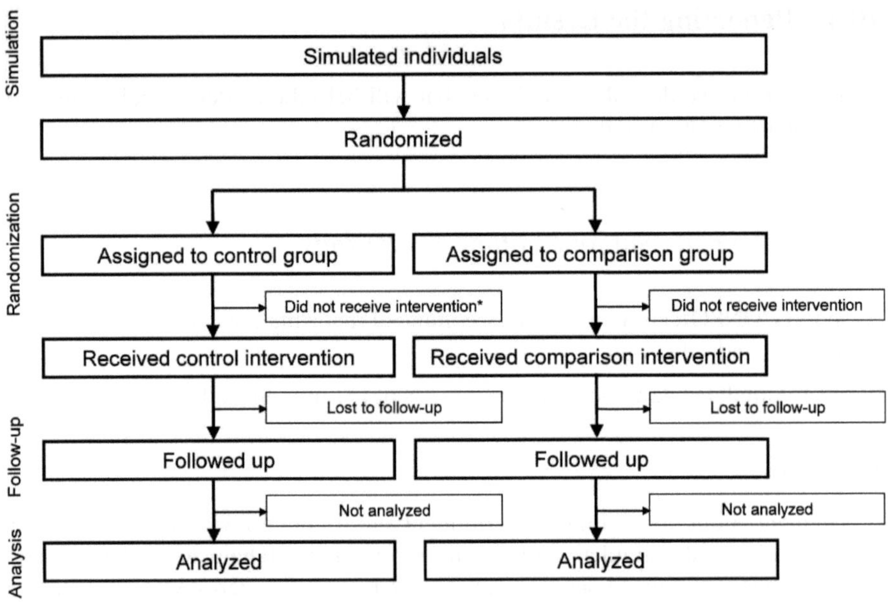

Fig. 10.1 Flow diagram for reporting the number of simulated individuals in control and comparison groups through the phases of a simulation study (∗e.g., a simulated patient is not booked for surgery in a study of methods of booking surgery)

group) of the numbers of runs and participants randomly assigned and analyzed for the primary outcome.

Explanation

Reporting the number of runs and simulated participants randomly assigned to experimental groups allows the reader to assess whether the planned number of simulation runs was performed. The assignment of simulated individuals (e.g., patients) through stages of the simulation study should be illustrated with a flow diagram (Fig. 10.1) to allow the reader to assess why some participants were not included in the analysis and how any such exclusions might affect interpretation of the results. If simulated clusters (e.g., modeled hospitals) are excluded through stages of the simulation study, a similar diagram should be developed for clusters.

Examples

The following sentences provide examples of reporting the number of simulation runs and the number of simulated individuals through a simulation study.

Methods–"The sample size for assessment of all main effects required 108 runs (36 runs for each scheduling method)" [145].

Results–"Regardless of the method of scheduling appointments, most of the referred patients had a surgical consultation by the end of the simulation (94% for individual-lists method, 94% for shortest list method, and 96% for pooled list method)" [145].

10.4.3 Baseline Data

Also in accordance with the CONSORT statement, we suggest reporting the baseline characteristics of the simulated clusters and individuals.

Item 15: Baseline information for each group at the cluster (hospital) and the individual (patient) levels, as applicable.

Explanation

If differences in experimental outcomes are to be attributed to the intervention, other factors (specifically, the baseline characteristics) should be similarly distributed between the experimental groups. Summary statistics of cluster-level and individual-level factors for each experimental group will allow the reader to the compare distributions of these factors. These statistics may be reported in a table.

Example

The following example reports baseline characteristics of simulated patients, in a simulation study.

Results–"The distribution of referrals by patient-level factors was also similar across scheduling methods . . . The majority of referrals were men (about 83%) and about 38% of patients were 60 to 69 years old. Most patients had multivessel disease (about 74%) and either major or minor concurrent conditions (about 50%)" [145].

10.4.4 Numbers Analyzed

As recommended in the CONSORT statement, we suggest reporting the number of simulation runs and simulated individuals that were analyzed.

Item 16: Numbers of simulation runs and simulated individuals for each experimental group included in the analysis.

Explanation

These values will represent the denominator in calculations of proportions. The numbers of clusters and individuals included in an analysis should correspond to the planned sample-size calculations. Reporting these numbers will help the reader to assess if the statistical power was acceptable or if it was lower than planned.

Example

The following paragraph reports the number of simulated patients that were analyzed in a simulation study.

Results–"In total, 200 experiments produced 287,144 patient trajectories: 143,469 for method 1 and 143,675 for method 2. At the end of simulation, 94.4% (method 1) and 96.4% (method 2) of trajectories on elective pathway had progressed through the appointment stage" [155].

10.4.5 Outcomes and Estimation

We recommend reporting the estimated effect size and its precision, as suggested in the CONSORT statement.

Item 17: For each primary and secondary outcome, a summary of results for each group, at the cluster (hospital) or individual (patient) level as applicable; for each primary and secondary outcome, the estimated effect size and its precision (e.g., 95% confidence interval); and for each primary outcome, an intracluster correlation coefficient.

Explanation

Reporting the estimated size of the effect and its 95% confidence interval will allow the reader to assess the statistical significance of the result, and to make decisions about whether the size of the effect is large enough to consider using the intervention in a real-world situation. In Part III of this book, we tend to report measures of precision as 95% confidence intervals, rather than a standard error. Reporting a standard error requires effort from the reader to compute a confidence interval or the confidence limits. Technically speaking, an interval specifies a range of values (e.g., 1.18–1.24), whereas limits specify the lower and upper boundaries of an interval (e.g., 1.18, 1.24). Also, reporting a p value does not allow the reader to assess the size of the effect or its precision.

Example

In the following example, the estimated effect size and its 95% confidence interval are reported.

Results–"After adjustment for hospital and patient factors, the weekly odds that a medium-priority patient on the wait list underwent the operation were 20% higher for pre-booking (OR 1.21, CI 1.18–1.24)" [144].

10.4.6 Adverse Events

The reporting of adverse events was recommended by CONSORT, and we also suggest that any adverse events generated by a simulation study be reported.

Item 19: All important adverse events in each experimental group.

Explanation

Reporting adverse events will help the reader to understand the types of events that have been modeled and that a simulated patient might experience. Information about whether the simulation model includes mechanisms to simulate adverse events affecting the flow of simulated patients through a care path will help the reader to interpret the results.

Example

The following excerpt describes simulated adverse events generated in a simulation study.

Results–"The proportion of elective procedures with high priority that took place within 1 week of the treatment decision was 96.4% for pre-booking and 88.9% for wait list booking; 3.2% and 5.6%, respectively, of such procedures were cancelled from the final operating room schedule" [144].

10.4.7 Limitations

The CONSORT statement also recommended reporting any limitations, and we similarly recommend that the limitations of a simulation study be reported.

Item 20: Trial limitations, addressing any sources of potential bias or imprecision, and, if relevant, risks associated with multiplicity of analyses.

Explanation

Reporting the limitations of the simulation study will help the reader to interpret the results and determine their applicability to the real world. In the CONSORT statement, this item was originally called "Interpretation," but it has been relabeled as "Limitations" in the 2010 revision [132].

Example

The following example reports the limitations of a simulation study.

Discussion–"However, our model also had several limitations. First, although we were able to account for the availability of surgeons for operations, we lacked information about shortages of other hospital staff, so our model did not consider fluctuations in their availability ..." [145].

10.4.8 Generalizability

Another important aspect recommended in the original statement is generalizability, and we also recommend reporting the generalizability of the findings of a simulation study to other contexts.

Item 21: Generalizability of the trial's findings to other clusters or other simulated patients (as relevant).

Explanation

It is important for the reader to understand the situations to which the results of the simulation study may be generalized. Moher et al. [109] provide a more detailed explanation of the importance of generalizability.

Example

The following example addresses the generalizability of the findings of a simulation study to other contexts.

Discussion–"The results may not be applicable to networks of hospitals where surgeons have admitting rights at more than one hospital, as performing surgery in other hospitals may further contribute to the unavailability of surgeons for appointments and operations" [156].

10.4.9 Overall Evidence

Similar to the CONSORT statement, we suggest reporting the interpretation of the results in the context of current evidence.

Item 22: General interpretation of the results in the context of current evidence.

Explanation

A general interpretation of the results helps the reader to understand how the simulation study contributes to existing knowledge.

Example

The following example interprets the results of a simulation study in the context of current evidence.

Discussion and Conclusions–"Higher cancellation rates after wait list booking may be attributable to a higher proportion of patients who need elective surgery being scheduled in the on-call slot with this method of booking, because of prioritization. Therefore, these patients are at higher risk of cancellation caused by the arrival of emergency patients or inpatients ... Others have used simulation experiments to explore the implications of different booking systems. Contrary to our results, they suggested that an increase in cancellations of scheduled cases may be an unintended consequence of pre-booking. However, their analysis ignored factors relevant to the underlying peri-operative process, including the weekly availability of specialists" [144].

10.5 Reporting with Effective Tables

Researchers use tables to report and summarize information, allowing the reader to readily understand the findings of a simulation study. Tables can be used to organize and display results more clearly and effectively than would be the case with descriptions in text. If devised effectively, tables also help the reader to compare results between experimental groups and to understand how certain derived results were calculated [91].

When planning the analysis of a simulation experiment, researchers create templates of tables for summarizing anticipated findings. Constructing a table template involves identifying the necessary components of the desired table (Box 10.1) [91]. For instance, column headings describe the information presented in the columns of the table. In a table showing the distribution of baseline characteristics between experimental groups, the first column heading might be "Characteristic," and the subsequent column headings might be the names of the experimental groups.

Box 10.1 Components of a table

- Table number enumerating the table in relation to other tables in the manuscript
- Table title describing the information presented
- Column headings describing the information presented in the columns
- Row headings describing the information presented in the rows
- Cell entries showing results of the study
- Horizontal lines marking boundaries of the table
- Footnote explaining each abbreviation used in the table
- Footnotes explaining selected entries in the table, keyed within the table

Another aspect of creating table templates is determining what footnotes are needed to help explain selected entries in the table. These footnotes may be used to provide definitions of terms, explain calculations, or report variables adjusted for in a regression analysis. Footnotes may be designated by the standard symbols ∗, †, ‡, §, ‖, ¶, ∗∗, ††, etc., but other schemes for designating footnotes are also possible.

Tables provide an effective way to display the information to be reported from simulation experiments based on a cluster randomized design, as suggested in the preceding sections of this chapter. In particular, researchers can use tables to summarize information on the distribution of cluster-level and individual-level characteristics across experimental groups (item 15 of Table 10.1). In such a table, the column headings describe the experimental groups, the row headings describe the characteristics, and the cells contain counts and percentages. Examples of tables showing baseline information across experimental groups appear in the case studies presented in Part III of this book (e.g., Tables 14.3, 14.4, and 16.4).

Researchers can also use tables to summarize results indicating the effect of an intervention (item 17 of Table 10.1). In such a table, the column headings describe the performance measure, the measure of effect size, and the intermediate statistics (e.g., total number of events) required to calculate these measures; the row headings describe the experimental groups; and the cells contain the estimates and their precision (e.g., 95% confidence intervals). These tables should be constructed in relation to the study question and anticipated interpretation of the estimates generated from the analyses. Examples of tables summarizing results to indicate the effect of an intervention appear in the case studies presented in Part III of this book (e.g., Tables 14.5 and 16.7). We constructed tables and report our results according to published guidelines for reporting statistics in medicine [91, 108, 109, 132].

Chapter 11
Evaluations at the Cluster Level

In Chap. 1, we discussed policy analysis involving the statistical comparison of performance measures across experimental groups. Statistical comparison determines whether an observed difference between groups should be interpreted as an effect of the intervention. Guided by the study question, evaluation of a policy may be performed at the level of the cluster or the individual, as discussed in Sect. 1.5 [140]. With the cluster as the unit of inference, we introduced two performance measures in Chap. 8. Evaluations at the cluster level, which typically assess whether a performance criterion is met, may involve comparing proportions. For example, this approach would be appropriate in determining whether booking surgery in advance reduces the proportion of hospitals that have surgical delays for high-priority elective procedures, relative to some other method of booking the procedures. Alternatively, evaluations at the cluster level may involve comparing averages. For example, comparisons of averages would be appropriate for studying whether use of a pooled list, rather than individual lists, for surgical consultation appointments decreases the average clearance time for the appointments lists.

In this chapter, we present methods for evaluating policy alternatives using simulation experiments with a cluster randomized design and performance measures at the level of the cluster. Here, the unit of randomization and the unit of analysis is the cluster. We discuss how to estimate and compare cluster-level measures while adjusting for potential confounders, using standard statistical methods. In addition, we discuss what to report from the cluster-level analysis.

11.1 Scenario Involving Proportions

As discussed in Chap. 8, cluster-level proportions summarize the performance of the system in several simulation runs, as measured by the fraction of clusters that satisfy a specified criterion. For example, researchers might want to determine the proportion of hospitals with delay of high-priority elective procedures, or the proportion of hospitals with cancellation of cases from the final operating room

B. Sobolev et al., *Health Care Evaluation Using Computer Simulation: Concepts, Methods, and Applications*, DOI 10.1007/978-1-4614-2233-4_11,

list because the patient was unfit for surgery. Whether the cluster-level proportion is suitable for assessing the effect of an intervention is related to the study hypothesis, the experimental outcome, and the corresponding measures of effect for comparisons across experimental groups (see Chap. 8). There are various scenarios in which the analysis of cluster-level proportions might arise.

In this chapter, we use the following scenario to illustrate the evaluation of system performance by analyzing cluster-level proportions. We will refer to this hypothetical situation as Scenario 11.1: A policy-maker must choose between continuing to use the existing method of booking elective surgeries, which happens to be wait-list booking, and switching to a new method, advance booking. He is particularly concerned with improving the hospital's performance by reducing cancellations of high-priority procedures. From experience, the policy-maker knows that other factors may affect cancellations, such as the booking method for surgical consultation appointments, the allocation of operating room slots, the clearance time for appointment lists, the clearance time for surgical wait lists, and the clearance time for inpatient surgical queues. Clearance times for backlogs in corresponding services are reported as the ratio of existing demand to capacity. He formulates the following study question: *Does the method of booking elective surgery affect whether a hospital can avoid cancellations of high-priority elective procedures, independent of other factors?* The study questions in the scenarios of Chap. 8 differ from the questions in the scenarios of this chapter. In Scenario 11.1, the policy-maker is interested in estimating the effect size, while adjusting for other factors which may affect the outcome of interest.

11.2 Preparing Data for Analysis of Proportions

To evaluate system performance on the basis of cluster-level proportions, a researcher requires data indicating whether a cluster has met a specific criterion. The researcher prepares simulated data for analysis by developing a data dictionary and creating an analytical data set. The variables in the data dictionary are determined by the study hypothesis. The structure of the analytical data set are determined by the unit of analysis and the data dictionary.

The data dictionary describes the variables related to the study question of interest. In particular, the data dictionary will include the name, description, data type, and categories or values of each variable. These components of the data dictionary are collaboratively developed by a research team, including health care researchers, statisticians, and database analysts, during the planning stages of the simulation experiment. For comparisons of cluster-level proportions, the data dictionary includes an indicator variable corresponding to the cluster-level outcome and a categorical variable corresponding to the experimental group. Other explanatory variables that could affect the outcome of interest are also listed.

The analytical data set for comparing cluster-level proportions has a specific structure. For an analysis at the cluster level, the data set is structured so that each

Table 11.1 Data dictionary of variables for estimating cluster-level performance measures in Scenarios 11.1 and 11.2

Variable	Description	Type	Categories or values
runid	Hospital identifier	Categorical	≥1
meth_app	Method of booking surgical consultation appointments	Categorical	1—Individual lists 2—Pooled list 3—Shortest list
meth_sx	Method of booking surgery	Categorical	1—Advance booking 2—Wait-list booking
or_slot	Allocation of operating room slots between elective and urgent procedures	Categorical	1—Weekly split 2—Daily split
ap_ct	Clearance time for appointment lists at start of simulation (weeks)	Numeric	1, 2, or 3
el_ct	Clearance time for surgical wait lists at start of simulation (weeks)	Numeric	3, 4, 5, or 6
ur_ct	Clearance time for inpatient surgical queues at start of simulation (weeks)	Numeric	0, 1, or 2
inocanc	Indicator for no cancellations of any high-priority elective procedures	Categorical	0—No 1—Yes
n_ptwt	No. of patients waiting during weeks when no surgical consultation appointments are available	Numeric	≥0

row represents a single cluster, the unit of analysis. For an analysis of cluster-level proportions, the columns of the analytical data set should contain, at a minimum, the variable representing the experimental group and the indicator variable representing whether the cluster has met the specific criterion, that is, the experimental outcome, the distribution of which will be summarized by a cluster-level proportion. Other potential variables in the simulated data set might include cluster-level factors that would affect the outcome. All of these variables are defined in the data dictionary.

Developing the data dictionary for Scenario 11.1 entails identifying the study variable, the experimental outcome, and pertinent environmental factors, as well as defining the type and coding for each variable. In this scenario, the study variable is the method of booking surgery (`meth_sx`) and the experimental outcome variable is an indicator of whether the hospital has no cancellations of high-priority elective procedures (`inocanc`). The data dictionary for this scenario also includes several environmental factors, such as the allocation of operating room slots (Table 11.1). With this data dictionary as a guide, the researcher can use simulation models to generate the analytical data set needed for evaluation purposes (Table 11.2).

The simulation experiment consists of runs of the model, with inputs representing proposed alternatives. Each run generates a cluster of patients, with data on the occurrence and timing of simulated events for each patient. Experimental outcomes

Table 11.2 Tab-delimited file containing the analytical data set for estimating cluster-level proportions in Scenario 11.1 (see Table 11.1 for data dictionary of variables in this data set)

runid	meth_app	meth_sx	or_slot	ap_ct	el_ct	ur_ct	inocanc
1	1	1	2	3	5	2	0
2	3	1	2	1	4	1	1
...							
144	2	1	1	3	6	0	0
145	1	2	1	2	3	0	0
146	2	2	2	1	6	1	0
...							
228	3	2	1	3	5	2	1

at the cluster level are then computed from the patient-level records. Each simulation run produces a binary response y_{ij} showing whether run $j = 1, \ldots, k$ in experimental group i meets a performance criterion, for example, whether a hospital modeled in the run has cancellations of some high-priority elective procedures for nonclinical reasons. The first row of the data set (Table 11.2) contains the variable names, and subsequent rows show the data values corresponding to those variables for a specific run. For example, according to the analytical data set for Scenario 11.1, hospital 1 (`runid` = `1`) used individual-lists booking for consultation appointments (`meth_app` = `1`) and advance booking for surgery (`meth_sx` = `1`). This hospital had no cancellations of high-priority elective procedures (`inocanc` = `0`).

If the experimental outcome for the cluster is based on individual-level data, then some effort must usually be expended in combining the simulated individual-level data into the required cluster-level variables before any cluster-level analysis can be performed. These combined observations are assumed to be independent across clusters. Statistical tests and confidence intervals will then be based on variation between clusters, not between individuals [49].

11.3 Adjusting Effect Size for Proportions

Once the cluster-level proportions have been estimated, standard statistical techniques can be applied to compare these proportions between experimental groups. For example, Pearson's χ^2 test indicates if there are differences in proportions at the cluster level. However, this test would not provide an estimate of the effect size. The crude odds ratio (see Sect. 8.3) provides an estimate of the effect size, but it does not allow adjustment for potential confounding factors.

Another method for estimating the crude odds ratio is simple logistic regression, which links the log odds of cluster j in group i meeting the performance criterion to a linear function of the experimental factors [77]:

$$\log\left(\frac{p_{ij}^{c}}{1 - p_{ij}^{c}}\right) = \beta_0 + \beta_1 I_{1ij}. \qquad (11.1)$$

In this equation, p^{c}_{ij} is the probability of cluster j in group i meeting the criterion, I_{1ij} is an indicator variable for the comparison group, coefficient β_0 is the log odds for the reference group, and coefficient β_1 is the difference in the log odds between the comparison group and the reference group. The exponential of regression coefficient $\exp(\beta_1)$ gives the crude odds ratio, where a value less than 1 indicates lower odds that a cluster will meet the performance criterion.

The logistic regression model in (11.1) can be extended to a multivariable model which adjusts for potential confounding factors:

$$\log\left(\frac{p^{\mathrm{c}}_{ij}}{1-p^{\mathrm{c}}_{ij}}\right) = \beta_0 + \beta_1 I_{1ij} + \cdots + \beta_r I_{rij}, \tag{11.2}$$

where I_{1ij} is the indicator variable for the comparison group and I_{2ij} to I_{rij} are other cluster-level variables. The regression coefficient β_1 in (11.2) is then the difference in the log odds between the comparison group and the reference group adjusted for the other factors. The exponential of this regression coefficient estimates the adjusted odds ratio.

The maximum likelihood estimate, $\hat{\beta}_1$, and its standard error, $\mathrm{SE}(\hat{\beta}_1)$, can be derived by statistical software. Then, the estimated effect of the intervention is odds ratio $= \exp(\hat{\beta}_1)$, and its $100(1-\alpha)\%$ confidence limits can be estimated as follows:

$$\begin{aligned} \mathrm{LCL} &= \exp[\hat{\beta}_1 - z_{\alpha/2}\mathrm{SE}(\hat{\beta}_1)], \\ \mathrm{UCL} &= \exp[\hat{\beta}_1 + z_{\alpha/2}\mathrm{SE}(\hat{\beta}_1)]. \end{aligned} \tag{11.3}$$

In Chap. 16, we describe in detail the results of a simulation experiment related to Scenario 11.1, evaluating the effect of surgical booking method—either wait-list booking or advance booking—on the proportion of hospitals with no cancellations of high-priority elective procedures. Using (8.2) and (8.3), we estimated hospital-level proportions and 95% confidence intervals for the wait-list booking and advance-booking methods as 5.6% (1.8–9.3%) and 2.8% (0.1–5.5%), respectively. These percentages indicate that a greater proportion of hospitals using the wait-list method of booking surgery had no cancellations of high-priority elective procedures.

We then used a multivariable logistic regression to estimate the effect of the method of booking surgery with adjustment for hospital-level variables. Several hospital-level variables likely to affect outputs of the simulation were entered into the regression model, in addition to the indicator variable for the method of booking surgery; see Table 11.3 (where subscripts for experimental group and cluster are suppressed). For each categorical variable in the regression analysis, a set of indicator variables was created. The number of indicator variables in each set was one less than the number of categories. For example, we entered one indicator variable, I_1, for the method of booking surgery, which took the value 1 for advance booking (i.e., `meth_sx = 1`) and the value 0 for wait-list booking

Table 11.3 Regression model for estimating the effect of the method of booking surgery on the proportion of hospitals having no cancellations of high-priority elective procedures

Question:	Does the method of booking elective surgery affect whether a hospital can avoid cancellations of high-priority elective procedures?
Model:	$\log\left(\frac{p}{1-p}\right) = \beta_0 + \beta_1 I_1 + \beta_2 I_2 + \beta_3 I_3 + \beta_4 I_4 + \beta_5 I_5 + \beta_6 I_6 + \beta_7 I_7 + \beta_8 I_8 + \beta_9 I_9 + \beta_{10} I_{10} + \beta_{11} I_{11}$
p	Proportion of hospitals with no cancellations of high-priority elective procedures
I_1	Indicator for advance vs. wait-list booking of surgery
I_2, I_3	Indicators for individual-lists and shortest-list vs. pooled-list booking of appointments
I_4	Indicator for daily vs. weekly split of operating room slots between elective and urgent procedures
I_5, I_6	Indicators for 2 or 3 vs. 1 week of clearance time for appointment lists at the start of simulation
I_7, I_8, I_9	Indicators for 4, 5, or 6 vs. 3 weeks of clearance time for surgical wait lists at the start of simulation
I_{10}, I_{11}	Indicators for 1 or 2 vs. 0 weeks of clearance time for inpatient surgical queues at the start of simulation

(i.e., `meth_sx = 2`). Also, we entered two indicator variables, I_2 and I_3, for the booking method for surgical consultations, which took the values $I_2 = 1$ and $I_3 = 0$ for the individual-lists method (i.e., `meth_app = 1`), the values $I_2 = 0$ and $I_3 = 1$ for the shortest-list method (i.e., `meth_app = 3`), and the values $I_2 = 0$ and $I_3 = 0$ for the pooled-list method (i.e., `meth_app = 2`).

The estimated regression coefficients corresponding to the model in Table 11.3 were

$$\log\left(\frac{p^{c}}{1-p^{c}}\right) = -2.23 - 0.81 I_1 - 1.50 I_2 + 0.57 I_3 - 0.79 I_4 - 1.42 I_5 + 0.66 I_6 - 0.30 I_7 - 0.71 I_8 - 0.29 I_9 - 0.27 I_{10} + 0.36 I_{11},$$

where the estimated regression coefficient for the method of booking surgery, $\hat{\beta}_1$, was about -0.811 with a standard error, $\mathrm{SE}(\hat{\beta}_1)$, of about 0.645. The effect of the intervention, as measured by an odds ratio, was estimated as $\exp(\hat{\beta}_1) = \exp(-0.811) \approx 0.44$, and its 95% confidence limits were estimated from (11.3) as

$$\mathrm{LCL} = \exp(-0.811 - 1.96 \times 0.645) \approx 0.13,$$

$$\mathrm{UCL} = \exp(-0.811 + 1.96 \times 0.645) \approx 1.57.$$

Therefore, the simulation study suggests the odds that a hospital would have no cancellations of high-priority elective procedures were 56% lower with the advance-booking method than with the wait-list booking method, after adjustment for hospital-related factors; however, this difference was not statistically significant (odds ratio = 0.44, 95% confidence interval 0.13–1.57) (see Sect. 8.3).

11.4 Reporting Results for Proportions

Appropriate reporting will help the reader interpret the results of a simulation experiment. In Chap. 10, we described the recommended items to report for a simulation study based on a cluster randomized design. Here, we elaborate on the results that should be reported from an analysis comparing cluster-level proportions.

The first item that should be reported is the estimated cluster-level proportion for each experimental group, since this is the performance measure of interest. Along with the estimated proportion, the number of clusters in each group (the denominator) and the number of clusters meeting the performance criterion in each group should also be explicitly reported (the numerator). Reporting absolute counts allows the reader to assess the number of simulated clusters in the experiment and whether the clusters were distributed equally between groups, as should be the case for a cluster randomized design. In addition, these counts allow the reader to understand how the proportions were calculated. For example, if a researcher simply reports that 10% of the clusters met the performance criterion, without providing absolute counts, the reader cannot tell whether the percentage represents 100 out of 1,000 clusters or just 1 out of 10 clusters. A reader might justifiably question the statistical power and smallest anticipated difference in a simulation experiment with just 10 runs for comparisons at the cluster level, but may be more confident about an experiment with 1,000 runs.

The second item that should be reported is the estimated odds ratio, along with its 95% confidence interval, which conveys information about statistical significance and precision. If the 95% confidence interval for an odds ratio does not span the value 1.0, then there is statistical evidence to support the conclusion that the interventions have different effects on the cluster-level proportions at the 5% significance level. However, statistical significance may not be clinically meaningful. Therefore, good reporting will allow the reader to assess not only the statistical significance but also the clinical significance. The magnitude of the odds for the comparison group relative to the odds for the reference group will help the reader to determine if the effect was clinically significant. The width of the corresponding confidence interval indicates the precision of the estimate, where a narrower interval indicates greater precision. The size of effect that is meaningful relates directly to the smallest anticipated difference, discussed in Sect. 7.3 and Appendix B.

The third item that should be reported consists of the unadjusted and adjusted odds ratios. These values allow the reader to assess the extent to which the estimated effect size changed after the researchers accounted for potential confounding factors. An odds ratio that does not change after adjustment for cluster-level factors could indicate that the intervention has an independent effect on the experimental outcome. A tabular format can be used to report these recommended items.

In Part III of this book, we use tables to report the results of comparisons of cluster-level proportions from various case studies. The results of a simulation experiment comparing the proportions of hospitals not canceling high-priority

Table 11.4 Preliminary table for reporting results on relation between methods of booking surgery and the proportion of hospitals without cancellation of high-priority procedures

meth_sx	sum_inocanc	nruns	prop	or	lcl	ucl
2	8	144	5.6	1.00		
1	4	144	2.8	0.44	0.13	1.57

procedures in relation to different methods of booking surgery (i.e., Scenario 11.1), are shown in a preliminary table (Table 11.4). The statistics reported in this preliminary table show the method of booking surgery (`meth_sx`), the number of hospitals with no cancellations of high-priority procedures (`sum_inocanc`), the number of hospitals in each group (`nruns`), the percentage of hospitals with no cancellations (`prop`), and the odds ratio for no cancellations (`or`), along with its corresponding lower and upper 95% confidence limits (`lcl` and `ucl`, respectively).

The results from this analysis of cluster-level proportions are reported in Table 16.6. From this table, the reader can readily see that hospitals were equally distributed between the methods of booking surgery, with 144 simulation runs per group. The table also shows that 5.6% of hospitals in the wait-list booking group and 2.8% of those in the advance-booking group had no cancellations of high-priority procedures. The value of 0.44 in column 5, the odds ratio, shows that, compared with the wait-list booking group, the odds for no cancellations of high-priority procedures were 56% lower among hospitals in the advance booking group. The confidence interval of 0.13–1.57 indicates that this effect was not statistically significant because it spans the value 1.0. Additional examples of reporting results from analyses of cluster-level proportions appear in Tables 14.7, 15.5, and 16.5.

11.5 Scenario Involving Averages

As discussed in Chap. 8, cluster-level averages summarize the performance of the cluster as a whole, as measured by an expected value of observations. For example, researchers might want to determine the average clearance time for appointments or the average weekly number of patients waiting for surgical consultation appointments during weeks when no appointments are available. Whether the cluster-level average is suitable for assessing the effect of an intervention is related to the study hypothesis, the experimental outcome, and the corresponding measures of effect for comparisons across experimental groups (see Chap. 8). There are various scenarios in which the analysis of cluster-level averages might arise.

In this chapter, we use the following scenario to illustrate the evaluation of system performance by analyzing cluster-level averages. We will refer to this hypothetical situation as Scenario 11.2: A health services researcher is studying alternatives for booking patients for their surgical consultation appointments. It seems that most hospitals have a separate wait list for each surgeon, with patients being served by the surgeon named in the referral on a first-come, first-served basis (i.e., the individual-list method). However, some hospitals have started to use a single, pooled wait list, whereby patients are still served on a first-come, first-served basis, but each patient's appointment is with the first available surgeon (i.e., the pooled-list method). The researcher would like to know if these two methods have a differential effect on how many patients are waiting for surgical consultation appointments during weeks when no appointments are available. From the literature, the researcher already knows that other factors may affect the number of these patients, such as the method of booking surgery, the allocation of operating room slots, the clearance time for appointment lists, the clearance time for surgical wait lists, and the clearance time for inpatient surgical queues. The hospital's management uses the ratio of existing demand to capacity to report clearance times for backlogs in corresponding services. She formulates the following study question: *Does the booking method for surgical consultation appointments affect the average number of patients on the appointment lists during weeks when no appointments are available, independent of other factors?* The study questions in the scenarios of Chap. 8 differ from the questions in the scenarios of this chapter. In Scenario 11.2, the researcher is interested in estimating the effect size, independent of other factors which may affect the outcome of interest.

11.6 Preparing Data for Analysis of Averages

To evaluate system performance on the basis of cluster-level averages, a researcher requires data suitable for calculating averages. The researcher prepares simulated data for analysis by developing a data dictionary and creating an analytical data set. Developing the study hypothesis guides in determining the variables to include in the data dictionary and the structure of the analytical data set (see Sect. 11.2). For comparisons of cluster-level averages, the data dictionary includes a continuous variable corresponding to the experimental outcome and a categorical variable corresponding to the experimental group. Other explanatory variables that could affect the outcome of interest are also listed.

The analytical data set for comparing cluster-level averages has a specific structure, which is similar to that of the data set for evaluating cluster-level proportions, as described in Sect. 11.2. Specifically, each row represents a cluster (the unit of analysis) and columns contain the variables listed in the data dictionary. For an analysis of cluster-level averages, the columns of the analytical data set should contain, at a minimum, the variable representing the experimental group and a continuous variable measuring some aspect of the cluster. Other potential variables in the simulated data set might include cluster-level factors that would affect the outcome.

Developing the data dictionary for Scenario 11.2 entails identifying the study variable, the experimental outcome, and pertinent environmental factors, as well as defining the type and coding for each variable. In this scenario, the study variable is the booking method for surgical consultation appointments (`meth_app`)

Table 11.5 Tab-delimited file containing the analytical data set for estimating cluster-level averages in Scenario 11.2 (see Table 11.1 for data dictionary of variables in this data set)

runid	meth_app	meth_sx	or_slot	ap_ct	el_ct	ur_ct	n_ptwt
1	1	1	2	3	5	2	43
2	1	2	2	1	4	1	38
...							
112	1	2	1	3	6	0	24
113	2	1	1	2	3	0	38
114	2	2	2	1	6	1	35
...							
224	2	2	1	3	5	2	25

because the researcher wants to compare the individual-lists and the pooled-list booking methods. The experimental outcome is the number of patients waiting for a surgical consultation appointment during weeks when no appointments are available (`n_ptwt`) (Table 11.1). The distribution of this outcome can be summarized by an average. The remaining variables in the data dictionary are environmental factors representing characteristics of the cluster that may affect the outcome.

With this data dictionary as a guide, the researcher can prepare the analytical data set needed for evaluation purposes (Table 11.5). The simulation experiment consists of runs of the model, with inputs representing proposed alternatives. Each simulation run j in experimental group i produces a continuous observation y_{ij}, the weekly number of patients waiting for an appointment during weeks when no appointments are available. The first row of the data set (Table 11.5) contains the variable names, and subsequent rows show the data values corresponding to those variables for a single cluster. For example, according to the analytical data set for Scenario 11.2, hospital 113 (`runid` = `113`) used the pooled-list booking method (`meth_app` = `2`) and the advance booking of surgery (`meth_sx` = `1`). This hospital had 38 patients on the appointment list during weeks when no appointments were available (`n_ptwt` = `38`).

The analytical data set for evaluating cluster-level proportions in Table 11.2 differs from the data set for evaluating cluster-level averages in Table 11.5. The data set in Table 11.2 includes the indicator outcome variable `inocanc`, whereas the data set in Table 11.5 shows the continuous outcome variable `n_ptwt`. In addition, the number of simulated hospitals differs between the analytical data sets because a different number of runs may be needed to detect anticipated differences in proportions than in averages.

11.7 Adjusting Effect Size for Averages

Once the cluster-level averages have been estimated, standard techniques can be used to compare these averages between experimental groups. For example, a two-sample t test indicates whether differences between averages at the cluster level are present and could generate a measure of the effect size for the intervention (i.e., the crude difference in averages between the two groups; see Sect. 8.7). However, this technique would not allow adjustment for potential confounding factors.

Linear regression methods are required to adjust for potential confounding factors, whereby the cluster-level average is modeled as a linear function of the study variable [159]. A simple linear regression model can provide an estimate of the crude difference in averages:

$$y_{ij} = \beta_0 + \beta_1 I_{1ij}, \tag{11.4}$$

where I_{1ij} is the indicator variable for the comparison group for run j of group i. This variable takes the value 0 for all runs in the reference group, and the value 1 for all runs in the comparison group. The regression coefficient β_1 is the crude difference in the averages between the two groups, which is the measure of effect size.

The linear regression model in (11.4) can be extended to adjust the effect of the intervention for other factors. This extension leads to a multivariable linear regression model:

$$y_{ij} = \beta_0 + \beta_1 I_{1ij} + \cdots + \beta_r I_{rij}, \tag{11.5}$$

where I_{1ij} is the indicator variable for the comparison group and I_{2ij} to I_{rij} are other cluster-level variables. The adjusted difference in averages between the experimental groups is estimated directly by β_1 in (11.5).

The maximum likelihood estimate, $\hat{\beta}_1$, and its standard error, $\text{SE}(\hat{\beta}_1)$, can be derived by statistical software. The regression estimate will have the 95% confidence limits calculated as follows:

$$\begin{aligned} \text{LCL} &= \hat{\beta}_1 - z_{\alpha/2}\text{SE}(\hat{\beta}_1), \\ \text{UCL} &= \hat{\beta}_1 + z_{\alpha/2}\text{SE}(\hat{\beta}_1). \end{aligned} \tag{11.6}$$

In Chap. 14, we describe in detail the results of a simulation experiment related to Scenario 11.2, evaluating the effect of the booking method for surgical consultation appointments—either individual lists or a pooled list—on the average number of patients waiting for appointments during weeks when no appointments are available. Using (8.10) and (8.11), we estimated hospital-level averages and 95% confidence intervals for the individual-lists and pooled-list booking methods as 38 (37–38) and 25 (25–26), respectively. These averages indicate that hospitals using the individual-lists method have, on average, more patients on the appointment lists during weeks when no appointments are available.

We then used a multivariable linear regression to estimate the effect of the booking method for surgical consultation appointments with adjustment for hospital-level variables. Several variables likely to affect outputs of the simulation were entered into the regression model, in addition to the indicator variable for the method

Table 11.6 Regression model for estimating the effect of the method of booking surgical consultation appointments on average weekly number of patients on appointment lists during weeks when no appointments are available

Question:	Does the method of booking surgical consultation appointments affect the average number of patients waiting for an appointment during weeks when no appointments are available?
Model:	$y = \beta_0 + \beta_1 I_1 + \beta_2 I_2 + \beta_3 I_3 + \beta_4 I_4 + \beta_5 I_5 + \beta_6 I_6 + \beta_7 I_7 + \beta_8 I_8 + \beta_9 I_9 + \beta_{10} I_{10}$
y	No. of patients waiting for an appointment during weeks when no appointments are available
I_1	Indicator for pooled-list vs. individual-lists booking of appointments
I_2	Indicators for advance vs. wait-list booking of surgery
I_3	Indicator for daily vs. weekly split of operating room slots between elective and urgent procedures
I_4, I_5	Indicators for 2 or 3 vs. 1 week of clearance time for appointment lists at the start of simulation
I_6, I_7, I_8	Indicators for 4, 5, or 6 vs. 3 weeks of clearance time for surgical wait lists at the start of simulation
I_9, I_{10}	Indicators for 1 or 2 vs. 0 weeks of clearance time for inpatient surgical queues at the start of simulation

of booking appointments; see Table 11.6 (where subscripts for experimental group and cluster are suppressed). The estimated regression coefficients corresponding to the model in Table 11.6 were

$$y = 37.6 - 12.3 I_1 - 0.5 I_2 + 0.4 I_3 - 0.4 I_4 + 0.6 I_5 + 0.2 I_6 - 0.1 I_7 - 0.2 I_8 + 0.4 I_9 - 0.3 I_{10},$$

where the estimated regression coefficient for the method of booking surgical consultation appointments, $\hat{\beta}_1$, was about -12.3 with a standard error, $\mathrm{SE}(\hat{\beta}_1)$, of about 0.4. Therefore, the estimated effect size of the pooled-list method, with adjustment for hospital-level variables, is -12.3, with 95% confidence limits

$$\mathrm{LCL} = -12.3 - 1.96 \times 0.4 \approx -13.1,$$

$$\mathrm{UCL} = -12.3 + 1.96 \times 0.4 \approx -11.5,$$

that were calculated from (11.6).

The effect size of 12.3 can be interpreted to mean that, on average, 12 (95% confidence interval 11.5–13.1) fewer patients are waiting for an appointment during weeks when no appointments are available in hospitals using the pooled-list method than in hospitals using the individual-lists method of booking surgical consultation appointments, independent of other factors (see Sect. 8.7).

11.8 Reporting Results for Averages

Appropriate reporting helps the reader to interpret the results of a simulation experiment. In Chap. 10, we described the recommended items to be reported for a simulation study based on a cluster randomized design. Here, we elaborate on what should be reported from an analysis comparing cluster-level averages.

The first item that should be reported is the estimated cluster-level average for each experimental group since this is the performance measure of interest. Along with the estimated average, an estimate of variability should also be provided, either as the standard deviation of the outcome of interest for each experimental group or as a confidence interval for the cluster-level average for each experimental group. Reporting the cluster-level averages for each group allows the reader to assess the magnitude of the performance measure, and reporting the variability for each group allows the reader to compare the spread of the observed outcomes and the precision of the estimated cluster average.

The second item that should be reported is the estimated difference in cluster-level averages, which is the measure of effect size, and its 95% confidence interval, which conveys information about statistical significance and precision. If the 95% confidence interval for the difference in averages does not span the value 0, then there is statistical evidence to support the conclusion that the interventions have different effects on the cluster-level averages at the 5% significance level. However, statistical significance may not be clinically meaningful. Therefore, good reporting will allow the reader to assess not only the statistical significance but also the clinical significance. The magnitude of the difference in averages between the comparison and reference groups will help the reader to determine if the effect was clinically significant. The width of the corresponding confidence interval indicates the precision of the estimate, where a narrower interval indicates greater precision. The size of effect that is meaningful relates directly to the smallest anticipated difference discussed in Sect. 7.3 and Appendix B.

The third item that should be reported consists of the unadjusted and adjusted differences. These values allow the reader to assess the extent to which the estimated effect size changed after the researchers accounted for potential confounding factors. A difference in averages or a regression coefficient that does not change after adjustment for cluster-level factors could indicate that the intervention has an independent effect on the experimental outcome. These recommended items to be reported in comparisons of cluster-level averages may be summarized in tabular format.

The distribution of a continuous variable can be efficiently conveyed through a box plot [91], which displays the minimum and maximum values, the 25th and 75th percentiles, and the median or average. Figure 11.1 shows a template for a typical box plot. The experimental groups appear along the horizontal axis, and the vertical axis shows the scale of the continuous experimental outcome variable, along with the units of measurement. Within the chart appears the box plot for each experimental group. The "whiskers" of the box plot extend from the minimum to the maximum observed value of the experimental outcome. In this example, the

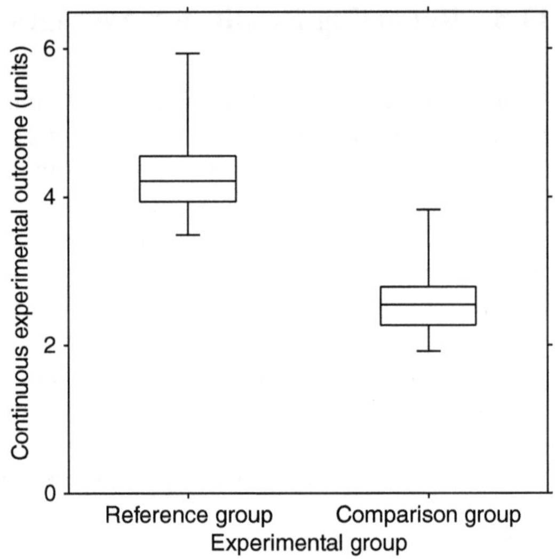

Fig. 11.1 Template for reporting results from an analysis of cluster-level averages as box plots, showing maximum and minimum values, 25th and 75th percentiles, and average for each group

Table 11.7 Preliminary table for relation between method of booking surgical consultation appointments and average weekly number of patients waiting for appointment in weeks when no appointments were available

meth_app	avg	sd	diff	lcl	ucl
1	37.6	3.6			
2	25.3	2.2	-12.3	-13.1	-11.5

whiskers for the box plot corresponding to the reference group extend from about 3.5 to about 5.9, and those for the comparison group extend from about 1.9 to about 3.8. The lower and upper horizontal edges of the box for each experimental group show the 25th and 75th percentiles, respectively. From the figure, these percentiles are about 3.9 and 4.6, respectively, for the reference group and about 2.3 and 2.8, respectively, for the comparison group. The horizontal line within the box usually represents the median but is sometimes used to show the average. In cases where the distribution of the experimental outcome is symmetric, the median and the average will be equivalent. In the example shown in Fig. 11.1, the horizontal line depicts the average, 4.3 for the reference group and 2.6 for the comparison group. In addition to displaying the estimate of the performance measure (i.e., the average) for each group, Fig. 11.1 also displays the magnitude of the effect size (i.e., the difference in averages). This is the vertical distance between the horizontal lines within each box, a value of about 1.7 (= 4.3 − 2.6).

In Part III of this book, we use tables and figures to report the results of comparisons of cluster-level averages from various case studies. The results of a simulation experiment comparing the average number of patients on the appointment lists during weeks when no appointments were available between two methods of booking these appointments (see Scenario 11.2) are shown in a preliminary table (Table 11.7). The statistics reported in this preliminary table show the method of booking appointments (`meth_app`), the average number of patients waiting (`avg`), the standard deviation of the number of patients waiting (`sd`), the difference in the averages between groups (`diff`), and its corresponding 95% confidence limits (`lcl` and `ucl`).

The results from this analysis of cluster-level averages are reported in Table 14.5. From this table, the reader can readily see that the average number of patients waiting among hospitals using the individual-lists method of booking was about 38, which is greater than the average of about 25 patients that was observed among hospitals using the pooled-list method. In addition, with a standard deviation of 3.6 weeks, the variation in clearance times seemed to be greater among hospitals using the individual-lists method. The value of −12.3 for the unadjusted difference indicates that, relative to the individual-lists group, the average number of patients waiting was about 12 less in the pooled-list group. The 95% confidence interval indicates that this effect size might have ranged between 11.5 and 13.1 patients.

The distribution of the average number of patients waiting is visually depicted in Fig. 14.1. Similar to the information in Table 14.5, the figure shows the cluster-level averages and offers information about the magnitude of the effect size. The box plots provide additional information about the variability by showing the minimum and maximum values, as well as the 25th and 75th percentiles. From this simulation experiment, there seems to be more variation in clearance times in the individual-lists group, which coincides with the larger standard deviation reported in Table 14.5. Additional examples of reporting results from analyses of cluster-level averages are shown in Tables 14.6, 14.21, and 14.22, and Fig. 14.1.

the standard deviation of the number of patients waiting (sd), the difference in the averages between groups (d), SE_d and its corresponding 95% confidence limits (LCL and UCL).

[illegible]

Chapter 12
Evaluations at the Individual Level

In this chapter, we present methods for evaluating policy alternatives using a simulation study with a cluster randomized design and the individual-level performance measures introduced in Chap. 9. Here, the unit of randomization is the cluster of simulated individuals, and the unit of analysis is the individual, which in the case of health care simulation would be the patient. Evaluations at the individual level often compare proportions of individuals in the experimental groups. For example, this approach would be appropriate in determining whether booking surgery in advance increases the proportion of patients undergoing an operation from wait lists each week. Evaluations may also compare the rates at which patients experience certain events. For example, comparisons of rates would be appropriate for studying whether use of a pooled wait list, rather than individual wait lists, for surgical consultation appointments increases the weekly rate of these appointments. We apply the methodological rigor of intervention research to assessing the effect of interventions in a simulation study. For example, the outcomes of simulated patients who are served in the same hospital may be more similar to each other than to the outcomes generated for patients in other hospitals in the simulation. Also, there may be other environmental factors or patient attributes that affect the outcome of interest. Therefore, we discuss how to compare individual-level measures using methods that adjust for similarities between outcomes and adjust for potential confounding factors. Finally, we discuss what to report from such analyses.

12.1 Scenario Involving Proportions

As discussed in Chap. 9, individual-level proportions quantify the fraction of simulated individuals experiencing an event of interest. For example, researchers might want to determine the proportion of patients whose elective procedure was canceled or the proportion of patients whose elective procedures were delayed after the recommended time. Whether the individual-level proportion is suitable

B. Sobolev et al., *Health Care Evaluation Using Computer Simulation: Concepts, Methods, and Applications*, DOI 10.1007/978-1-4614-2233-4_12,

for assessing the effect of an intervention is related to the study hypothesis, the experimental outcome, and the corresponding measures of effect (see Chap. 9). The analysis of individual-level proportions might arise in various scenarios.

In this chapter, we use the following scenario to illustrate the evaluation of system performance by analyzing individual-level proportions. We will refer to this hypothetical situation as Scenario 12.1: A surgeon has noticed that the waiting times for his patients are exceeding the benchmark times. His outpatient clinic uses the individual-lists method of booking surgical consultation appointments, and he would like to understand whether the pooled-list method of booking these appointments could help him to meet the benchmark times for a greater number of patients. From experience, the surgeon knows that other factors may affect waiting times, such as the method of booking surgery, the allocation of operating room slots, the clearance time for appointment lists, the clearance time for surgical wait lists, and the clearance time for inpatient surgical queues. Clearance times for backlogs in corresponding services are reported as the ratio of existing demand for capacity. He formulates the following study question: *Does the method of booking surgical consultation appointments affect the probability that a patient's access to surgery will be delayed after the recommended time, independent of other factors?* The study questions in the scenarios of Chap. 9 differ from the questions in the scenarios of this chapter. In Scenario 12.1, the surgeon is interested in estimating the effect of booking method, while adjusting for other factors which may affect the outcome of interest.

12.2 Preparing Data for Analysis of Proportions

To evaluate system performance on the basis of individual-level proportions, a researcher requires data indicating whether an individual has experienced the event of interest. This contrasts with cluster-level proportions, for which the researcher needs data indicating whether a group of individuals (i.e., a cluster) has met a specific criterion (see Chap. 11). The researcher prepares simulated data for analysis by developing a data dictionary and creating an analytical data set. The study hypothesis helps in determining the variables to be included in the data dictionary and the structure of the data set (see Sect. 9.1).

The data dictionary describes the variables related to the study question, specifically variables used to evaluate individual-level proportions. In particular, the data dictionary will include the name, description, type, and categories or values of each variable. These components of the data dictionary are collaboratively developed by a research team, including health care researchers, statisticians, and database analysts, during the planning stages of the simulation experiment. For comparisons of individual-level proportions between experimental groups, the data dictionary includes an indicator variable corresponding to each individual's response and a categorical variable relating to the experimental group. Other explanatory variables that could affect the outcome of interest are also listed.

The analytical data set for comparing individual-level proportions has a specific structure, in which each row represents a single individual (the unit of analysis) and columns contain the variables listed in the data dictionary. The columns should contain, at a minimum, the variable representing the experimental group to which the individual belongs and the indicator variable representing whether the individual has experienced the event of interest, the distribution of which will be summarized by a proportion. Other potential variables in the simulated data set might include both cluster-level and individual-level factors that could potentially affect the outcome.

Developing the data dictionary for Scenario 12.1 necessitates identifying the study variable, the experimental outcome, and pertinent environmental factors, as well as defining the type and coding for each variable. In this scenario, the study variable is the method of booking appointments (`meth_app`), and the experimental outcome variable is an indicator variable for whether the patient's surgery was performed after the recommended time (`isxafter`). The data dictionary for this scenario also includes several other variables measured at the level of the patient (e.g., sex) and at the level of the hospital (e.g., allocation of operating room slots) (see Table 12.1).

Using the data dictionary, the researcher can prepare the analytical data set needed for evaluating simulation experiments. The simulation experiment consists of runs of the model, with inputs representing experimental groups. Each run generates a cluster of individuals with data on the occurrence of simulated events for each individual. The first row of the data set contains the variable names, and subsequent rows show the values of those variables for a single individual (see Table 12.2). For example, according to the data set for Scenario 12.1, patient 1 was a woman (`sex` = `1`) at least 80 years of age (`agegrp` = `5`) who was registered on a surgical wait list with low priority (`ur_bk` = `3`) and whose surgery was performed after the recommended time (`isxafter` = `1`). This simulated patient received care in hospital 1, which used the individual-lists method of booking surgical consultations (`meth_app` = `1`) and which booked surgery in advance (`meth_sx` = `1`).

12.3 Adjusting Effect Size for Proportions

Once the proportions have been estimated, statistical techniques are used to compare these proportions across experimental groups. The techniques presented here allow for adjustment of other factors that may affect the outcome of interest and account for correlation between individual outcomes in each simulation run. In particular, for binary outcomes, we use multivariable logistic regression and generalized estimating equations.

To begin, the effect of the intervention on the proportions of individuals experiencing the event of interest can be estimated by means of simple logistic regression:

Table 12.1 Data dictionary of variables for estimating individual-level performance measures in Scenarios 12.1 and 12.2

Variable	Description	Type	Categories or values
Hospital level			
runid	Hospital identifier	Categorical	≥1
meth_app	Method of booking surgical consultation appointments	Categorical	1—Individual lists 2—Pooled list
meth_sx	Method of booking surgery	Categorical	1—Advance booking 2—Wait-list booking
or_slot	Allocation of operating room slots between elective and urgent procedures	Categorical	1—Weekly split 2—Daily split
ap_ct	Clearance time for appointment lists at start of simulation (weeks)	Numeric	1, 2, or 3
el_ct	Clearance time for surgical wait lists at start of simulation (weeks)	Numeric	3, 4, 5, or 6
ur_ct	Clearance time for inpatient surgical queues at start of simulation (weeks)	Numeric	0, 1, or 2
Patient level			
pid	Patient identifier	Categorical	≥1
agegrp	Age group (years)	Categorical	1—<50 2—50 to 59 3—60 to 69 4—70 to 79 5—≥80
sex	Sex	Categorical	0—Male 1—Female
anatom	Coronary anatomy affected	Categorical	1—Left main 2—Multivessel 3—Limited
comor	Comorbidity	Categorical	1—Major conditions* 2—Other conditions† 3—None
ur_bk	Priority at registration on surgical wait list	Categorical	1—High priority 2—Medium priority 3—Low priority 99—Not applicable‡
ctreg	Clearance time for elective surgery at time of registration (weeks)	Numeric	≥0
isxafter	Timing of surgery	Categorical	0—Within recommended time 1—After recommended time
isx	Indicator variable for access to surgery	Categorical	0—No 1—Yes
wtime_sx	Time from registration to surgery (weeks)	Numeric	≥0

*Congestive heart failure, diabetes mellitus, chronic obstructive pulmonary disease, rheumatoid arthritis, cancer

†Peripheral vascular disease, cerebrovascular disease, dementia, peptic ulcer disease,

‡Patient did not receive surgical consultation appointment

Table 12.2 Tab-delimited file containing the analytical data set for estimating individual-level proportions in Scenario 12.1 (see Table 12.1 for data dictionary of variables in this data set)

runid	meth_app	meth_sx	or_slot	ap_ct	el_ct	ur_ct	pid	agegrp	sex	anatom	comor	ur_bk	ctreg	isxafter
1	1	1	1	2	4	1	1	5	1	1	2	3	3.4	1
1	1	1	1	2	4	1	2	2	0	3	2	2	2.2	0
...														
1	1	1	1	2	4	1	819	1	1	2	1	3	4.0	0
2	1	2	2	1	3	0	820	2	0	2	3	2	1.2	0
2	1	2	2	1	3	0	821	4	0	3	1	1	0.6	1
...														
2	1	2	2	1	3	0	1,642	4	1	1	2	3	3.0	0
...														
112	1	2	2	3	6	2	90,913	5	0	2	1	3	2.8	1
112	1	2	2	3	6	2	90,914	3	0	1	3	2	1.0	1
...														
112	1	2	2	3	6	2	91,728	3	0	2	3	3	2.6	0
113	2	1	2	2	6	1	91,729	4	0	1	2	3	3.7	0
113	2	1	2	2	6	1	91,730	3	1	3	1	2	1.8	1
...														
113	2	1	2	2	6	1	92,562	3	0	1	2	2	2.5	0
114	2	2	1	3	5	0	92,563	5	1	2	3	2	0.8	0
114	2	2	1	3	5	0	92,564	1	0	2	1	3	1.3	1
...														
114	2	2	1	3	5	0	93,385	3	0	3	1	1	0.4	1
...														
224	2	2	1	1	4	2	182,710	2	0	3	2	3	3.4	0
224	2	2	1	1	4	2	182,711	5	1	1	1	2	2.8	0
...														
224	2	2	1	1	4	2	183,550	4	1	2	3	2	0.8	0

$$\log\left(\frac{p_{ijl}}{1-p_{ijl}}\right) = \beta_0 + \beta_1 I_{1ijl}, \tag{12.1}$$

where p_{ijl} is the probability that y_{ijl} equals 1 and the group indicator I_{1ijl} is 1 if individual l in run j belongs to the comparison group and 0 otherwise. The exponential of the regression coefficient, $\exp(\beta_1)$, gives the crude odds ratio for the comparison group relative to the reference group. A value less than 1 indicates lower odds that an individual will experience the event.

In a multivariable analysis, the logistic regression model in (12.1) can be expanded to control for cluster-level and individual-level factors:

$$\log\left(\frac{p_{ijl}}{1-p_{ijl}}\right) = \beta_0 + \beta_1 I_{1ijl} + \cdots + \beta_r I_{rijl}, \tag{12.2}$$

where I_{1ijl} is an indicator for the comparison group and I_{2ijl} to I_{rijl} are other explanatory variables. The regression coefficient β_1 is the difference in the log odds between the comparison group and the reference group adjusted for other factors in the analysis. The exponential of this regression coefficient estimates the adjusted odds ratio. The multivariable logistic regression model in (12.2) does not account for correlation of observations within a simulation run, so the generalized estimating equation method is used to estimate the model parameters while allowing for such correlation [94].

The maximum likelihood estimate, $\hat{\beta}_1$, and its standard error, $\mathrm{SE}(\hat{\beta}_1)$, can be estimated by means of statistical software. Then, the estimated effect of the intervention is given by $\exp(\hat{\beta}_1)$, and its $100(1-\alpha)\%$ lower and upper confidence limits can be estimated as follows:

$$\begin{aligned} \mathrm{LCL} &= \exp\left[\hat{\beta}_1 - z_{\alpha/2}\mathrm{SE}(\hat{\beta}_1)\right], \\ \mathrm{UCL} &= \exp\left[\hat{\beta}_1 + z_{\alpha/2}\mathrm{SE}(\hat{\beta}_1)\right]. \end{aligned} \tag{12.3}$$

In Chap. 14, we describe in detail the results of a simulation study related to Scenario 12.1, evaluating the effect of the booking method for surgical consultation appointments—either individual lists or pooled list—on the probability that elective surgery will be performed after the recommended time. Using (9.2) and (9.4), we estimated the patient-level proportions (expressed as percentages) and 95% confidence intervals for the individual-lists and pooled-list methods as 1.0% (0.9–1.0%) and 1.5% (1.4–1.5%), respectively. These percentages indicate that a greater proportion of patients who were treated in hospitals using the pooled-list method of booking these appointments had surgery delayed after the recommended time. We then used logistic regression and generalized estimating equations to evaluate the effect of the method of booking appointments with adjustment for some other variables. Several hospital-level and patient-level factors likely to affect the outputs of the simulation were entered into the regression model, in addition to the indicator variable for the method of booking appointments; see Table 12.3 (where subscripts for experimental group, cluster, and patient are suppressed).

Table 12.3 Regression model for estimating the effect of the method of booking surgical consultation appointments on proportion of patients undergoing surgery after the recommended time

Question:	Does the method of booking surgical consultation appointments affect the probability that a patient's surgery will be performed after the recommended time?
Model:	$\log\left(\frac{p}{1-p}\right) = \beta_0 + \beta_1 I_1 + \beta_2 I_2 + \beta_3 I_3 + \beta_4 I_4 + \beta_5 I_5 + \beta_6 I_6 + \beta_7 I_7 + \beta_8 I_8 + \beta_9 I_9 + \beta_{10} I_{10} + \beta_{11} I_{11} + \beta_{12} I_{12} + \beta_{13} I_{13} + \beta_{14} I_{14} + \beta_{15} I_{15} + \beta_{16} I_{16} + \beta_{17} I_{17} + \beta_{18} I_{18} + \beta_{19} I_{19} + \beta_{20} I_{20} + \beta_{21} I_{21} + \beta_{22} X_{22}$
p	Proportion of patients undergoing surgery after the recommended time
I_1	Indicator for pooled-list vs. individual-lists booking of appointments
I_2	Indicator for advance vs. wait-list booking of surgery
I_3	Indicator for daily vs. weekly split of operating room slots between elective and urgent procedures
I_4, I_5	Indicators for 2 or 3 vs. 1 week of clearance time for appointment lists at the start of simulation
I_6, I_7, I_8	Indicators for 4, 5, or 6 vs. 3 weeks of clearance time for surgical wait lists at the start of simulation
I_9, I_{10}	Indicators for 1 or 2 vs. 0 weeks of clearance time for inpatient surgical queues at the start of simulation
I_{11}	Indicator for female sex of patient
$I_{12}, I_{13}, I_{14}, I_{15}$	Indicators for <50, 50–59, 70–79, or ≥80 vs. 60–69 years age group
I_{16}, I_{17}	Indicators for high or low vs. medium priority at time of registration on surgical wait list
I_{18}, I_{19}	Indicators for multivessel or limited vs. left main coronary anatomy affected
I_{20}, I_{21}	Indicators for major conditions or other conditions vs. none
X_{22}	Clearance time for elective surgery at time of registration on the surgical wait list (weeks)

For each categorical variable, a set of indicator variables was created for the regression analysis. The number of indicator variables in each set was one less than the number of categories. For example, we created one indicator variable, I_1, for the method of booking surgical consultation appointments, which took the value 1 for the pooled-list method (i.e., `meth_app = 2`) and the value 0 for the individual-lists method (i.e., `meth_app = 1`). The estimated regression coefficients corresponding to the model in Table 12.3 were

$$\log\left(\frac{p}{1-p}\right) = -5.79 + 0.32I_1 - 1.91I_2 + 1.03I_3 + 0.20I_4 + 0.59I_5 + 0.14I_6 + 0.05I_7 + 0.27I_8 - 0.01I_9 + 0.10I_{10} + 0.01I_{11} - 0.00I_{12} + 0.04I_{13} - 0.02I_{14} + 0.05I_{15} + 2.36I_{16} - 0.99I_{17} - 0.03I_{18} - 0.17I_{19} - 0.06I_{20} - 0.02I_{21} + 0.92X_{22},$$

where the estimated regression coefficient for the method of booking appointments, $\hat{\beta}_1$, was about 0.3224 with a standard error of about 0.0839. The effect of the intervention, as measured by an odds ratio $\exp(\hat{\beta}_1)$, was $\exp(0.3224) \approx 1.38$, with the following 95% confidence limits

$$\begin{aligned} \text{LCL} &= \exp(0.3224 - 1.96 \times 0.0839) \approx 1.17, \\ \text{UCL} &= \exp(0.3224 + 1.96 \times 0.0839) \approx 1.63. \end{aligned}$$

Therefore, the simulation study suggested the odds that a patient's surgery would be delayed after the recommended time were 38% higher with the pooled-lists method than with the individual-lists method, after adjustment for hospital-level and patient-level factors (see Sect. 9.1).

12.4 Reporting Results for Proportions

In Chap. 10, we recommended items for reporting on a simulation study based on a cluster randomized design. Here, we elaborate on the results that should be reported from an analysis comparing individual-level proportions.

The first item is the estimated proportion of individuals for each experimental group since this is the performance measure of interest. Along with the estimated proportion, the number of individual in each group (the denominator) and the number of individuals experiencing the event of interest (the numerator) should also be explicitly reported. Reporting absolute counts allows the reader to assess the number of simulated individuals in the study and whether they were distributed approximately equally across groups, as should be the case for a cluster randomized design. In addition, these counts allow the reader to understand how the proportions were calculated. For example, if a researcher simply reports that 5% of the individuals experienced the event of interest, without providing counts, the reader cannot tell whether the percentage represents 5,000 out of 100,000 observations or just 5 out of 100. A reader might justifiably question the statistical power and smallest anticipated difference in a simulation experiment with just 100 individuals, but may be more confident about an experiment with 100,000 individuals.

The second item is the estimated odds ratio, along with its confidence interval, which conveys information about statistical significance and precision. If the 95% confidence interval for an odds ratio does not span the value 1.0, then there is statistical evidence to support the conclusion that the interventions have different effects on the individual-level proportions at the 5% significance level. However, statistical significance may not be meaningful in the clinical context. The magnitude of the odds for the comparison group relative to the odds for the reference group will help the reader to determine if the effect was clinically significant. The width of the corresponding confidence interval indicates the precision of the estimate, where a narrower interval indicates greater precision.

The third item consists of the unadjusted and adjusted odds ratios. These values allow the reader to assess the extent to which the estimated effect size changed

Table 12.4 Preliminary table for reporting results on relation between methods of booking surgical consultation appointments and undergoing surgery after the recommended time, among patients with medium priority at registration

meth_app	sum_isxafter	npts	prop	or	lcl	ucl
1	439	56,357	0.8	1.00		
2	641	56,895	1.1	1.40	1.24	1.59

after the researchers accounted for potential confounding factors. An odds ratio that does not change after adjustment for cluster-level and individual-level factors could indicate that the intervention has an independent effect on the experimental outcome. Finally, a measure of correlation between individual observations should be reported, to allow the reader to assess the degree of similarity among the simulated individuals. These recommended items to be reported in comparisons of individual-level proportions may be summarized in tabular format.

In Part III of this book, we use tables to report the results of comparisons of individual-level proportions from various case studies. The results of a simulation study comparing two methods of booking consultation appointments in terms of the proportions of patients with medium priority at the time of registration whose elective surgery was performed after recommended time (see Scenario 12.1), are shown in a preliminary table (Table 12.4). The statistics reported in this table show the number of patients with surgery delayed after the recommended time (`sum_isxafter`), the number of patients in each group (`npts`), the percentage of patients with delayed surgery (`prop`), and the odds ratio (`or`), along with the corresponding lower and upper 95% confidence limits (`lcl` and `ucl`, respectively).

The results from this analysis are reported in Table 14.15. The statistics in this table show that patients were approximately equally distributed between the two experimental groups, with about 57,000 patients per group. The rows of the table represent the two groups that were compared, and the reader can readily see that 0.8% of patients in the individual-lists group and 1.1% of those in the pooled-list group had their surgery after the recommended time. The value of 1.40 in the last column, the odds ratio, shows that, compared with the individual-lists group, the odds of surgery after the recommended time for an individual patient with medium priority at the time of registration were 40% higher in the pooled-list group. The confidence interval of 1.24–1.59 indicates that the actual effect size may have ranged from 24% to 59%. Additional examples of reporting results from analyses of patient-level proportions appear in Tables 14.15, 14.15, 14.26, 15.7, 15.8, 16.10, 16.11, 16.12, 16.13, 16.14, and 16.15.

12.5 Scenario Involving Rates

As discussed in Chap. 9, rates quantify the number of events over a specified time interval. For example, researchers might want to determine the weekly rate of clinic appointments or the weekly rate of elective surgery. Whether the event rate is suitable for assessing the effect of an intervention at the individual level is related to the study hypothesis, the experimental outcome, and the corresponding measures of effect (see Chap. 9). There are several scenarios in which the analysis of individual-level rates might arise. In this chapter, we use the following scenario to illustrate the evaluation of system performance by analyzing individual-level rates. We will refer to this hypothetical situation as Scenario 12.2: A hospital manager has noticed that the wait times for high-priority elective surgery are exceeding the recommended times. The hospital she manages uses the wait-list method of booking elective surgery, but she would switch to another method of scheduling if surgical waiting times could be reduced. In particular, the manager has been asked to consider booking elective surgery in advance. From experience, she knows that other factors may also affect surgical waiting times. These include the method of booking surgical consultation appointments, the allocation of operating room slots. There is also empirical evidence that the clearance times for appointment lists, surgical wait lists, and inpatient surgical queues lengthen the wait time. She formulates the following study question: *Does the method of booking elective surgery affect the weekly rate at which high-priority elective procedures are performed, independent of other factors?* The study questions in the scenarios of Chap. 9 differ from the questions in the scenarios of this chapter. In Scenario 12.2, the hospital manager is interested in estimating the effect size, while adjusting for other factors which may affect the outcome of interest.

12.6 Preparing Data for Analysis of Rates

Evaluating performance on the basis of rates requires data indicating whether the event of interest has occurred as well as data on when it occurred. This contrasts with the situation for proportions, for which only the first of these data types is required. The researcher prepares simulated data on the occurrence and timing of the event for analysis by developing a data dictionary and creating an analytical data set. The study hypothesis guides in determining the variables to be included in the data dictionary and the structure of the data set during the planning stages of the simulation experiment (see Sect. 9.5). For comparisons of individual-level rates between experimental groups, the data dictionary includes an indicator variable that shows whether an individual has experienced the event of interest and another variable that records the time to the event, if it occurred, or the time the individual was last observed, if the event did not occur. The data dictionary also includes a categorical variable relating to the experimental group, as well as other explanatory variables that could affect the occurrence of the outcome.

The analytical data set for comparing individual-level rates has a structure similar to that of the data set for evaluating individual-level proportions. As described in Sect. 12.2, each row represents a single individual (the unit of analysis) and columns contain the variables listed in the data dictionary. The columns should contain, at a minimum, the variable representing the experimental group to which the individual belongs, the indicator variable representing whether the patient has experienced the event of interest, and the variable representing the timing of the event. The latter two together make up the experimental outcome. Other potential variables in the data set might include both cluster-level and individual-level factors that would affect the outcome.

Developing the data dictionary for Scenario 12.2 entails specifying the study variable, the experimental outcome, and pertinent environmental factors, as well as defining the type and coding for each variable. In this scenario, the data dictionary includes a variable for the method of booking elective surgery (i.e., the study variable, `meth_sx`) and variables for the experimental outcome, namely, `isx`, an indicator variable for undergoing surgery, and `wtime_sx`, the number of weeks from registration on the wait list to surgery or removal from the list without surgery (see Table 12.1 above).

As discussed in the previous sections, the simulation experiment consists of runs of the model, with inputs corresponding to various model configurations. Each run generates a cluster of individuals with data on the occurrence and timing of simulated events for each individual. Using the data dictionary, the researcher can prepare the analytical data set needed for the evaluation of simulation experiments. The first row of the data set contains the variable names, and subsequent rows show the data values corresponding to those variables for a single individual. For example, according to the analytical data set for Scenario 12.1 presented in Table 12.5, patient 1 was a man (`sex = 0`) 50 to 59 years of age (`agegrp = 2`) who was registered on the surgical wait list with medium priority (`ur_bk = 2`). The patient underwent surgery (`isx = 1`) after 6 weeks on the wait list (`wtime_sx = 6`). The hospital where this simulated patient received care was using the individual-lists method for booking consultation appointments (`meth_app = 1`), and the surgery itself was booked in advance (`meth_sx = 1`).

The analytical data set for evaluating individual-level proportions in Table 12.2 differs slightly from the data set for evaluating individual-level rates in Table 12.5. The data set in Table 12.2 shows the indicator outcome variable (`idelay`), whereas the data set in Table 12.5 indicates both indicator and continuous outcome variables (`isx` and `wtime_sx`).

12.7 Adjusting Effect Size for Rates

Once the rates have been estimated, statistical techniques are used to compare these rates across experimental groups. These techniques can adjust for potential confounding factors and account for correlation between individual outcomes generated in each simulation run. When the time at risk is discrete, the event rate becomes the conditional probability of the event among those who are at risk just before each time t. The time at risk is the period in which an individual may experience the event of interest. For example, in studies on access to elective surgery,

Table 12.5 Tab-delimited file containing the analytical data set for estimating patient-level rates in Scenario 12.2 (see Table 12.1 for data dictionary of variables in this data set)

runid	meth_app	meth_sx	or_slot	ap_ct	el_ct	ur_ct	pid	agegrp	sex	anatom	comor	ur_bk	ctreg	isx	wtime_sx
1	1	1	1	2	4	1	1	2	0	1	2	2	3.4	1	6
1	1	1	1	2	4	1	2	2	0	3	2	2	2.2	1	3
...															
1	1	1	1	2	4	1	819	1	1	2	1	3	4.0	1	4
2	1	2	2	1	3	0	820	2	0	2	3	2	1.2	0	2
2	1	2	2	1	3	0	821	4	0	3	1	1	0.6	1	1
...															
2	1	2	2	1	3	0	1,642	4	1	1	2	3	3.0	1	4
...															
112	1	2	2	3	6	2	90,913	5	0	2	1	3	2.8	1	12
112	1	2	2	3	6	2	90,914	3	0	1	3	2	1.0	0	8
...															
112	1	2	2	3	6	2	91,728	3	0	2	3	3	2.6	1	13
113	2	1	2	2	6	1	91,729	4	0	1	2	3	3.7	0	10
113	2	1	2	2	6	1	91,730	3	1	3	1	2	1.8	1	6
...															
113	2	1	2	2	6	1	92,562	3	0	1	2	2	2.5	1	5
114	2	2	1	3	5	0	92,563	5	1	2	3	2	0.8	1	7
114	2	2	1	3	5	0	92,564	1	0	2	1	3	1.3	0	11
...															
114	2	2	1	3	5	0	93,385	3	0	3	1	1	0.4	1	2
...															
224	2	2	1	1	4	2	182,710	2	0	3	2	3	3.4	1	10
224	2	2	1	1	4	2	182,711	5	1	1	1	2	2.8	0	9
...															
224	2	2	1	1	4	2	183,550	4	1	2	3	2	0.8	1	6

time to admission is inherently discrete and is best measured as the number of new scheduling cycles from registration for surgery to admission to hospital because only scheduling generates elective admissions [139]. In this example, the time at risk is the period from registration on a wait list for elective surgery to removal from the wait list because of surgery performed or some other reason.

The odds ratios derived from a simple discrete-time survival regression model,

$$\log\left(\frac{p_{ijlt}}{1-p_{ijlt}}\right) = \beta_{0t} + \beta_1 I_{ijl}, \tag{12.4}$$

measures the effect of an intervention on the proportion of individuals experiencing events per unit time among those remaining at risk [3, 139]. In this equation, p_{ijlt} is the conditional probability of individual l in run j of experimental group i experiencing an event at time t, and the group indicator I_{ijl} is 1 if patient l in run j belongs to the comparison group and 0 otherwise. The coefficient β_{0t} represents the log odds of the event occurring at time t in the reference group. The exponential of the regression coefficient $\exp(\beta_1)$ gives the crude ratio of odds for the comparison group relative to the reference group, where a value less than 1 indicates a lower event rate.

In a multivariable analysis, the discrete-time survival regression model in (12.4) can be expanded to control for cluster-level and individual-level factors:

$$\log\left(\frac{p_{ijlt}}{1-p_{ijlt}}\right) = \beta_{0t} + \beta_1 I_{ijl} + \ldots + \beta_r I_{rijl}, \tag{12.5}$$

where I_{1ijl} is an indicator for the comparison group and I_{2ijl} to I_{rijl} are additional explanatory variables. The regression coefficient β_1 is the adjusted difference in the log odds between the comparison group and the reference group adjusted for both other factors in the analysis and the time at risk. The exponential of this regression coefficient gives the adjusted ratio of odds.

As in Sect. 12.3, generalized estimating equations are used to estimate the standard error of the regression coefficient, $\mathrm{SE}(\hat{\beta})$, because this method accounts for correlation of individuals within the same cluster [95]. The maximum likelihood estimate, $\hat{\beta}_1$, and its standard error, $\mathrm{SE}(\hat{\beta}_1)$, can be estimated by means of statistical software. Then, the effect of the intervention is given by $\exp(\hat{\beta}_1)$, and its 100 $(1-\alpha)\%$ lower and upper confidence limits can be estimated as follows:

$$\mathrm{LCL} = \exp\left[\hat{\beta}_1 - z_{\alpha/2}\mathrm{SE}(\hat{\beta}_1)\right],$$

$$\mathrm{UCL} = \exp\left[\hat{\beta}_1 + z_{\alpha/2}\mathrm{SE}(\hat{\beta}_1)\right]. \tag{12.6}$$

In Chap. 16, we describe in detail the results of a simulation study related to Scenario 12.2, evaluating the effect of the method of booking surgery—either wait-list booking or advance booking—on the weekly rate of high-priority elective surgery. Using (9.16) and (9.18), we estimated the surgery rates and 95% confidence

Table 12.6 Regression model for estimating the effect of the method of booking surgery on weekly proportion of patients undergoing surgery from wait lists

Question:	Does the method of booking surgery affect the weekly rate at which high-priority elective procedures are performed?
Model:	$\log\left(\frac{p_t}{1-p_t}\right) = \beta_{0t} + \beta_1 I_1 + \beta_2 I_2 + \beta_3 I_3 + \beta_4 I_4 + \beta_5 I_5 + \beta_6 I_6 + \beta_7 I_7 + \beta_8 I_8 + \beta_9 I_9 + \beta_{10} I_{10} + \beta_{11} I_{11} + \beta_{12} I_{12} + \beta_{13} I_{13} + \beta_{14} I_{14} + \beta_{15} I_{15} + \beta_{16} I_{16} + \beta_{17} I_{17} + \beta_{18} I_{18} + \beta_{19} I_{19} + \beta_{20} I_{20} + \beta_{21} X_{21} + \beta_{22} X_{22}$
p_t	Probability of undergoing surgery among patients remaining on wait lists at week t
I_1	Indicator for advance vs. wait-list booking of surgery
I_2, I_3	Indicators for individual lists or shortest list vs. pooled list booking of appointments
I_4	Indicator for daily vs. weekly split of operating room slots between elective and urgent procedures
I_5, I_6	Indicators for 2 or 3 vs. 1 week of clearance time for appointment lists at the start of simulation
I_7, I_8, I_9	Indicators for 4, 5, or 6 vs. 3 weeks of clearance time for surgical wait lists at the start of simulation
I_{10}, I_{11}	Indicators for 1 or 2 vs. 0 weeks of clearance time for inpatient surgical queues at the start of simulation
I_{12}	Indicator for female sex of patient
I_{13}, I_{14}, I_{15}, I_{16}	Indicators for <50, 50–59, 70–79, or ≥80 vs. 60–69 years age group
I_{17}, I_{18}	Indicators for multivessel or limited vs. left main coronary anatomy affected
I_{19}, I_{20}	Indicators for major conditions or other conditions vs. none
X_{21}	Clearance time for elective surgery at time of registration on the surgical wait list (weeks)
X_{22}	No. of additional surgeries performed without wait-list registration

intervals for the wait-list booking and advance booking methods as 75.8 procedures per 100 patient-weeks (73.9–77.7) and 92.5 procedures per 100 patient-weeks (90.2–94.8), respectively. These rates indicate that a higher number of patients undergo surgery over a given time interval in hospitals using the advance booking of surgery than in hospitals using the wait-list booking method. We then used the discrete-time survival regression in (12.5) to estimate the effect of booking with adjustment for other hospital-level and patient-level variables that likely affect access to surgery. All variables listed in Table 12.6 were entered into the regression model, along with the indicator variable for the method of booking surgery. As before, we entered one indicator variable, I_1, for the method of booking surgery, which took the value 1 for advance booking (i.e., `meth_sx` = `1`) and the value 0 for wait-list booking (i.e., `meth_sx` = `2`).

The estimated regression coefficients corresponding to the model are listed below, where subscripts for experimental group, run, and patient are suppressed:

$$\log\left(\frac{p_t}{1-p_t}\right) = \beta_{0t} + 0.83I_1 + 0.10I_2 - 0.06I_3 - 0.90I_4 - 0.09I_5 - 0.11I_6$$

$$-0.13I_7 - 0.11I_8 - 0.04I_9 - 0.00I_{10} + 0.08I_{11} - 0.00I_{12}$$

$$+0.01I_{13} - 0.14I_{14} - 0.09I_{15} - 0.07I_{16} + 0.03I_{17} - 0.02I_{18}$$
$$- 0.09I_{19} - 0.06I_{20} - 5.01X_{21} - 0.24X_{22},$$

where $\hat{\beta}_{0t}$ ranged from 1.65 to 3.92 for different weeks t on the wait list. The estimated regression coefficient for the method of booking surgery, $\hat{\beta}_1$, was about 0.833 with a standard error, SE($\hat{\beta}_1$), of about 0.058. The effect of the intervention, as measured by exp($\hat{\beta}_1$), was exp(0.833) $\approx$ 2.30 (95% confidence interval 2.05–2.58). The confidence limits were estimated from (12.6). Therefore, we can conclude that the weekly rate of high-priority procedures scheduled with the advance booking method is 2.3 times of that with wait-list booking method, after adjustment for hospital and patient factors (see Sect. 9.5).

12.8 Reporting Results for Rates

In Chap. 10, we described items recommended for reporting in simulation studies based on a cluster randomized design. Here, we elaborate on what should be reported from an analysis comparing individual-level rates.

The first item that should be reported is the estimated performance measure for each experimental group, which is an individual-level rate in this case. Along with the estimated rate, the total duration of time over which all simulated individuals were observed (the denominator), and the number of individuals who experienced the event of interest (the numerator) should also be explicitly reported for each group. Reporting the observed figures allows the reader to assess how long the simulated individuals were followed in the experiment and how many events occurred in each group. In addition, raw values help the reader to understand how the rates were calculated.

The second item is the estimated weekly (or monthly or yearly) odds ratio, which is the measure of effect size, and its confidence interval. The width of the corresponding confidence interval indicates the precision of the estimate, where a narrower interval indicates greater precision. If the 95% confidence interval for a weekly odds ratio does not include the value 1.0, then there is statistical evidence to support the conclusion that the interventions have different effects on the weekly proportions at the 5% significance level. The magnitude of the weekly odds for the comparison group relative to the odds for the reference group will help the reader to determine if the effect is clinically meaningful. The size of effect that is meaningful relates directly to the smallest anticipated difference discussed in Sect. 7.3 and Appendix B.

The third item presents the unadjusted and adjusted relative weekly odds. Their values allow the reader to assess the extent to which the estimated effect size changed after the researchers accounted for potential confounding factors. A weekly odds ratio that does not change after adjustment for cluster-level and individual-level factors could indicate that the intervention has an independent effect on

Table 12.7 Preliminary results for reporting results on relation between methods of booking surgery and weekly proportion of patients undergoing surgery, among high-priority patients at registration

meth_sx	sum_isx	sum_wttime_sx	rate	lcl_rate	ucl_rate	or	lcl	ucl
2	5,987	7,898	75.8	73.9	77.7	1.00		
1	6,278	6,788	92.5	90.2	94.8	2.30	2.05	2.58

the experimental outcome. Finally, a measure of correlation between individual observations should be reported, to allow the reader to assess the degree of similarity among the simulated individuals. These recommended items to be reported in comparisons of individual-level rates may be summarized in tabular format.

In Part III of this book, we use tables to report the results of comparisons of individual-level rates from various case studies. The results of a simulation study comparing the weekly rate of surgery among high-priority patients between two methods of booking surgery are shown in a preliminary table (Table 12.7). The statistics reported in this table show that more patients had their operation over a shorter total duration of time, which led to higher weekly surgery rates, in hospitals using the advance booking method than in hospitals using the wait-list booking method (`sum_isx` = `6,278` and `sum_wttime_sx` = `6,788` for `meth_sx` = 1 vs. `sum_isx` = `5,987` and `sum_wttime_sx` = `7,898` for `meth_sx` = 2). Further results from this analysis are reported in Table 16.7. In this table, the reader can readily see that the weekly rate of surgery was 75.8 per 100 patient-weeks in the wait-list booking group and 92.5 per 100 patient-weeks in the advance booking group. The last column shows that compared with the wait-list booking group, the weekly odds of having an operation were about 2.3 times higher in the advance booking group. The 95% confidence interval indicates that this effect size might have ranged from 2.05 to 2.58 times higher. Additional examples of reporting results from analyses of patient-level rates are shown in Tables 14.9, 14.10, 14.12, 14.13, 14.14, 14.24, 14.25, 15.6, 16.8, and 16.9.

Part III
Applications

Chapter 13
Simulation Model for Surgical Service

In this chapter, we describe in detail the discrete-event simulation model of patient flow developed for policy evaluation in the case studies presented in Chaps. 14 to 19. In particular, we describe the modeled perioperative process of cardiac surgical care, the requirements of the model, and technical details about implementation of the model.

13.1 Modeled Process

We based development of the discrete-event simulation model of patient flow on a previous description of cardiac surgical services at a tertiary care hospital in British Columbia, Canada, one of the four hospitals delivering adult open-heart surgical services to the province's four million residents [93]. In Chap. 3, we presented a thorough review of the process of cardiac surgical care. Below, we summarize that review into a narrative of surgical services for a setting with three surgeons, whose weekly availability for operations depends on their schedules for consultations, planned operations, on-call duties, and vacation. Through the hospital, the three surgeons have access to an outpatient clinic for consultations and a dedicated operating room. The use of clinic and operating room time is managed through the periodic assignment of clinic and operating room slots to the surgeons [18].

We modeled three care paths following angiography—elective, inpatient, and emergency—that patients with established coronary artery disease are likely to experience, according to initial presentation and subsequent decisions leading to the operation. The elective path applies to patients for whom surgical consultation and subsequent operation can be safely delayed. This path starts with referral for a consultation appointment with a surgeon in the outpatient clinic. The inpatient path applies to patients admitted to hospital directly from the catheterization laboratory when urgent surgical assessment is necessary. The emergency path applies to patients requiring immediate surgical intervention.

B. Sobolev et al., *Health Care Evaluation Using Computer Simulation: Concepts, Methods, and Applications*, DOI 10.1007/978-1-4614-2233-4_13,

Patients referred for a consultation appointment with a surgeon in the outpatient clinic are kept on the appointment list with a designated priority (high or low) until an opening for a consultation becomes available. After the consultation, the office of the consulting surgeon registers on the surgeon's priority wait list the names of patients who require coronary revascularization, designating the required procedure as having high, medium, or low priority, according to the affected coronary anatomy and symptoms. The hospital's booking office books patients into operating room slots assigned to the consulting surgeon according to their priority and the date of registration. A draft operating room list with the scheduled operations for the upcoming week is generated every Friday. The draft list includes the procedures that have been booked from the wait lists and those booked for inpatients already waiting in hospital. The list is finalized the following Monday and may be subsequently changed to reflect the arrival of inpatients and emergency patients. The availability of the three surgeons for operations and consultations is coordinated through their weekly schedules such that, in any given week, one surgeon is on call (assessing inpatients and performing urgent operations), one performs planned operations, and one conducts outpatient surgical consultations. During weeks when one surgeon is on vacation, the two remaining surgeons alternate call and planned duties and no consultations are scheduled.

13.2 Modeling Requirements

We identified and modeled 10 perioperative clinical and managerial activities occurring in a clinic setting (Table 13.1) and 16 activities occurring in hospital (Table 13.2). The modeling requirements used in the design and development of the discrete-event simulation model are based on the functions of the perioperative activities. These requirements, and the modeled activities that implement each requirement, are summarized in Table 13.3.

13.2.1 Case Mix of Patients

We modeled three types of patients according to the three care paths: elective patients, inpatients, and emergency patients. Each simulated patient was assigned the following attributes according to historical data for 1991 to 2000 from a population-based patient registry [142]:

- Sex: male or female.
- Age group: <50, 50–59, 60–69, 70–79, or ≥80 years of age.
- Coronary anatomy affected: left main, multivessel, or limited.
- Comorbidity at registration: major conditions, other conditions, or none.

Table 13.1 Modeled activities occurring in an outpatient setting

Activity	Function
Outpatient clinic	
Referral of patients for surgical consultation in outpatient clinic	Patients presenting with symptoms are sent for consultation with surgeon in outpatient clinic
Registration of elective patients on appointment list	Details of referred patients are registered
Booking of outpatient surgical consultation appointments	Time and duration of consultation appointments are determined
Outpatient consultations with cardiac surgeon	Indication for operation is assessed (by cardiac surgeon)
Registration on a surgical wait list	Details of patients who require and decide to undergo the operation are registered
Advance booking of elective operations	Projected dates of operations within the upcoming 36-week period are determined
Referral of elective patients for preoperative assessment	Elective patients requiring operation are referred for a preoperative assessment in preadmission clinic
Preadmission clinic	
Booking of preoperative assessments	Time and duration of preoperative assessments are determined
Preoperative assessments	Patients' suitability for operation is determined (by anesthesiologist)
Booking of patients for additional preoperative assessments	Time and duration of subsequent preoperative assessments are determined

Major conditions were congestive heart failure, diabetes mellitus, chronic obstructive pulmonary disease, rheumatoid arthritis, and cancer. Other conditions were peripheral vascular disease, cerebrovascular disease, dementia, peptic ulcer disease, hemiplegia, renal disease, and liver disease.

13.2.2 Surgeons' Duty Rotation

We modeled three surgeons who coordinate their weekly duties such that one surgeon is on call and performs some operations (on-call duty), one surgeon is in clinic and assesses patients registered on appointment lists (office duty), and one surgeon performs the majority of operations (operating room duty). When one of the surgeons is on vacation, the two remaining surgeons alternate on-call and operating room duties, leaving the office duty unfilled; as such, no surgical consultation

Table 13.2 Modeled activities occurring in hospital

Activity	Function
Clinical activities	
Referral of patients requiring urgent surgical assessment (inpatients)	Patients requiring urgent assessment after angiography are referred (by cardiologist)
In-hospital assessment of patients requiring urgent operation (inpatients)	Suitability of patients for admission to hospital as inpatients is determined (by on-call surgeon)
Registration of inpatients for surgery	Details are registered for patients who must undergo the operation and who are admitted directly to hospital
In-hospital preoperative assessment of elective patients	Suitability of patients for operation is determined in hospital one day before operation (by anesthesiologist)
Scheduling of OR time	Inpatients and elective patients waiting for operation are identified and registered on a draft OR list; hospital resources are reserved
Updating of OR time	Final OR list is created, listing the current week's scheduled operations
Arrival of emergency patients	Patients requiring emergency operation are sent for procedure
Cancellation of scheduled operations by emergency arrivals	Emergency patients requiring surgery immediately replace previously scheduled patients on the OR list
Cancellation of scheduled operations by inpatients	Inpatients requiring surgery replace previously scheduled patients on the OR list
Rescheduling of canceled operations	Patients whose surgery was canceled and who are still waiting for the operation are identified, and hospital resources are reserved
Surgical procedures	Operation is performed, during which time patients have access to OR resources
Postoperative treatment	Patients recover in the CS-ICU
Discharge from hospital	Patients are prepared for postoperative care at home or in rehabilitation or community facilities
Supporting activities	
Auditing of wait lists	Names of patients who died or whose condition deteriorates while waiting for the operation are removed from surgical waiting list
Assignment of clinic and OR slots to surgeons	Clinic and OR slots are assigned to surgeons according to duty rotation and vacation schedule for upcoming 18-week period
Assignment of preoperative assessment slots in the PAC	Preoperative assessment slots in the PAC are assigned for upcoming weeks

Abbreviations: OR = operating room, CS-ICU = cardiac surgery intensive care unit, PAC = preadmission clinic

Table 13.3 Modeling requirements and modeled activities that implement each requirement

Requirement	Modeled activities
Case mix of patients	Referral of patients for surgical consultation in outpatient clinic
	Referral of patients requiring urgent surgical assessment (inpatients)
	Arrival of emergency patients
Surgeon's duty rotation	Assignment of clinic and OR slots to surgeons
Assignment of clinic and OR slots	Assignment of clinic and OR slots to surgeons
Booking of outpatient surgical consultations	Referral of patients for surgical consultation in outpatient clinic
	Registration of elective patients on appointment list
	Booking of outpatient surgical consultation appointments
	Outpatient consultations with cardiac surgeon
Assessment by on-call surgeon	Referral of patients requiring urgent surgical assessment (inpatients)
	In-hospital assessment of patients requiring urgent operation (inpatients)
	Registration of inpatients for surgery
Booking of elective operations	Registration on a surgical wait list
	Advance booking of elective operations
	Scheduling of OR time
	Updating of OR time
	Rescheduling of canceled operations
	Surgical procedures
Preoperative assessment of elective patients in PAC and in hospital	Referral of elective patients for preoperative assessment
	Booking of preoperative assessments
	Preoperative assessments
	Booking of patients for additional preoperative assessments
	In-hospital preoperative assessment of elective patients
	Assignment of preoperative assessment slots in the PACs
Booking inpatients and emergency operations	Scheduling of OR time
	Updating of OR time
	Arrival of emergency patients
	Cancellation of scheduled operations by emergency arrivals
	Cancellation of scheduled operations by inpatients
	Rescheduling of canceled operations
	Surgical procedures
Managing postoperative treatment	Postoperative treatment
	Discharge from hospital
Auditing of wait lists	Auditing of wait lists

Abbreviations: OR = operating room, PAC = preadmission clinic, CS-ICU = cardiac surgery intensive care unit appointments are scheduled during vacation periods. A surgeon returning from vacation resumes with on-call duty. The duty rotation and vacation schedule of surgeons is planned for 18 weeks in advance, as shown in Table 13.4.

13.2.3 Assignment of Clinic and Operating Room Slots

We modeled 16 clinic slots per week for surgical consultations. The surgeon on office duty is assigned eight clinic slots on Monday and another eight slots on Tuesday. We modeled three operating room slots per weekday. The surgeon on on-call duty is assigned one of the three operating room slots available every weekday and performs surgeries on weekends if necessary. The surgeon on operating room duty is assigned the remaining two operating room slots available every weekday. Weekly operating room slots may be designated for elective or urgent procedures.

13.2.4 Booking of Outpatient Surgical Consultations

We modeled three alternative methods of booking surgical consultation appointments in the outpatient clinic: pooled list, individual lists, and shortest list. A thorough comparison of these methods is presented in Chap. 14. With the individual-lists method, consultations are booked with the surgeon named in the referral. With the pooled-list method, consultations are booked with the first available surgeon. With the shortest-list method, patients are placed on the appointment list of the surgeon who has the fewest patients waiting. In the model, the draft clinic schedule for the following week is generated on Fridays and is based on the assignment of clinic slots to the surgeon who is on office duty. On Mondays, the draft clinic schedule becomes the current clinic schedule and is used for the surgical consultations of the current week.

13.2.5 Assessment by On-call Surgeon

Patients admitted to hospital directly from the catheterization laboratory because of their requirement for urgent surgical assessment (i.e., patients on the inpatient care path) are assessed by the on-call surgeon on the day of arrival. After assessment, these inpatients are assigned a surgical priority, either high or low, according to the affected coronary anatomy and symptoms. A certain proportion of the low-priority inpatients are discharged with a promise to be readmitted for their operation.

Table 13.4 Duty rotation of three surgeons over an 18-week period, according to the service and vacation schedule

	Weeks																	
Surgeon	1	2	3	4	5	6	7	8	9	10	11	12	13	14	15	16	17	18
1	OR	OF	OC	V	V	V	OC	OR	OF	*	*	*	†	‡	‡	*	*	*
2	OF	OC	OR	*	*	*	†	‡	‡	V	V	V	OC	OR	OF	*	*	*
3	OC	OR	OF	*	*	*	†	‡	‡	*	*	*	†	‡	‡	V	V	V

Abbreviations: OR = operating room duty, OF = office duty, OC = on-call duty, V = vacation

*Surgeons not on vacation alternate between OR and OC duties with starting duty assigned randomly

†OR if last duty was OC, OF if last duty was OR

‡Duty rotation according to the first duty assigned after vacation period

13.2.6 Booking of Elective Operations

We modeled two methods of booking elective patients for their operations: wait-list booking and advance booking. A thorough comparison of these methods is presented in Chap. 16.

With wait-list booking, elective patients are registered on the priority wait list of the consulting surgeon without a projected date of operation. A surgical priority, high, medium, or low, is assigned to each patient according to the urgency of the operation. The surgeons' wait lists store patient information until the operation can be scheduled. Attempts to schedule patients for their operations are made periodically until an appropriate operating room slot is available. A draft operating room list for the following week is generated every Friday. It contains the scheduled operations of elective patients selected from wait lists, low-priority inpatients waiting in hospital, and patients who were previously discharged with a promise to readmit. On Mondays, the draft operating room list becomes the current operating room list, with the scheduled operations for the current week.

With advance booking, elective patients are registered on a wait list with a projected date of operation. The projected date of operation is the date of the next available operating room slot assigned to the consulting surgeon on the projected list for the upcoming 36-week period after the surgical consultation. Similar to the situation for wait-list booking, a draft operating room list is generated every Friday and is used as the basis for the next week's list, generated the following Monday. The draft list contains the operations of elective patients from the coming week's projected list, as well as the operations of inpatients waiting in hospital and patients who were previously discharged with a promise to readmit.

With both booking methods, the current operating room list may be modified unexpectedly by the arrival of emergency patients and inpatients, who are given preferential access to operating room slots, which causes cancellation of previously booked operations.

13.2.7 Preoperative Assessment of Patients in Preadmission Clinic and in Hospital

With the advance method of booking surgery, elective patients are assigned a date for a preoperative assessment in the preadmission clinic at the same time as the projected date for the operation is assigned. We modeled two methods of booking elective patients for this presurgical assessment: the all-screened method and the some-screened method. With the all-screened method, all elective patients are assessed in the preadmission clinic before being admitted for the operation. Elective patients are scheduled for their preoperative assessment within the 3-week period before the projected date of the operation. If no clinic slots are available within that period, the operation is canceled on the projected operating room list and rescheduled so that a new date for a preoperative assessment in the preadmission clinic can be determined.

With the some-screened method, an attempt is made to book elective patients for a preoperative assessment in the preadmission clinic within the 3-week period before the projected date of the operation. If no clinic slots are available within that period, these elective patients are admitted to hospital one day before the projected date of operation and the preoperative assessment is performed in the hospital. It is expected that some of the elective patients admitted in this way will require further tests after the in-hospital assessment. In these cases, the operation is canceled on the current operating room list and then rescheduled, so that a new date for preoperative assessment in the preadmission clinic can be determined.

With both methods, some elective patients may be deemed unsuitable for the operation on the basis of the initial preoperative assessment in the preadmission clinic, and they may require an additional assessment. In these cases, the operation is canceled on the projected operating room list and then rescheduled, so that a date for the additional assessment (in the preadmission clinic) can be determined. These additional assessments in the preadmission clinic are booked differently for the two methods of screening patients. With the all-screened method, if no slots in the preadmission clinic are available for the additional assessment within the 3-week period before the projected date of the operation, the operation is canceled on the projected operating room list and then rescheduled, so that a date for the additional assessment can be determined. With the some-screened method, if no slots in the preadmission clinic are available for the additional assessment within the 3-week period before the projected date of the operation, these elective patients are admitted to hospital one day before the projected date of surgery for an in-hospital preoperative assessment.

13.2.8 Booking of Operations for Inpatients and Emergency Patients

High-Priority Inpatients

Two attempts are made to book each high-priority inpatient for the operation. The first attempt involves booking this type of inpatient two days after admission to hospital, into a slot assigned to the on-call surgeon and designated for inpatients. If that attempt is unsuccessful, because no slots are available, the second attempt involves booking this type of inpatient into a weekend slot assigned to the on-call surgeon. If both attempts are unsuccessful, these inpatients are booked into the first available slot the following week. All booking attempts for high-priority inpatients may cause the cancellation of an already-booked operation of lower surgical priority.

Low-Priority Inpatients

Every Friday, an attempt is made to book low-priority inpatients into operating room slots designated for inpatients. If two attempts to make such a booking are unsuccessful, the inpatient is discharged from hospital with a promise of readmission for the operation at a later date.

Patients Discharged with a Promise to Readmit

Every Friday, an attempt is made to rebook patients who have previously been discharged with a promise to readmit into operating room slots designated for inpatients. High- and low-priority inpatients are always booked for their operations before any "promise-to-readmit" patients are booked.

Emergency Patients

Emergency patients are booked for their operations on the day of arrival at the hospital, which may cause cancellation of an already-booked operation of lower surgical priority.

13.2.9 Postoperative Treatment

After their operations, all patients are admitted to the cardiac surgery intensive care unit for postoperative treatment. Scheduled operations listed on the current operating room list may be canceled if no beds are available in this unit for recovery. Available beds in the main hospital intensive care unit may be used for emergency patients if all of the cardiac surgery intensive care unit beds are unavailable.

13.2.10 Auditing of Wait Lists

A certain proportion of elective patients waiting to be booked for an operation may die, or their condition may deteriorate. These patients are removed from the wait lists. Patients removed because of deteriorating condition are admitted to hospital as emergency patients or high-priority inpatients, according to their surgical priority. The decision to admit an elective patient to hospital is made by the wait-list coordinator.

13.3 Modeling Assumptions

In developing the model requirements, we made the following simplifying assumptions:

General Assumptions:

1. For each simulation week, the random numbers of referrals for surgical consultations, of emergency patients, and of inpatients are drawn from Poisson distributions, to allow for fluctuations in demand for service.
2. Simulated patients differ by sex, age group, affected coronary anatomy, and comorbidity. The distribution of referrals by patient attributes is based on historical data obtained from a patient registry for the period 1991 to 2000 [142].

3. The surgeons' service and vacation schedules are planned according to an 18-week cycle, and the booking horizon is 36 weeks. Each surgeon is on vacation for 3 of every 18 weeks.
4. The progress of patients needing elective surgery from their consultation priority groups to the corresponding surgical priority groups is governed by binomial probability distributions, as is the progress of patients needing urgent operations from expedited consultation to operation (as either inpatients or outpatients).

Surgical Consultations:

1. Referred patients have high or low priority for surgical consultation. Patients with high priority are scheduled before those with low priority, and those with the same priority are scheduled by their respective referral times.
2. Sixteen consultation appointments are available each week, and all patients attend their appointments.
3. All patients assessed in the outpatient clinic are deemed to be suitable candidates for surgery and are registered on the consulting surgeon's priority wait list.
4. Elective patients with a high priority for consultation are assigned a high priority for the operation.
5. A certain proportion of elective patients with a low priority for consultation are assigned a medium priority for the operation, and the remaining elective patients with low priority for consultation are assigned a low priority for the operation.
6. All inpatients are assessed by the on-call surgeon on the day of admission to hospital.

Booking of Operations:

1. With wait-list booking, elective patients with high priority for their operations are booked before those with low priority, and patients with the same priority are booked by their respective dates of registration.
2. With wait-list booking, patients with any priority may be booked into any urgent slots available to the consulting surgeon, so long as no inpatients are waiting in hospital.
3. With advance booking, patients with high and medium priority are eligible for booking into both elective and urgent slots available to the consulting surgeon, whereas those with low priority may be booked only into elective slots available to the consulting surgeon.
4. Each week, seven operating room slots are available for elective surgery and eight for urgent procedures. Two methods for allocating operating room slots over weekdays are modeled: a weekly or a daily split between elective and urgent procedures.
5. Emergency patients and high-priority inpatients are booked on the current operating room list immediately. They are booked into urgent slots, if such are available; otherwise, previously booked operations may be canceled to accommodate these cases.
6. Low-priority inpatients are booked for surgery on the current operating room list if urgent slots are available; otherwise, they are booked into available urgent slots the following week.

Preoperative Assessment:

1. Twenty appointments for preoperative assessments are available at the preadmission clinic each week, and all patients attend their appointments.
2. Inpatients and previous inpatients who were discharged with a promise to readmit are assessed in hospital on the day of the operation.
3. All emergency patients are deemed suitable for the operation and do not undergo a preoperative assessment.

Cancellation of Scheduled Operations:

1. The scheduled operation of an elective patient may be canceled by the arrival of an emergency patient or a high-priority inpatient.
2. The scheduled operation of a high-priority inpatient may be canceled by the arrival of an emergency patient.
3. The scheduled operation of a low-priority inpatient may be canceled by the arrival of an emergency patient or a high-priority inpatient.
4. The scheduled operation of a patient whose surgery was previously canceled with a promise to readmit may be canceled by the arrival of an emergency patient or a high-priority inpatient.
5. The scheduled operation of an emergency patient cannot be canceled.
6. Canceled high- and medium-priority elective operations are rebooked as inpatient operations after the operations of all previously registered inpatients have been booked.
7. Canceled low-priority elective operations are rebooked as "promise-to-readmit" operations after the operations of all previously registered "promise-to-readmit" patients have been booked.
8. Canceled high-priority inpatient operations are rebooked as high-priority inpatient operations ahead of the operations for any previously registered high-priority inpatients.
9. Canceled low-priority inpatient operations are rebooked as low-priority inpatient operations ahead of the operations for any previously registered low-priority inpatients.
10. Canceled "promise-to-readmit" operations are rebooked as "promise-to-readmit" operations ahead of the operations for any previously registered "promise-to-readmit" patients.

Postoperative Treatment:

1. After their surgery, patients recover in the cardiac surgery intensive care unit, for an average of one day.
2. Four beds are available in the cardiac surgery intensive care unit. Two additional beds from the main hospital intensive care unit may be used for emergency patients if no cardiac surgery intensive care beds are available.
3. If no cardiac surgery intensive care beds are available for recovery from a planned operation, the operation is canceled.

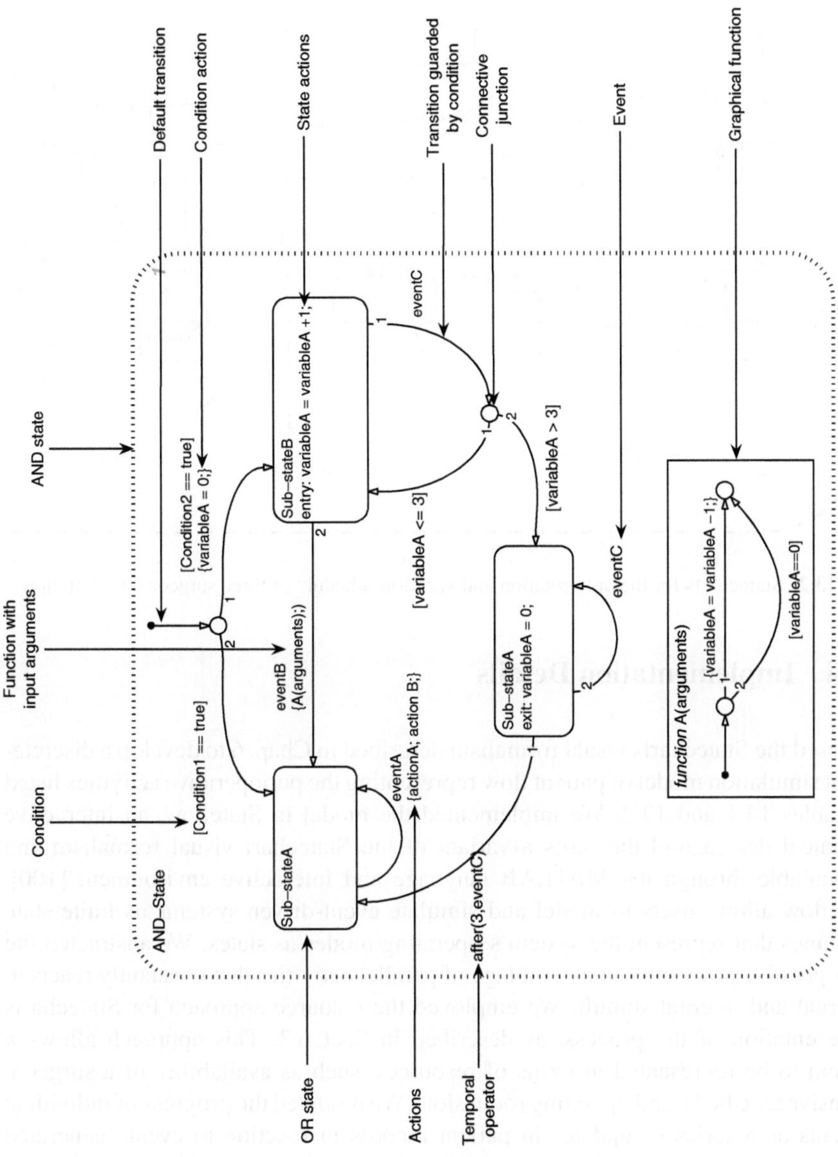

Fig. 13.1 Semantics of Statecharts in Stateflow

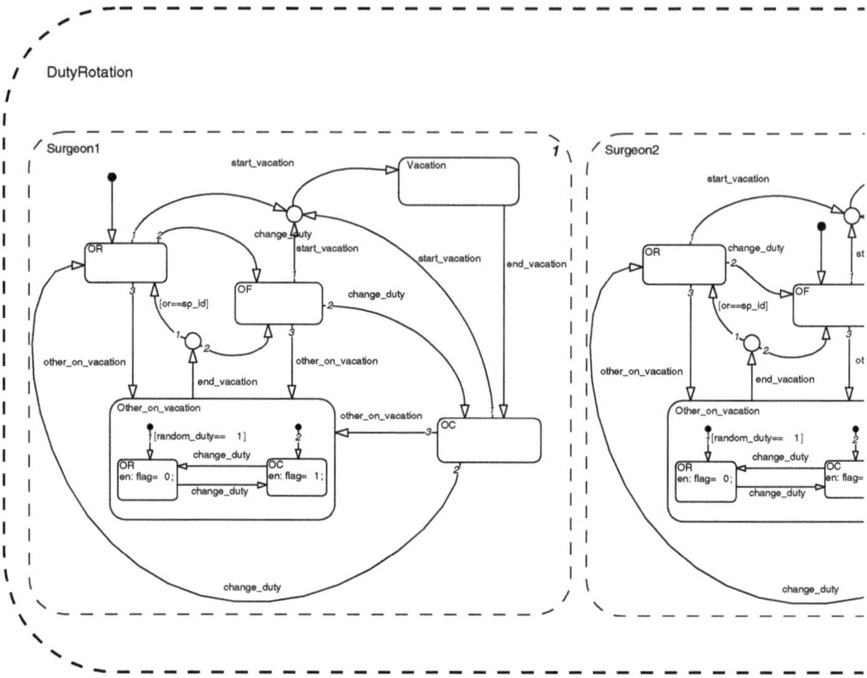

Fig. 13.2 Statecharts for the duty rotation and vacation schedule of three surgeons, in Stateflow

13.4 Implementation Details

We used the Statecharts visual formalism described in Chap. 6 to develop a discrete-event simulation model of patient flow representing the perioperative activities listed in Tables 13.1 and 13.2. We implemented the model in Stateflow, an interactive graphical design tool that uses a variant of the Statechart visual formalism and is available through the MATLAB language and interactive environment [100]. Stateflow allows users to model and simulate event-driven systems as finite-state machines that represent the system's operating modes as states. We abstracted the perioperative process as an assemblage of parallel activities that constantly reacts to external and internal stimuli. We employed the resource approach for Statecharts representation of the process, as described in Sect. 6.3. This approach allows a system to be represented in terms of resources, such as availability of a surgeon, intensive care beds, and operating room slots. We modeled the progress of individual patients as a series of updates in patient records in reaction to events generated asynchronously by the modeled activities. We employed graphical functions to implement algorithms and actions executed by the modeled activities, and we used dynamic tables to store the occurrence and timing of simulation events.

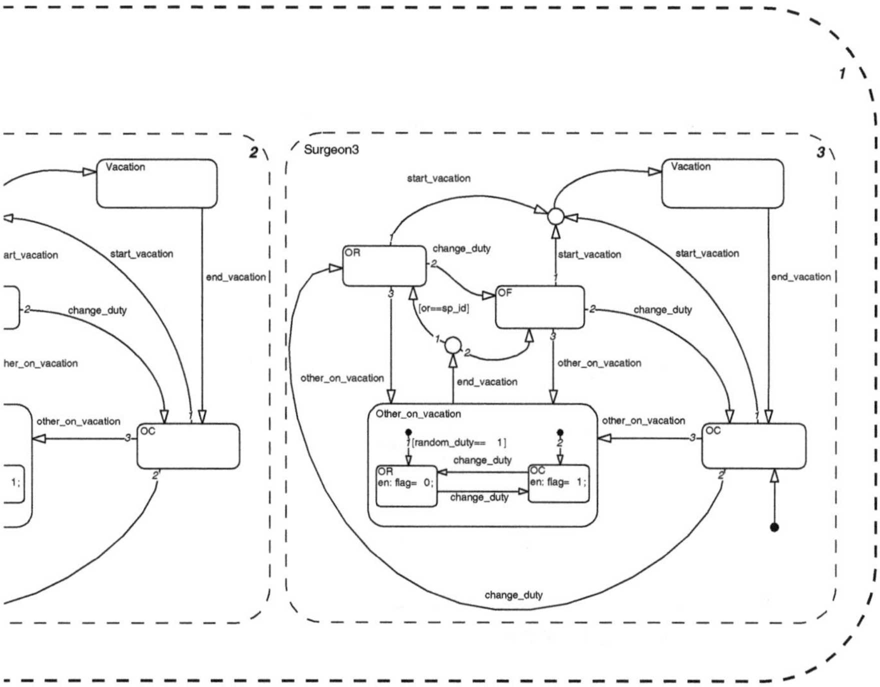

Fig. 13.2 (continued)

13.4.1 Statecharts in Stateflow

Stateflow follows the semantics of the Statechart visual formalism to define states, events, transitions between states, actions, and conditions, as outlined in Chap. 6 and illustrated in Fig. 13.1. In addition, Stateflow employs an event-scheduling mechanism that allows the use of temporal operators (`before`, `after`, `at`, and `every`) to specify scheduling logic for transition and state actions. As an example, Fig. 13.2 shows the Statechart implementing the duty rotation and vacation schedule of the modeled three-surgeon surgical service. Figure 13.3 shows the Statecharts representing an appointment list.

13.4.2 Graphical Functions in Stateflow

Graphical functions in Stateflow provide the means for graphically programming an algorithm and tracking its behavior during a simulation. These functions offer the capability to broadcast events that trigger transitions in various machines. The functions may be called by machines and other graphical functions with

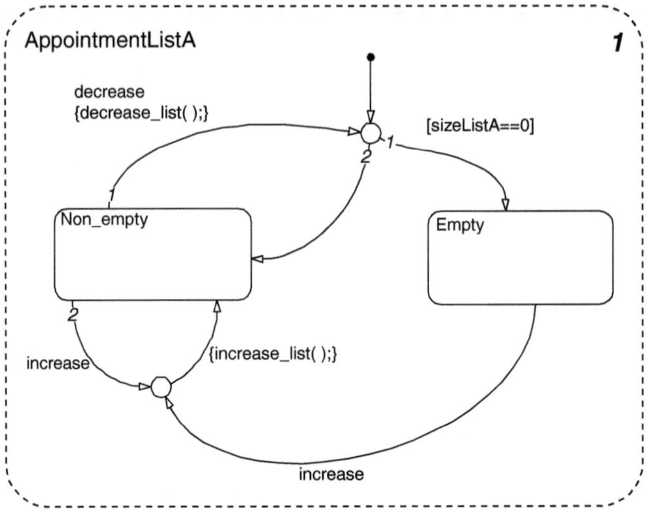

Fig. 13.3 Statecharts for an appointment list, in Stateflow

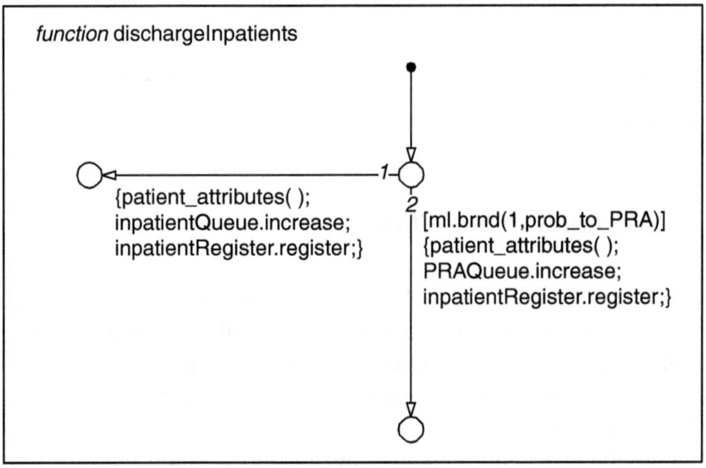

Fig. 13.4 Graphical function for discharging a portion of inpatients from hospital with a promise to readmit

argument values represented by the input variables to the function. They may also return values represented by output variables of the function. We used graphical functions to implement algorithms (such as the algorithms for booking operations or appointments at the preadmission clinic) and as extensions to actions executed by the machines. As an example, Fig. 13.4 shows a graphical function to implement the action of discharging a proportion of low-priority inpatients from hospital with a promise to readmit.

Table 13.5 Values of input parameters for the discrete-event simulation model of a cardiac surgical service

Input parameter	Values
Priority group	
Outpatient surgical consultation	High, low
Elective operation	High, medium, low
Urgent operation	High, low, promise to readmit
Arrival rate (patients per week)	
High priority for surgical consultation	0.5
Low priority for surgical consultation	6.5
Inpatients	5.8
Emergency	0.5
Probability of progression (elective operation)	
High priority for consultation to high priority for operation	1
Low priority for consultation to medium priority for operation	0.76
Low priority for consultation to low priority for operation	0.24
Probability of progression (urgent operation)	
High priority for assessment to high priority for operation	1
Low priority for assessment to low priority for operation	0.5
Low priority for assessment to promise-to-readmit status	0.5
Capacity	
No. of surgeons	3
Weekly no. of outpatient consultations	16*
Weekly no. of slots for elective operations	7
Weekly no. of slots for urgent operations	8
Weekly no. of consultations in the preadmission clinic	20
No. of beds in cardiac surgery intensive care unit	4
Horizon for advance booking (weeks)	36

*Eight on Monday, eight on Tuesday

13.4.3 Input Parameters

Input parameters are used as inputs to the model for its execution. They may represent various aspects of the model, such as patient arrival rates, branching probabilities, control logic, the probability that an event will occur, and the availability of resources. More specifically, input parameters are used to generate random numbers, control loops, and if-then-else statements; to compute preexisting records in appointment and wait lists upon initialization of the model; to generate assignments of clinic and operating room slots to surgeons; and to specify bed availability in the intensive care unit. Table 13.5 shows the values of the input parameters of the model, including number of priority groups, referral rates, probabilities of progression, and capacities.

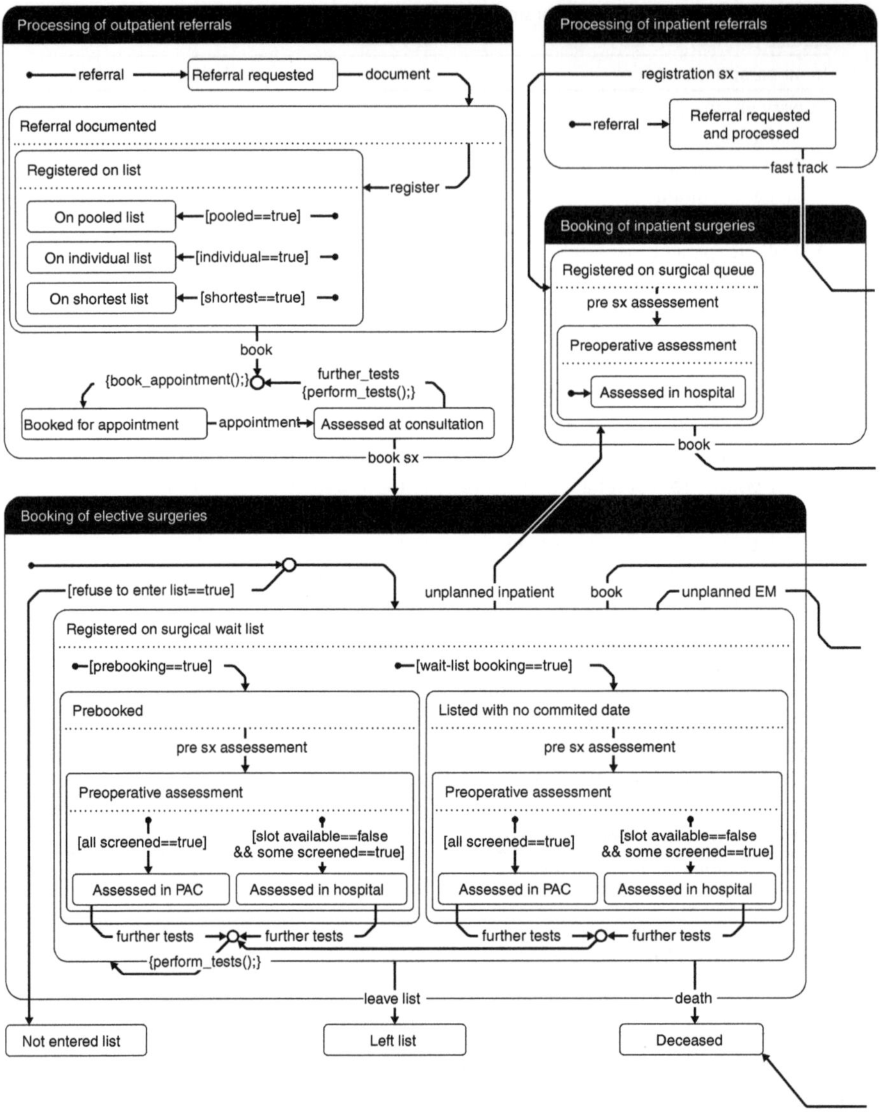

Fig. 13.5 Statecharts diagram of patient flow in the process of cardiac surgical care listed in Tables 13.1 and 13.2 (OR = operating room, PAC = preadmission clinic, CS_ICU = cardiac surgery intensive care unit)

13.4.4 Internal Queues

Internal queues are dynamic tables used to store patient records in coordination with the modeled perioperative activities. During a simulation run, some modeled activities react to events generated by other modeled activities by updating internal

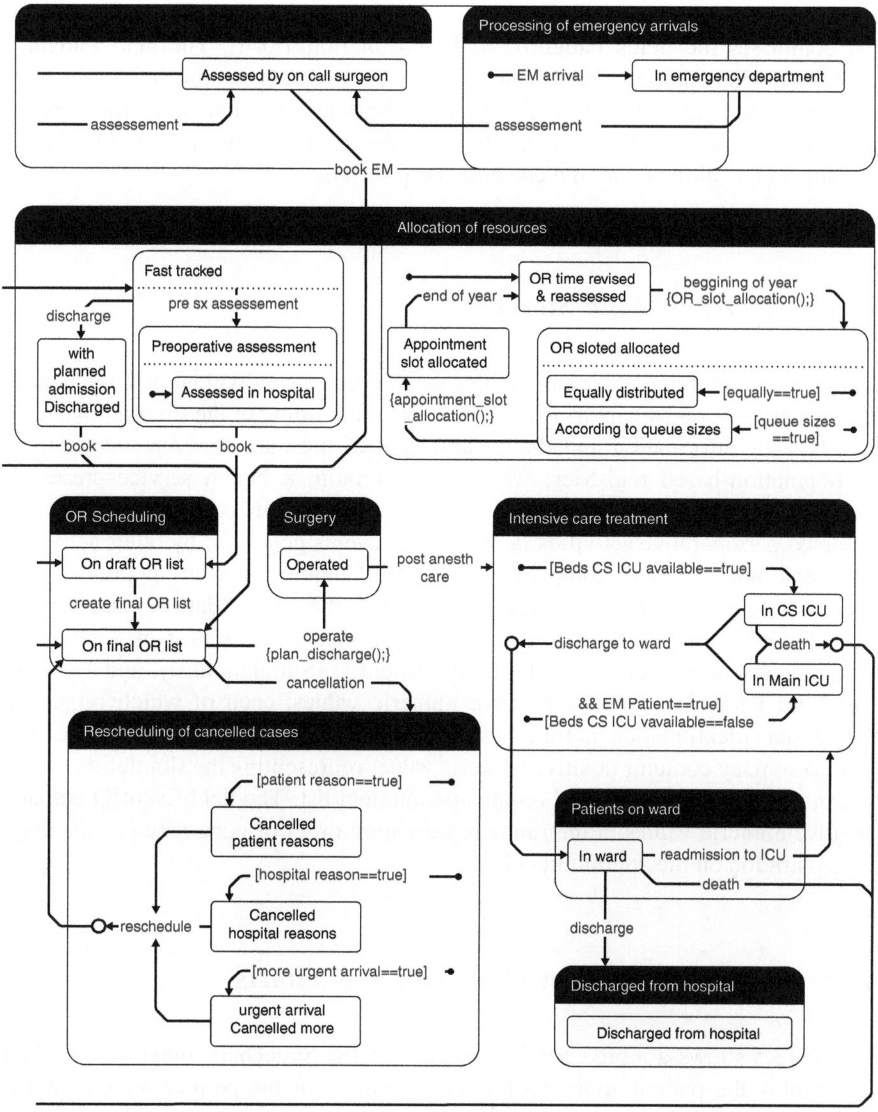

Fig. 13.5 (continued)

queues. For example, appointment lists are represented in the model by a set of internal queues. The activity of referring an elective patient for consultation with a surgeon in the outpatient clinic will cause the addition of a patient record to the pertinent internal queue. Completion of the consultation will cause removal of the corresponding patient record from the pertinent internal queue.

Each internal queue comprises a number of fields, which are populated with specific categories or ranges of values dictated by the type of data contained in the field.

For example, the internal queue representing a particular surgeon's appointment list comprises the fields PatientID and ConsultationPriority. The field PatientID contains positive numeric values, each of which represents the unique identification number associated with a particular patient. The field ConsultationPriority contains a numeric value of either 1 or 2, where a value of 1 signifies a low consultation priority and a value of 2 a high consultation priority.

13.4.5 External Data Stores

External data stores are dynamic tables used to collect individual paths generated through simulation by capturing the occurrence and timing of the simulation events. The type of information and the organization of the data stored resemble those of population-based registries, which are common in health services research. As with the internal queues, data stores are updated in coordination with the modeled perioperative activities in reaction to events generated by other activities. Each external data store comprises a number of fields, which are populated with specific categories or ranges of values dictated by the type of data contained in the field. For example, the external data store representing registration of a patient on an appointment list comprises the fields PatientID, SimulationDay, and EventID. The field PatientID contains positive numeric values, each of which represents the unique identification number associated with a particular patient. The field SimulationDay contains positive numeric values representing the simulation day on which a patient was registered on the appointment list. The field EventID contains positive numeric values in the range representing order of occurrence of the event of registration on the appointment list.

13.5 Describing Patient Flow with Statecharts

Figure 13.5 shows a more complex example of the Statecharts diagram, in which we employ the patient approach for representation of the perioperative activities listed in Tables 13.1 and 13.2. This diagram represents the flow of patients in terms of the states that patients may occupy in the process of surgical care. The diagram shows the three care paths following angiography—elective, inpatient, and emergency—that patients with established coronary artery disease are likely to experience, as described in Sect. 13.1. Appendix C provides detailed tables that specify the states, transition labels, and events of the Statecharts diagram for patient flow. Tables C.1 to C.5 list the states and substates that patients may occupy in the process shown in Fig. 13.5, a description of their functionality, and their associated events and conditions. Tables C.6 to C.8 list the corresponding events shown and a description of their occurrences. Table C.9 lists the functions shown in Fig. 13.5 and a description of their functionality.

Chapter 14
Booking Consultation Appointments

In this chapter, we first compare two methods of booking consultation appointments in a surgical service with several specialists, both in terms of the average clearance time for the appointment list, which is of interest to hospitals, and the weekly appointment rate, which is of interest to patients. We then expand the comparison by contrasting a third method to the original two methods. We used discrete-event simulation of patient flow described in detail in the previous chapter. In the simulation study, we apply a cluster randomized design, in which the unit of allocation was the hospital and the units of analysis were both the simulated hospital and the simulated patient. Our results suggest that clearance times were shorter in hospitals where patients waited for surgical consultations in a single queue and that within each week a larger proportion of patients were likely to have an appointment if they were in a single queue.

14.1 The Simulation Study

14.1.1 Background

The management of outpatient surgical consultations constitutes an important aspect of planning activities in a surgical service [158]. The booking process used for these appointments determines the appointment date for any patient referred for consultation about an operation [84]. Within a regional network of hospitals, a variety of methods may be used for booking surgical consultations, but a better understanding is needed of the implications of these different methods for managing access to elective surgery.

B. Sobolev et al., *Health Care Evaluation Using Computer Simulation: Concepts, Methods, and Applications*, DOI 10.1007/978-1-4614-2233-4_14,

Box 14.1 What is already known and what this study adds on booking consultations

What is already known

- The time between referral and consultation depends on the method of booking appointments, the number and type of referrals, and the availability of surgeons for appointments [72, 106].
- The most common method of booking appointments is to place patients on the appointment list of the surgeon named in the referral, that is, the individual-lists method.
- In services where any one of a group of surgeons may see patients, pooling referrals on a single appointment list (i.e., the pooled-list method) has been suggested as a way to reduce the time to consultation with a specialist [125].

What this study adds

- This simulation study shows the effects of using the pooled-list method of booking surgical consultation appointments on the flow of patients from referral to consultation and from consultation to operation in the context of cardiac surgical services.

14.1.2 The Study Rationale

The purpose of this simulation study was to estimate the effects of various methods of booking surgical consultation appointments on the flow of patients from referral to consultation and from consultation to surgery in the context of cardiac surgical services. We compared two appointment methods—assigning patients either to individual lists for specific surgeons or to a pooled list—in terms of the following performance measures: average number of patients waiting for a surgical consultation appointment, average clearance time for appointment lists [39], proportion of hospitals with delay of high-priority elective procedures, weekly rate of surgical consultation appointments [143], weekly rate of surgery [139], and proportion of patients undergoing surgery after the recommended time. In particular, we were interested in whether the pooled-list method would reduce the average number of patients waiting, the average clearance time, and the proportion of hospitals with delay of high-priority elective procedures; whether it would increase the proportion of patients having appointments each week and the proportion of patients undergoing an operation from wait lists each week; and whether it would decrease the proportion of patients undergoing surgery after the recommended time. Box 14.1 summarizes the study rationale.

14.1.3 The Management Alternatives

We considered two methods of booking surgical consultation appointments: the individual-lists system and the pooled-list system. With the individual-lists system, consultations are booked with the surgeon named in the referral. This method ensures that each patient is seen by the surgeon chosen by the referring physician. With the pooled-list system, consultations are booked with the first available surgeon [156].

14.1.4 Study Questions

The following study questions were of interest for this simulation study:

- Are there fewer patients waiting for surgical consultation appointments with the pooled-list method than with the individual-lists method?
- Are clearance times for appointment lists shorter in services with the pooled-list method than in services with the individual-lists method?
- Is there a lower chance that a hospital will have delayed high-priority elective procedures with the pooled-list method than with the individual-lists method?
- Is the time to appointment shorter with the pooled-list method than with the individual-lists method?
- Is the time to surgery shorter with the pooled-list method than with the individual-lists method?
- Is there a lower chance of undergoing elective surgery after the recommended time with the pooled-list method than with the individual-lists method?

14.2 The Simulation Model

We used a discrete-event simulation model of patient flow representing the process of cardiac surgical care, as described in Chap. 13. In particular, we modeled three care paths that patients are likely to experience: the elective path, which applies to patients for whom surgical consultation and subsequent operation can be safely delayed; the inpatient path, which applies to patients admitted to hospital directly from the catheterization laboratory when urgent surgical assessment is necessary; and the emergency path, which applies to patients requiring immediate surgical intervention.

14.2.1 Modeling Requirements

We studied a service where three cardiac surgeons had admitting privileges at a single hospital and used a shared clinic for outpatient consultations. In this setting, the surgeons' availability for operations depended on their schedules for consultations, planned operations, on-call duties, and vacations. Sixteen consultation appointments, seven operating room slots for planned operations (elective pathway), and eight slots for urgent cases (inpatient pathway) were available each week. Emergency cases could cause the cancellation of planned operations. Patients referred for consultation with a surgeon were kept on the appointment list with a designated priority (high or low) until an opening for an appointment became available.

After each consultation, the office of the consulting surgeon registered on a wait list the name of any patient who needed coronary revascularization, designating the required procedure as high, medium, or low priority according to the affected coronary anatomy and the patient's symptoms. The hospital's booking office assigned patients to the operating room slots that had been allocated to the consulting surgeon, according to the priority of each case and the date of registration on the wait list. We considered two methods of booking elective operations: wait-list booking and advance booking. With wait-list booking, a patient is registered on the priority wait list of the consulting surgeon without a projected date of operation. Attempts to book each patient for the operation are made periodically until an appropriate operating room slot is available. With advance booking, the hospital's booking office schedules each patient in advance for the next available operating room slot available to the consulting surgeon in the upcoming 36-week period.

14.2.2 Modeling Assumptions

The complete list of assumptions of the discrete-event simulation model appears in Sect. 13.3. For the reader's convenience, the modeling assumptions related to the management of outpatient surgical consultations are repeated here.

Surgical Consultations

1. Referred patients have high or low priority for surgical consultation. Patients with high priority are scheduled before those with low priority, and those with the same priority are scheduled by their respective referral times.
2. Sixteen appointments are available each week, and all patients attend their appointments.
3. All patients assessed in the outpatient clinic are deemed to be suitable candidates for surgery and are registered on the consulting surgeon's priority wait list.
4. Elective patients with a high priority for consultation are assigned a high priority for the operation.
5. A certain proportion of elective patients with a low priority for consultation are assigned a medium priority for the operation, and the remaining elective patients with low priority for consultation are assigned a low priority for the operation.
6. All inpatients are assessed by the on-call surgeon on the day of admission to hospital.

Table 14.1 Configurations of the discrete-event simulation model for two methods of booking surgical consultation appointments, allowing variation in methods of booking elective operations

Configuration	Appointments	Elective operations
A	Individual lists	Wait-list booking
B	Individual lists	Advance booking
C	Pooled list	Wait-list booking
D	Pooled list	Advance booking

14.2.3 Configurations of the Model

We developed four configurations of the discrete-event simulation model to implement the two methods of booking appointments and the two methods of booking elective operations (Table 14.1). In configurations A and B, which used the individual-lists method of booking appointments, there were three priority lists, with surgeon-specific referral rates represented by three internal queues. During each simulated week, the model booked patients waiting on the appointment list of the surgeon who was available for the clinic that week. In configurations C and D, which used the pooled-list method, there was a single priority list for appointments, with an aggregated referral rate represented by a single internal queue. During each simulated week, the model booked patients waiting on the pooled list for an appointment with the surgeon who was available for the clinic that week.

14.2.4 Input Parameters

The input parameters for the model (listed in Table 13.5) corresponded to the workload and capacities of the cardiac surgery service in one hospital in British Columbia. The random numbers of weekly referrals of patients on the elective pathway for surgical consultation and of patients on the inpatient and emergency pathways for operations had a Poisson distribution. The progression of patients waiting for elective surgery from their respective appointment-priority groups to their respective surgical-priority groups was governed by binomial probability distributions, as was the progression of patients from urgent assessment to inpatient surgery. Within every six-week period, one of the three surgeons took 3 weeks of vacation. During these vacation periods, no appointments could be booked, as explained in Sect. 13.2.

14.2.5 Output Data

During each simulation run, patient records were stored in internal queues, such as appointment lists, whereas the occurrence and timing of simulation events, such as registrations and cancellations, were stored in external data stores. After a simulation run, individual patient paths were re-created by importing records from the data stores into a relational database and then linking the data stores by the combination of run and patient identification numbers that uniquely specified all rows in each data store. We then used the re-created paths for individual patients to construct the output data according to our predetermined data dictionaries. We developed one data dictionary for the analytical data set for elective cases (see Table D.1 in Appendix D) and another data dictionary for the analytical data set for inpatient cases (Table D.2 in Appendix D). The data set for elective cases contained information on our study population, including hospital characteristics, patient attributes, and outcomes. The data set for inpatient cases was used to compute the weekly number of inpatient or emergency procedures, which was used for adjustment in regression analysis.

14.3 Plan of Experiment

14.3.1 Primary Study Factor

Our primary study factor was the method of booking surgical consultation appointments, which in this simulation study had two categories: individual appointment lists and pooled appointment list, that is, simulation runs had either category 1 or category 2 for `meth_app` defined in Table D.1. This study factor was represented by one indicator variable for the two methods of booking appointments, where we defined the individual-lists method as the reference group.

14.3.2 Performance Measures

We were interested in performance measures at the level of both the hospital and the patient. In particular, we considered the following hospital-level performance measures:

- Average weekly number of patients on the appointment lists for surgical consultation during weeks when no appointments were available.
- Average clearance time for the appointment lists (in weeks).
- Proportion of hospitals with delay of any high-priority elective procedures.

The patient-level performance measures include:

- Weekly rate of appointments among referrals.
- Weekly rate of surgery among patients remaining on wait lists.
- Proportion of wait-listed patients undergoing surgery after the recommended time.

14.3.3 Experimental Responses

We computed the performance measures from experimental responses (i.e., output data) generated by the individual simulation runs, with each run representing one simulated hospital. The following hospital-level experimental responses were generated:

- For each hospital, the weekly numbers of patients waiting for the appointments during weeks when no appointments were available (continuous variable).
- For each hospital, the clearance times in weeks for appointment lists (continuous variable).
- For each hospital, whether any high-priority elective procedures were delayed (indicator variable).

The patient-level experimental responses were:

- For each patient, whether the patient received an appointment (indicator variable) and the number of weeks from referral to appointment or removal from the list (continuous variable).
- For each patient, whether the patient underwent planned surgery (indicator variable) and the number of weeks from registration to surgery or removal from the list (continuous variable).
- For each patient, whether surgery was performed after the recommended time (indicator variable).

14.3.4 Hospital-Level and Patient-Level Factors

In this study, we varied five experimental hospital-level factors that might have affected the experimental responses, namely, method of booking surgery, allocation of operating room slots, and clearance times for appointment lists, surgical wait lists, and inpatient surgical queues at the start of the simulation. We also varied five patient-level factors that might have affected time to surgical consultation appointment, namely, sex, age group, coronary anatomy affected, comorbidity, and priority of elective referral. We varied three other patient-level factors that might have affected time to surgery: priority of registration on the surgical wait list, clearance time at time of registration on the wait list, and weekly number of inpatient and emergency procedures [141].

14.3.5 Measure of Effect Size

To compare the effects of the methods of booking surgical consultation appointments on the performance measures at the hospital level, we used the following measures of effect size corresponding to those measures:

- Difference in average weekly number of patients waiting for surgical consultation appointments during weeks when no appointments were available.
- Difference in average clearance time for appointment lists (in weeks).
- Odds ratio for delay of any high-priority elective procedures.

Similarly, we used the following measures of effect size to compare the effects of the booking methods on the performance measures at the patient level:

- Ratio of weekly odds for receiving an appointment among referrals.
- Ratio of weekly odds for undergoing surgery among patients remaining on wait lists.
- Odds ratio for undergoing surgery after the recommended time.

14.3.6 Design of Experiment

We used a cluster randomized design, in which the unit of allocation was a simulated hospital. As described in Sect. 7.3, a simulated hospital was produced by one run of the simulation model. The number of simulation runs was chosen to detect the anticipated effects of the booking methods with high probability (see Appendix B). We performed provisional runs of the simulation model, with 30 hospitals per experimental group, to estimate the magnitude of each performance measure in the reference group and to estimate the measures of variability and correlation needed for computing the number of simulation runs. For comparison of the two methods of booking surgical consultation appointments, we calculated that 112 simulation runs per experimental group would be needed. This estimate was based on the maximum estimated number of runs across the hospital-level and patient-level performance measures of interest, as described below. All calculations assumed a two-sided test with 0.05 significance level and 90% power. We used the Fedorov algorithm to ensure optimal distribution of the experimental factors across the runs [55]. This algorithm randomly assigned each group of patients from simulation runs with the specified combination of values of the hospital-level factors to an experimental group.

Number of Runs for Cluster-Level Evaluations

We determined the number of runs needed to detect the anticipated difference in each hospital-level (i.e., cluster-level) performance measure in four calculations. First, we calculated the number of runs needed to detect a difference in the average weekly number of patients waiting for surgical consultation appointments during weeks when no appointments were available. According to provisional runs of the simulation model, the hypothesized value of this average was 37.6 patients (standard deviation [SD] = 4.1) with the individual-lists method. We estimated the number of simulation runs needed to detect a reduction in this average of eight patients. The magnitude of the difference corresponded to half the number of appointments available each week. Using (8.15), the required number of simulation runs (rounding up to the nearest integer) is as follows:

$$k = \frac{2(4.1)^2(1.96 + 1.28)^2}{8^2} \approx 6.$$

The formula in (8.15) is based on the normal approximation for a large number of runs. Because the estimated number of simulation runs was small, we also determined the number of runs according to the t distribution, which has no simple formula and requires the aid of a computer. With this method, the estimated number of simulation runs was larger: seven runs per experimental group.

Second, we estimated the number of runs needed to detect a difference in the average weekly clearance time for appointment lists. The provisional runs showed that the hypothesized average weekly clearance time for appointments was 5.2 weeks (SD = 0.52) with the individual-lists method (the reference method). The number of simulation runs needed to detect a reduction of 1 week in this average clearance time was estimated. Using (8.15), the required number of simulation runs (rounding up to the nearest integer) is as follows:

$$k = \frac{2(0.52)^2(1.96 + 1.28)^2}{1^2} \approx 6.$$

Again, because the formula in (8.15) is based on the normal approximation for a large number of runs, we also determined the number of runs based on the t distribution. With this method, the estimated number of simulation runs was seven per experimental group.

Third, we estimated the number of runs needed to detect a difference in the proportion of hospitals with delay of any high-priority elective procedures. According to the provisional runs, the hypothesized proportion of hospitals with delay of any high-priority elective procedures was 0.367 with the individual-lists method. The number of simulation runs needed to detect a decrease of 0.20 in this proportion was estimated. Using (8.8), the required number of simulation runs (rounding up to the nearest integer) is as follows:

$$k = \left[\frac{1.96\sqrt{2(0.267)(1-0.267)} + 1.28\sqrt{0.367(1-0.367) + 0.167(1-0.167)}}{0.167 - 0.367} \right]^2$$

$$\approx 101.$$

Finally, for the purpose of the regression analysis, we determined the number of runs to generate an adequate number of observations per regression variable. Our primary experimental factor was represented by one variable for methods of booking surgical consultation appointments. In addition, we used two variables for clearance times for appointment lists at the start of simulation, three variables for clearance times for surgical wait lists at the start of simulation, two variables for clearance times for inpatient surgical queues at the start of simulation, one variable for methods of booking surgery, and one variable for allocation of operating room slots. Therefore, with a total of 10 variables, we estimated that 50 ($=10 \times 10/2$) observed events per booking method would be needed, allowing for 10 events per regression variable [73]. From provisional runs of the model, the event of a hospital having a delay for any high-priority procedures occurred about 45% of the time. Therefore, we estimated that we would need at least 112 runs ($\approx 50/0.45$) per method of booking surgical consultation appointments.

Number of Runs for Individual-Level Evaluations

We next calculated the number of runs needed to detect the anticipated difference in each patient-level (i.e., individual-level) performance measure in four calculations. For analyses at the patient level, the dependence between experimental responses within each hospital necessitated adjustment for within-hospital correlation [140].

First, we estimated the number of runs needed to detect a difference in surgical consultation appointment rates among referrals. Given the results of provisional runs of the simulation model, we assumed an average of 2,931 patient-weeks per simulation run and a coefficient of variation of 0.03 [74]. The hypothesized weekly rate of appointments was 20 per 100 patient-weeks with the individual-lists method (i.e., the reference method). We estimated that 14 runs per booking method would allow us to detect a 10% increase in the weekly appointment rate between groups of patients [49]. It may be undesirable to assume an equal number of patient-weeks across hospitals and identical coefficients of variation between experimental groups. We therefore used the Hayes method in (9.24) to estimate the number of runs (rounding up to the nearest integer), as follows:

$$k = 1 + \frac{(1.96 + 1.28)^2}{(0.20 - 0.20 \times 1.10)^2} \times \left(\frac{0.20}{3{,}611} + \frac{0.20 \times 1.10}{2{,}200} + 0.0003084 \right) \approx 14.$$

Second, we calculated the number of runs required to detect a difference in rates of surgery among registered patients. From the provisional runs, we assumed an average of 1,823 patient-weeks per simulation run and a coefficient of variation of 0.14. The hypothesized weekly rate of surgery was 32 per 100 patient-weeks with the individual-lists method (i.e., the reference method). We estimated that 35 runs per booking method would allow us to detect a 10% increase in the weekly surgery rate between groups of patients [49]. Again, we used the Hayes method to avoid the assumption of an equal number of patient-weeks across hospitals and identical coefficients of variation between experimental groups. Using (9.24), the number of runs (rounding up to the nearest integer) is

$$k = 1 + \frac{(1.96 + 1.28)^2}{(0.32 - 0.32 \times 1.10)^2} \times \left(\frac{0.32}{1{,}720} + \frac{0.32 \times 1.10}{1{,}861} + 0.002845 \right) \approx 35.$$

Third, we estimated the number of runs required to detect a difference in the proportion of patients whose elective procedures were performed after the recommended time. The hypothesized proportion of patients with delayed surgery was 0.10 among patients whose consultation appointments were booked with the reference method (i.e., the individual-lists method). We estimated that seven runs per booking method would allow us to detect a 0.05 decrease in this proportion between groups of patients [49]. We used (9.9) to estimate the intracluster correlation coefficient:

$$\hat{\rho} = \frac{0.09032 - 0.01052}{0.09032 + (716.5 - 1)(0.01052)} \approx 0.01048.$$

Then, using (9.14), we calculated the inflation factor:

$$\text{IF} = 1 + (717 - 1) \times 0.01048 \approx 8.5.$$

Therefore, because of the clustered nature of the experimental design, we determined that we would need almost nine times more patients in our experiment with randomization at the level of runs (i.e., hospitals) than in an experiment with randomization at the level of individual patients. Using (9.13), we then computed the number of runs per experimental group (rounding up to the nearest integer):

$$k = \frac{(1.96 + 1.28)^2[0.10(1 - 0.10) + 0.05(1 - 0.05)]}{717(0.05 - 0.10)^2} 8.5 \approx 7.$$

Finally, for the purpose of the regression analysis, we determined the number of runs needed to generate an adequate number of observations per regression variable. As described above, the primary study factor was represented by one variable for methods of booking surgical consultation appointments In addition, we used two variables for clearance times for appointment lists at the start of simulation, three variables for clearance times for surgical wait lists at the start of simulation, two variables for clearance times for inpatient surgical queues at the

Table 14.2 Number of simulation runs required to compare two methods of booking surgical consultation appointments with 0.05 significance level and 90% power, per experimental group

Performance measure	Reference value	Effect size	No. of runs
Hospital level			
Average weekly number of patients waiting for appointments during weeks when no appointments available (standard deviation)	37.6 (4.1)	8-patient decrease	7
Average clearance time for appointments in weeks (standard deviation)	5.2 (0.52)	1-week decrease	7
Proportion of hospitals with delay of any high-priority procedures	0.367	0.20 decrease	101*
Patient level			
Appointment rate per 100 patient-weeks	20	10% increase	14
Surgery rate per 100 patient-weeks	32	10% increase	34
Proportion of patients with surgery after recommended time	0.10	0.05 decrease	7

*112 runs required to allow 10 events per regression variable in cluster-level evaluation

start of simulation, one variable for methods of booking surgery, and one variable for allocation of operating room slots. The patient-level variables consisted of one variable for sex, four variables for age groups, two variables for categories of coronary anatomy affected, two variables for categories of comorbidity, two variables for priorities at registration, one time-dependent continuous variable for the weekly number of inpatient and emergency procedures, and one time-dependent continuous variable for wait-list clearance time at registration. Therefore, with a total of 23 variables, we estimated that 115 ($=23 \times 10/2$) observed events per booking method would be needed, allowing for 10 events per regression variable [73]. Provisional runs of the model indicated that delay of surgery occurred about 1.1% of the time, and there were about 717 patients per hospital. Therefore, we estimated that we would need at least 16 runs ($\approx 115/[0.0105 \times 717]$) per method of booking appointments.

The estimates of the number of simulation runs required for each performance measure are summarized in Table 14.2. To ensure adequate power to detect clinically significant differences between the two experimental groups in each performance measure, the minimum number of simulation runs per experimental group had to meet the requirements for the performance measure with the largest number of simulation runs required. Therefore, the minimum number of simulation runs was 112.

14.4 Evaluation of Experiment

Analyses were conducted at the level of both the hospital and the patient. For analyses at the hospital level, we report differences between the two methods of booking surgical consultation appointments in terms of the average weekly number of patients waiting for appointments during weeks when no appointments were available, the average clearance time for appointment lists, and the odds of delay for high-priority elective procedures. For analyses at the patient level, we report differences between the two booking methods in terms of the weekly odds that a patient will have an appointment, the weekly odds that a patient will undergo elective surgery, and the odds that the surgery will be performed after the recommended time.

14.4.1 Statistical Instruments

To compare graphically the performance of booking methods for surgical consultation appointments at the level of the hospital, we used box plots to show the distribution of the average weekly number of patients waiting for appointments during weeks when no appointments were available and the distribution of average clearance time.

We used linear regression methods to model the relation between the booking method and the average weekly number of patients waiting for appointments during weeks when no appointments were available, or the average clearance time. We used logistic regression methods to model the probability of delay of any high-priority elective procedures in relation to the method of booking consultation appointments. We used multivariable regressions to adjust the effects of booking methods for hospital-level factors. In particular, we included sets of indicator variables as described in the previous section.

The coefficients derived from linear regression measured the effects of using the pooled-list method on the average weekly number of patients waiting for appointments during weeks when no appointments were available and the average clearance times for appointment lists, relative to the individual-lists method (i.e., the reference method) [159]. The average clearance time was estimated as the average of observed clearance times over 18 cycles for each run. The odds ratios derived from logistic regressions measured the effects of using the pooled-list method on the probability that any high-priority procedures would be delayed at a given hospital, relative to hospitals using the reference booking method [139].

To assess patient-level performance, we plotted the access curves from referral to appointment and from registration to surgery, by method of booking appointments and by priority group. We used discrete-time survival regression methods to model the relation between method of booking appointments and time to appointment or time to elective surgery, with adjustment for hospital-level and patient-level factors (see Table D.1 in Appendix D). We used logistic regression models, with adjustment for correlation between patients, to model the relation between the method of booking appointments and the probability of undergoing surgery after the recommended time. In these regression models, we adjusted for hospital-level and patient-level variables by including sets of indicator variables as described in the previous section.

The odds ratios derived from discrete-time survival regressions measured the effects of using the pooled-list method on the weekly proportion of patients on the appointment lists who received their surgical consultation appointments and who underwent the operation, relative to the individual-lists method [139]. The odds ratios derived from logistic regressions measured the effects of using the pooled-list method on the odds that a patient's surgery would be delayed relative to the individual-lists method.

14.4.2 Hospital and Patient Characteristics

The 224 simulation runs generated a total of 160,325 referrals for elective procedures, 167,207 urgent cases, and 12,107 emergency cases over six 18-week cycles of assignment of clinic and operating time starting on the arbitrarily chosen date of September 1, 2008. On average, the simulation model generated 345 elective referrals, 359 urgent cases, and 26 emergency arrivals per modeled hospital in one year. The modeled surgical services performed 666 procedures per year on average.

By design, there was a similar distribution of hospitals' characteristics across booking methods (Table 14.3). The distribution of referrals by patient-level factors was also similar across booking methods (Table 14.4). The majority of referrals were for men (83.6%), and 37.6% of the patients were 60–69 years old. Most patients had multivessel disease (73.6%) and either major or minor concurrent conditions (49.5%).

At the time of referral, 92.9% of the patients had low priority for the consultation. Regardless of the method of booking surgical consultation appointments, most of the referred patients had a consultation by the end of the simulation (94.1% for the individual-lists method and 95.8% for the pooled-list method). The rest of the patients were still waiting for an appointment because their referral times were close to the end of the simulation period. At the time of registration on a surgical wait list, 70.5% of patients had medium priority for the operation. The waiting time for elective surgery was less than half a week for 67.6% of the patients booked through the individual-lists method, but for only 54.2% with the pooled-list method.

Of all the patients who were registered on a surgical wait list, 78.4% underwent the planned procedure. The reasons for removal from the lists without surgery were similar across booking methods: 8.0% of planned procedures were canceled because no beds were available in the intensive care unit for recovery after surgery, and 9.1%

Table 14.3 Characteristics of simulated hospitals, by method of booking surgical consultation appointments

Characteristic	Booking method; no. (%) of hospitals	
	Individual lists ($n = 112$)	Pooled list ($n = 112$)
Method of booking surgery		
Wait-list booking	56 (50.0)	56 (50.0)
Advance booking	56 (50.0)	56 (50.0)
Allocation of operating room slots between elective and urgent procedures		
Weekly split	56 (50.0)	56 (50.0)
Daily split	56 (50.0)	56 (50.0)
Clearance time for appointment lists at start of simulation (weeks)		
1	37 (33.0)	37 (33.0)
2	38 (33.9)	38 (33.9)
3	37 (33.0)	37 (33.0)
Clearance time for surgical wait lists at start of simulation (weeks)		
3	28 (25.0)	28 (25.0)
4	28 (25.0)	28 (25.0)
5	28 (25.0)	28 (25.0)
6	28 (25.0)	28 (25.0)
Clearance time for inpatient surgical queues at start of simulation (weeks)		
0	38 (33.9)	38 (33.9)
1	37 (33.0)	37 (33.0)
2	37 (33.0)	37 (33.0)

of planned procedures were canceled because an inpatient was admitted for surgery. Another 4.5% of patients were removed from the list for other reasons, or they remained on the wait list at the end of the simulation.

14.4.3 Number of Patients on Appointment Lists

On average, 38 patients per week were waiting for surgical consultation appointments during weeks when no appointments were available in hospitals using the individual-lists method, whereas about 25 patients were waiting in hospitals using the pooled-list method (Fig. 14.1). The average weekly number of patients was about 12 fewer with the pooled-list method than with the individual-lists method (Table 14.5).

Table 14.4 Characteristics of simulated patients referred for surgical consultation, by method of booking surgical consultation appointments

Characteristic	Booking method; no. (%) of referrals			
	Individual lists ($n = 84,774$)		Pooled list ($n = 84,551$)	
Age group (years)				
<50	6,133	(7.2)	6,045	(7.1)
50–59	19,405	(22.9)	19,410	(23.0)
60–69	31,862	(37.6)	31,878	(37.7)
70–79	24,743	(29.2)	24,560	(29.0)
≥80	2,631	(3.1)	2,658	(3.1)
Sex				
Male	70,931	(83.7)	70,678	(83.6)
Female	13,843	(16.3)	13,873	(16.4)
Coronary anatomy affected				
Left main	14,166	(16.7)	14,223	(16.8)
Multivessel*	62,448	(73.7)	62,166	(73.5)
Limited†	8,160	(9.6)	8,162	(9.7)
Comorbidity				
Major conditions‡	18,845	(22.2)	18,980	(22.4)
Other conditions§	23,081	(27.2)	22,888	(27.1)
None	42,848	(50.5)	42,683	(50.5)
Priority of elective referral				
High	5,933	(7.0)	6,046	(7.2)
Low	78,841	(93.0)	78,505	(92.8)
Method of booking surgery				
Wait-list booking	42,412	(50.0)	42,211	(49.9)
Advance booking	42,362	(50.0)	42,340	(50.1)
Allocation of operating room slots between elective and urgent procedures				
Weekly split	42,268	(49.9)	42,384	(50.1)
Daily split	42,506	(50.1)	42,167	(49.9)
Clearance time for appointment lists at start of simulation (weeks)				
1	28,161	(33.2)	27,677	(32.7)
2	28,800	(34.0)	28,736	(34.0)
3	27,813	(32.8)	28,138	(33.3)
Clearance time for surgical wait lists at start of simulation (weeks)				
3	21,210	(25.0)	21,160	(25.0)
4	21,172	(25.0)	21,226	(25.1)
5	21,205	(25.0)	21,004	(24.8)
6	21,187	(25.0)	21,161	(25.0)

(continued)

Table 14.4 (continued)

	Booking method; no. (%) of referrals	
	Individual lists	Pooled list
Clearance time for inpatient surgical queues at start of simulation (weeks)		
0	28,725 (33.9)	28,795 (34.1)
1	28,125 (33.2)	27,877 (33.0)
2	27,924 (32.9)	27,879 (33.0)

∗Two- or three-vessel disease with proximal left anterior descending (PLAD) artery

†Two-vessel disease with no PLAD or one-vessel disease with PLAD

‡Congestive heart failure, diabetes mellitus, chronic obstructive pulmonary disease, rheumatoid arthritis, cancer

§Peripheral vascular disease, cerebrovascular disease, dementia, peptic ulcer disease, hemiplegia, renal disease, liver disease

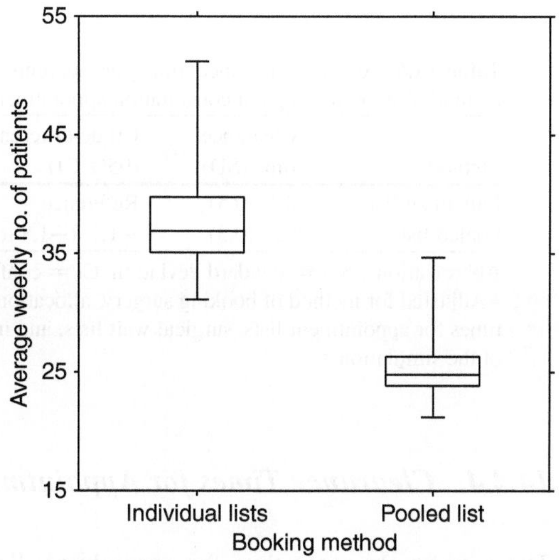

Fig. 14.1 Number of patients waiting for surgical consultation appointments during weeks when no appointments were available, by method of booking appointments

Table 14.5 Average weekly number of patients on appointment lists when no appointments were available, in relation to method of booking surgical consultation appointments

Method	No. of patients waiting (SD)	Crude difference (95% CI)	Adjusted difference (95% CI)∗
Individual lists	37.6 (3.6)	Reference	Reference
Pooled list	25.3 (2.2)	−12.3 (−13.1 to −11.5)	−12.3 (−13.1 to −11.5)

Abbreviations: SD = standard deviation, CI = confidence interval

∗Adjusted for method of booking surgery, allocation of operating room slots, clearance times for appointment lists, surgical wait lists, and inpatient surgical queues at the start of the simulation

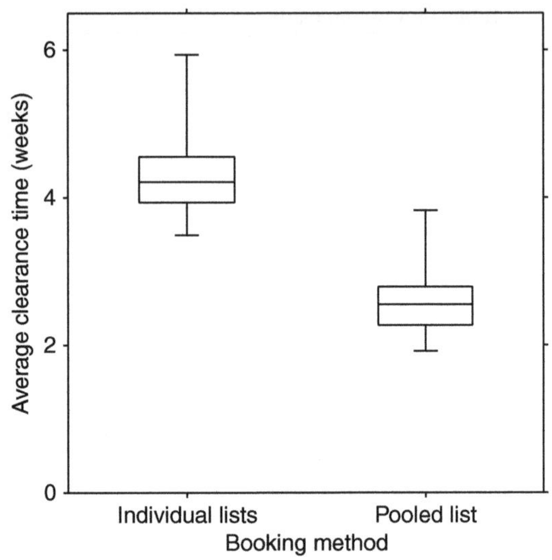

Fig. 14.2 Clearance time for appointment lists, by method of booking surgical consultation appointments

Table 14.6 Average clearance time for appointment lists in weeks, in relation to method of booking surgical consultation appointments

Method	Clearance time (SD)	Crude difference (95% CI)	Adjusted difference (95% CI)*
Individual lists	4.3 (0.5)	Reference	Reference
Pooled list	2.6 (0.3)	−1.7 (−1.8 to −1.6)	−1.7 (−1.8 to −1.6)

Abbreviations: SD = standard deviation, CI = confidence interval
*Adjusted for method of booking surgery, allocation of operating room slots, clearance times for appointment lists, surgical wait lists, and inpatient surgical queues at the start of the simulation

14.4.4 Clearance Times for Appointment Lists

The average clearance time for appointment lists was shorter when a pooled list was used than when individual lists were used (2.6 weeks vs. 4.3 weeks) (Fig. 14.2). After adjustment for hospital-level factors, the average clearance time was about 1.7 weeks shorter for the pooled-list method than for the individual-lists method (Table 14.6).

14.4.5 Proportion of Hospitals with Delay of Surgery

The proportion of hospitals with delays of any high-priority elective procedures was higher among hospitals using the pooled-list method than among those using the individual-lists method (about 55% vs. about 39%) (Table 14.7). The likelihood of a hospital having delays of high-priority elective procedures was over four times

Table 14.7 Proportion of hospitals with delay of any high-priority elective procedures, in relation to method of booking surgical consultation appointments

Method	% (no. of hospitals with delays/ total no. of hospitals)	Odds ratio (95% CI)*
Individual lists	39.3 (44/112)	1.0
Pooled list	54.5 (61/112)	4.4 (1.8–11.0)

Abbreviation: CI = confidence interval
*Adjusted for method of booking surgery, allocation of operating room slots clearance times for appointment lists, surgical wait lists, and inpatient surgical queues at the start of the simulation

Table 14.8 Weekly rate of surgical consultation appointments, in relation to method of booking surgical consultation appointments

Method	Appointment rate* (95% CI)	Ratio of weekly odds (95% CI)†
Individual lists	19.9 (19.8–20.0)	1.0
Pooled list	33.8 (33.6–34.1)	4.3 (4.3–4.4)

Abbreviation: CI = confidence interval
*Per 100 patient-weeks, calculated as the number of appointments divided by the total time in patient-weeks
†Adjusted for method of booking surgery, allocation of operating room slots, clearance times for appointment lists, surgical wait lists, and inpatient surgical queues at the start of the simulation, age, sex, coronary anatomy affected, comorbidities, priority at referral, and week from referral

greater with the pooled-list booking method than with the individual-lists method, after adjustment for hospital-level factors (Table 14.7).

14.4.6 Weekly Rate of Appointments

Among all patients referred for surgical consultation, the average weekly number of appointments was about 34 per 100 patients waiting for consultation in hospitals using the pooled-list method of booking and about 20 per 100 patients waiting for consultation in hospitals using the individual-lists method (Table 14.8). More than half of patients in hospitals using the pooled-list method received their appointments within 3 weeks, whereas the time required for more than half of patients in hospitals using the individual-lists method to receive their appointments was longer, at 5 weeks. After adjustment for hospital-level and patient-level factors, the weekly odds that a patient would receive an appointment were about 4.3 times greater with the pooled-list method than with the individual-lists method (Table 14.8).

We also evaluated the effect of booking method for each priority group at the time of referral for a surgical consultation. Among patients with high-priority at referral, the average weekly number of appointments was greater with the pooled-list method than with the individual-lists method (about 42 vs. about 24 per 100 patients remaining on the list) (Table 14.9). High-priority patients whose appointments were booked by the individual-lists method had longer waiting times (with about half

Table 14.9 Weekly rate of surgical consultation appointments among patients with high priority at referral, in relation to method of booking surgical consultation appointments

Method	No. of appointments	No. of patient-weeks	Appointment rate* (95% CI)	Ratio of weekly odds (95% CI)†
Individual lists	5,636	23,178	24.3 (23.7–25.0)	1.0
Pooled list	5,817	13,953	41.7 (40.6–42.8)	3.6 (3.4–3.8)

Abbreviation: CI = confidence interval
*Per 100 patient-weeks, calculated as the number of appointments divided by the total time in patient-weeks
†Adjusted for method of booking surgery, allocation of operating room slots, clearance times for appointment lists, surgical wait lists, and inpatient surgical queues at the start of the simulation, age, sex, coronary anatomy affected, comorbidities, and week from referral

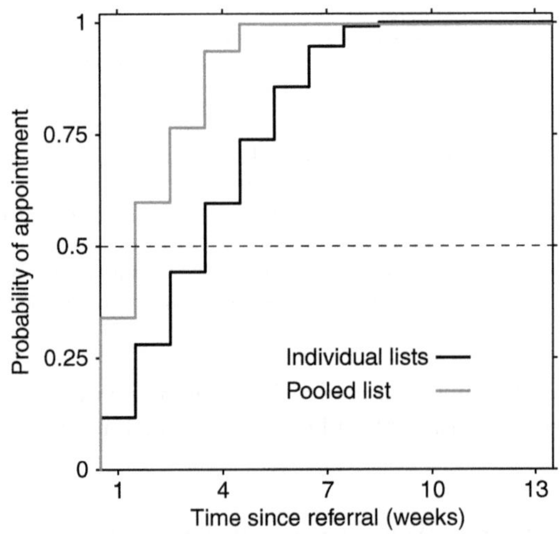

Fig. 14.3 Probability of surgical consultation within a certain time since referral among patients with high priority at referral, by method of booking appointments

having their appointments within 4 weeks) than those booked by the pooled-list method (with about half having their appointments within 2 weeks) (Fig. 14.3).

After adjustment for hospital-level and patient-level factors, the weekly odds that a high-priority patient on the wait list would have his or her appointment were 3.6 times greater with the pooled-list method than with the individual-lists method (Table 14.9). The effect of method of booking appointments was similar after additional adjustment for correlation between patients in the same hospital (odds ratio = 3.6, 95% confidence interval [CI] 3.4–3.8).

Among patients with low priority at the time of referral, the average weekly number of appointments was also greater with the pooled-list method than the individual-lists method (about 33 vs. about 20 per 100 patients remaining on the list) (Table 14.10). Low-priority patients who were booked in hospitals using the individual-lists method had longer waiting times (with about half having their appointments within 5 weeks) than those booked by the pooled-list method (with about half having their appointments within 3 weeks) (Fig. 14.4).

Table 14.10 Weekly rate of surgical consultation appointments among patients with low priority at referral, in relation to method of booking surgical consultation appointments

Method	No. of appointments	No. of patient-weeks	Appointment rate∗ (95% CI)	Ratio of weekly odds (95% CI)†
Individual lists	74,099	377,498	19.6 (19.5–19.8)	1.0
Pooled list	75,157	225,482	33.3 (33.1–33.6)	4.4 (4.3–4.4)

Abbreviation: CI = confidence interval

∗Per 100 patient-weeks, calculated as the number of appointments divided by the total time in patient-weeks

†Adjusted for method of booking surgery, allocation of operating room slots, clearance times for appointment lists, surgical wait lists, and inpatient surgical queues at the start of the simulation, age, sex, coronary anatomy affected, comorbidities, and week from referral

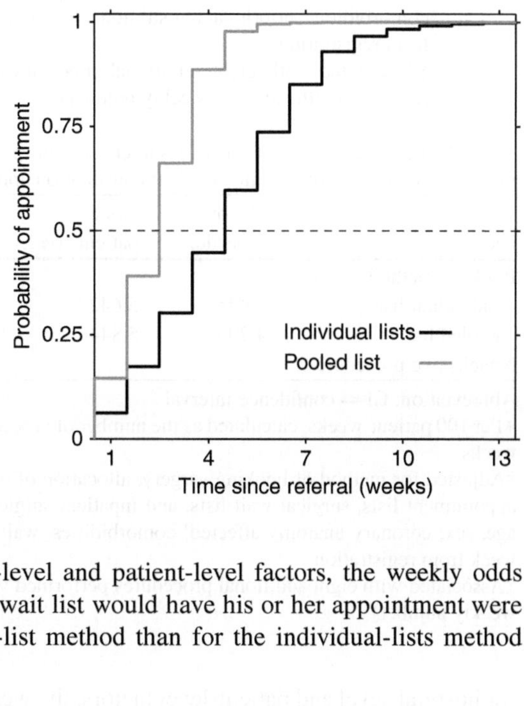

Fig. 14.4 Probability of surgical consultation within a certain time since referral among patients with low priority at referral, by method of booking appointments

After adjustment for hospital-level and patient-level factors, the weekly odds that a low-priority patient on the wait list would have his or her appointment were 4.4 times greater for the pooled-list method than for the individual-lists method (Table 14.10).

14.4.7 Weekly Rate of Surgery

Once a patient had a consultation, he or she was registered on a surgical wait list and assigned to one of three priority groups. Among all patients registered on the list, about half underwent surgery within 2 weeks of registration. The average weekly number of operations was lower with the pooled-list method of booking surgical consultation appointments than with the individual-lists method, about 29 vs. about 32 per 100 patients remaining on the list (Table 14.11). After adjustment

Table 14.11 Weekly rate of elective surgery, in relation to method of booking surgical consultation appointments

Factor	Surgery rate∗ (95% CI)	Ratio of weekly odds (95% CI)†
Booking method		
Individual lists	31.7 (31.4–31.9)	1.00
Pooled list	29.3 (29.1–29.5)	0.87 (0.86–0.88)
Nonelective procedures‡		0.41 (0.40–0.42)

Abbreviation: CI = confidence interval

∗Per 100 patient-weeks, calculated as the number of procedures divided by the total time in patient-weeks

†Adjusted for method of booking surgery, allocation of operating room slots, clearance times for appointment lists, surgical wait lists, and inpatient surgical queues at the start of the simulation, age, sex, coronary anatomy affected, comorbidities, priority at registration, clearance times at registration, and week from registration

‡Associated with eight additional procedures performed without wait-list registration (the average weekly number)

Table 14.12 Weekly rate of elective surgery among patients with high priority at registration, in relation to method of booking surgical consultation appointments

Factor	No. of procedures	No. of patient-weeks	Surgery rate∗ (95% CI)	Ratio of weekly odds (95% CI)†
Booking method				
Individual lists	4,645	5,642	82.3 (80.0–84.7)	1.00
Pooled list	4,799	5,844	82.1 (82.1–84.4)	0.92 (0.83–1.03)
Nonelective procedures‡				0.15 (0.12–0.17)

Abbreviation: CI = confidence interval

∗Per 100 patient-weeks, calculated as the number of procedures divided by the total time in patient-weeks

†Adjusted for method of booking surgery, allocation of operating room slots, clearance times for appointment lists, surgical wait lists, and inpatient surgical queues at the start of the simulation, age, sex, coronary anatomy affected, comorbidities, wait-list clearance times at registration, and week from registration

‡Associated with eight additional procedures performed without wait-list registration (the average weekly number)

for hospital-level and patient-level factors, the weekly odds that a patient on the wait list for elective surgery would undergo the operation were 13% lower in the pooled-list group than the individual-lists group (Table 14.11). Accounting for correlation between patients within the same hospital gave similar results (odds ratio = 0.85, 95% CI 0.83–0.87).

We also evaluated the effect of consultation booking method for each individual priority group at registration. In the high-priority group, the average weekly number of operations was similar, regardless of the booking method (about 82 procedures for every 100 patients remaining on the wait lists) (Table 14.12). High-priority patients also had similar waiting times, regardless of the booking method (with over half having their operations within 1 week) (Fig. 14.5).

Fig. 14.5 Probability of undergoing surgery within a certain time since registration among patients with high priority at registration, by method of booking appointments

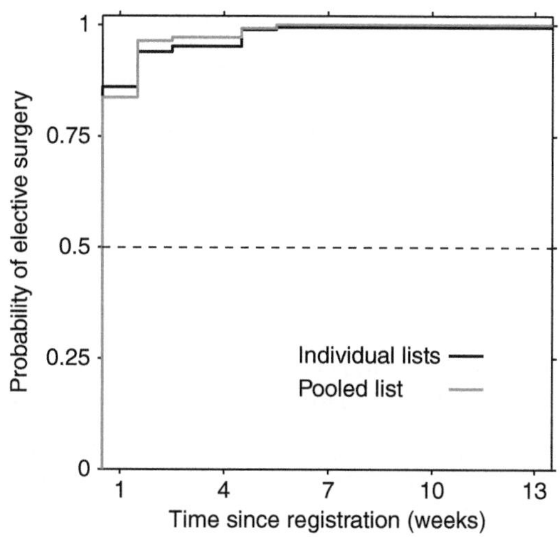

We adjusted the effect of consultation booking method on the odds of undergoing an operation for a variety of hospital-level and patient-level factors. After these adjustments, the weekly odds that a high-priority patient on the wait list for elective surgery would undergo the operation were similar either with the pooled-list or with the individual-lists method (Table 14.12). After adjustment for correlation between patients within the same hospital, the ratio of weekly odds of undergoing the operation did not change (odds ratio = 0.93, 95% CI 0.76–1.13).

In the medium-priority group, the average weekly number of operations was slightly higher in hospitals using the individual-lists method than in hospitals using the pooled-list method (Table 14.13). Regardless of the booking method, over half of the medium-priority patients waiting for elective surgery had their operations within 2 weeks (Fig. 14.6).

After adjustment for hospital-level and patient-level factors, the weekly odds that a medium-priority patient would undergo the operation were 13% lower in hospitals using the pooled-list method than in hospitals using the individual-lists method (Table 14.13). After adjustment for correlation between patients within the same hospital, the ratio of weekly odds of undergoing the operation did not change (odds ratio = 0.86, 95% CI 0.83–0.88).

Trends for the low-priority group were similar to those for the medium-priority group. Low-priority patients had longer waiting times with the pooled-list method than with the individual-lists method (with half having their operations within 4 vs. 3 weeks) (Fig. 14.7). The weekly odds of undergoing the operation were 16% lower among patients booked for surgical consultation by the pooled-list method than by the individual-lists method (Table 14.14). After adjustment for correlation between patients within the same hospital, the weekly odds of undergoing the operation were 38% lower with the pooled-list method than with the individual-lists method (odds ratio = 0.62, 95% CI 0.55–0.70).

Table 14.13 Weekly rate of elective surgery among patients with medium priority at registration, in relation to method of booking surgical consultation appointments

Factor	No. of procedures	No. of patient-weeks	Surgery rate* (95% CI)	Ratio of weekly odds (95% CI)†
Booking method				
Individual lists	43,563	127,186	34.3 (33.9–34.6)	1.00
Pooled list	43,597	136,235	32.0 (31.7–32.3)	0.87 (0.85–0.88)
Nonelective procedures‡				0.37 (0.36–0.38)

Abbreviation: CI = confidence interval

*Per 100 patient-weeks, calculated as the number of procedures divided by the total time in patient-weeks

†Adjusted for method of booking surgery, allocation of operating room slots, clearance times for appointment lists, surgical wait lists, and inpatient surgical queues at the start of the simulation, age, sex, coronary anatomy affected, comorbidities, wait-list clearance times at registration, and week from registration

‡Associated with eight additional procedures performed without wait-list registration (the average weekly number)

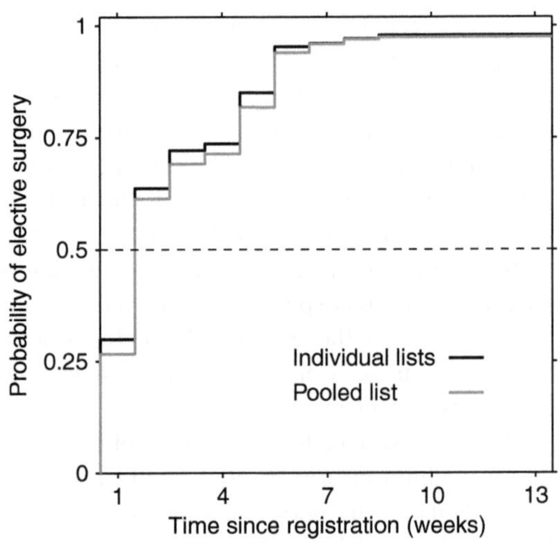

Fig. 14.6 Probability of undergoing surgery within a certain time since registration among patients with medium priority at registration, by method of booking appointments

14.4.8 Proportion of Surgeries After the Recommended Time

As described above, each patient was assigned to one of three priority groups at the time of registration on the surgical wait list. A patient was classified as having high priority if the recommended time to surgery was within three days, medium priority if the suggested time was within six weeks, and low priority if the recommended time was within 12 weeks. A patient who waited longer than the recommended time was considered to have delayed access to surgery.

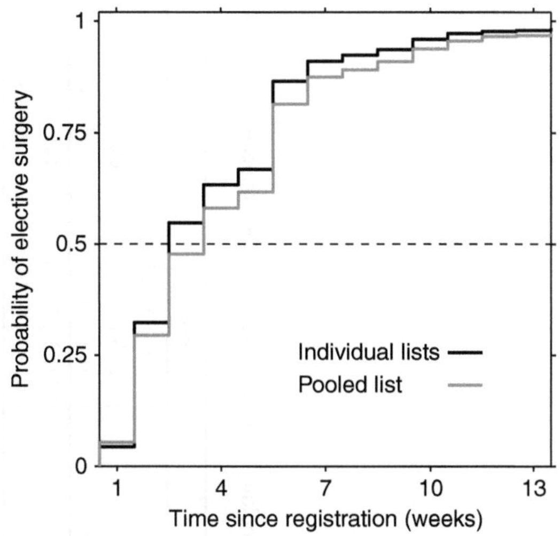

Fig. 14.7 Probability of undergoing surgery within a certain time since registration among patients with low priority at registration, by method of booking appointments

Table 14.14 Weekly rate of elective surgery among patients with low priority at registration, in relation to method of booking surgical consultation appointments

Factor	No. of procedures	No. of patient-weeks	Surgery rate* (95% CI)	Ratio of weekly odds (95% CI)†
Booking method				
Individual lists	14,557	65,210	22.3 (22.0–22.7)	1.00
Pooled list	14,888	73,752	20.2 (19.9–20.5)	0.84 (0.82–0.86)
Nonelective procedures‡				0.47 (0.45–0.48)

Abbreviation: CI = confidence interval

*Per 100 patient-weeks, calculated as the number of procedures divided by the total time in patient-weeks

†Adjusted for method of booking surgery, allocation of operating room slots, clearance times for appointment lists, surgical wait lists, and inpatient surgical queues at the start of the simulation, age, sex, coronary anatomy affected, comorbidities, wait-list clearance times at registration, and week from registration

‡Associated with eight additional procedures performed without wait-list registration (the average weekly number)

A greater percentage of high-priority elective procedures were delayed among patients booked in hospitals using the pooled-list method of booking surgical consultation appointments rather than the individual-lists method. The odds of delayed access to surgery were 45% higher with the pooled-list method (Table 14.15).

Similar results were observed for both the medium-priority and low-priority patients waiting for elective surgery. Relative to the individual-lists method, the odds of delayed access to surgery were 40% higher with the pooled-list method for medium-priority patients (Table 14.15) and 49% higher with the pooled-list method for low-priority patients, respectively (Table 14.15).

Table 14.15 Probability of undergoing surgery after the recommended time in relation to method of booking surgical consultation appointments, by priority at registration

	High priority		Medium priority		Low priority	
Method	% (no. of delayed procedures/total no. of procedures)	Odds ratio (95% CI)*	% (no. of delayed procedures/total no. of procedures)	Odds ratio (95% CI)*	% (no. of delayed procedures/total no. of procedures)	Odds ratio (95% CI)*
Individual lists	4.8 (271/5,636)	1.00	0.8 (439/56,357)	1.00	0.3 (52/17,742)	1.00
Pooled list	6.8 (398/5,817)	1.45 (1.22–1.73)	1.1 (641/56,895)	1.40 (1.24–1.59)	0.8 (139/18,262)	1.49 (1.05–2.11)

Abbreviation: CI = confidence interval

*Adjusted for method of booking surgery, allocation of operating room slots, clearance times for appointment lists, surgical wait lists, and inpatient surgical queues at the start of the simulation, age, sex, coronary anatomy affected, comorbidities, and wait-list clearance times at registration

14.5 Three-Way Comparison

In this section, we describe an expanded version of the study, in which we added a third option for booking surgical consultation appointments: placing patients on the list of the surgeon with the fewest patients waiting (the shortest-list method). Again, we used discrete-event simulation with a cluster randomized design, in which the unit of allocation was the hospital and the units of analysis were both the hospital and the patient. Our results suggest that clearance times were shorter in hospitals where patients waited for appointments in a single queue and that each week a larger proportion of patients were likely to have an appointment if they were in a single queue.

14.5.1 The Study Rationale

The analysis described earlier in this chapter suggested that the method of booking surgical consultation appointments may influence the time between consultation and surgery. For example, pooling referrals (i.e., placing all patients on one appointment list and booking appointments with the first available surgeon) seemed to reduce the time to consultation but increased the time to surgery for patients with nonurgent needs.

In surgical services where patients may see any one of a group of surgeons, directing patients to the shortest queue has long been considered a suitable alternative to the single-queue system of appointments [52]. This system differs in one important respect from a system of booking each appointment with the specific surgeon named in the referral, which is that a patient may have to see a surgeon other than the one who was recommended by the referring specialist. As argued by Murray and Berwick for the primary care setting [114], adopting this appointment system in a surgical services setting presents the patient with a trade-off between the value of consulting with the surgeon recommended by the referring physician and the value of early consultation, which might not be with the surgeon originally recommended.

The objective of this experiment was to estimate the effects of three methods of booking surgical consultation appointments—individual lists, pooled list, and shortest list—on the flow of patients from referral to consultation and from consultation to surgery in the context of cardiac surgical services. Box 14.2 summarizes the study rationale.

Box 14.2 What is already known and what this study adds on options for booking consultations

What is already known

- Placing the patient's name on the appointment list of the surgeon specified in the referral (i.e., the individual-lists method) is the most common method of booking appointments in surgical services where patients may see any one of a group of surgeons [156].
- Placing all patients' names on one appointment list and booking each appointment with the first available surgeon (i.e., the pooled-list method) reduces the time to consultation but increases the time to surgery for patients with nonurgent needs.
- In services where any one of a group of surgeons may see patients, directing patients to the surgeon with the shortest queue (i.e., the shortest-list method) has long been considered a suitable alternative to the single-queue system of appointments [52].

What this study adds

- This simulation study shows the effects of using the shortest-list method of booking surgical consultation appointments on the flow of patients from referral to consultation and from consultation to operation in the context of cardiac surgical services.

14.5.2 The Management Options

In this expanded study, we considered three methods of booking surgical consultation appointments. Two of the methods were compared in the study described earlier in this chapter (see Sects. 14.1–14.4): the individual-lists method and pooled-list method. The third method was the shortest-list method, whereby patients are placed on the list of the surgeon who has the fewest patients waiting.

14.5.3 Study Questions

The following study questions were of interest for this simulation experiment:

- Are there fewer patients waiting for surgical consultation appointments with the shortest-list method than with the individual-lists and pooled-list methods?
- Are clearance times for appointment lists shorter with the shortest-list method than clearance times with the individual-lists and pooled-list methods?
- Is there a lower chance that a hospital will have delayed high-priority elective procedures with the shortest-list method than with the individual-lists and pooled-list methods?
- Is the time to appointment shorter with the shortest-list method than with the individual-lists and pooled-list methods?
- Is the time to surgery shorter with the shortest-list method than with the individual-lists and pooled-list methods?

Table 14.16 Additional configurations of the discrete-event simulation model for comparing three methods of booking surgical consultation appointments

Configuration	Appointments	Elective operations
E	Shortest list	Wait-list booking
F	Shortest list	Advance booking

- Is there a lower chance of undergoing elective surgery after the recommended time with the shortest-list method than with the individual-lists and pooled-list methods?

14.5.4 Configurations of the Model

We developed two additional configurations of the discrete-event simulation model to implement the shortest-list method for booking surgical consultation appointments and the two methods of booking elective operations (Table 14.16). In these configurations of the model (configurations E and F), there were three priority lists with an aggregated referral rate represented by a single internal queue. Each patient referred for consultation was placed on the priority list of the surgeon with the fewest patients waiting. During each simulated week, the model booked patients waiting on the appointment list of the surgeon who was available for the clinic that week. For this expanded simulation experiment, all model requirements, modeling assumptions, and input parameters were identical with those described in Sect. 14.2.

14.5.5 Output Data

With one exception, the data dictionaries for comparing the three methods of booking appointments were identical with those used in the previous analysis (as listed in Tables D.1 and D.2 in Appendix D). The exception was the entry for the booking method, which was modified to take one of three values corresponding to the three methods of booking appointments.

14.5.6 Primary Study Factor

The primary study factor was the method of booking surgical consultation appointments, which in this study had three categories: individual appointment lists, pooled appointment list, and shortest appointment list. This study factor was represented by two indicator variables for the three methods of booking appointments, where we defined the pooled-list method as the reference group. These indicator variables were calculated from the variable `meth_app` in Table D.1 in Appendix D.

14.5.7 Performance Measures, Responses, Factors, and Effect-Size Measures

The performance measures at the hospital and patient levels remained the same as in the simulation experiment described earlier in this chapter. As a result, the experimental responses, hospital-level and patient-level factors, and measures of effect size were also unchanged (see Sect. 14.3).

14.5.8 Design of Experiment

Similar to the previous study for comparing two methods of booking surgical consultation appointments, we used a cluster randomized design, in which the unit of allocation was the simulation run, as described in Sect. 7.3. Each simulation run represented a simulated hospital. The number of simulation runs was chosen to detect the anticipated effects of the booking methods with high probability. With three methods of booking, we used the smallest anticipated difference between the shortest-list and pooled-list methods and between the individual-lists and pooled-list methods to determine the number of runs. In Part II of this book, we showed that calculations for patient-level performance measures require some information about the comparison groups, such as the anticipated number of patient-weeks that will be observed during the experiment. Therefore, if the calculations required information about the comparison groups (i.e., the individual-lists or shortest-list experimental groups), we performed two calculations: one for the comparison between the individual-lists group and the pooled-list group (i.e., the reference group) and the other for the comparison between the shortest-list group and the pooled-list group. We performed provisional runs of the simulation model, with 30 hospitals per experimental group, to estimate the magnitude of each performance measure in the reference group and to estimate the measures of variability and correlation needed for estimating the number of runs.

For comparison of the three methods of booking surgical consultation appointments, we calculated that 128 simulation runs per experimental group would be needed. This estimate was based on the maximum estimated number of runs across the hospital-level and patient-level performance measures of interest, as described below. All calculations assumed a two-sided test with 0.05 significance level and 90% power. Again, we used the Fedorov algorithm to ensure optimal distribution of the experimental factors across the runs [55].

Number of Runs for Cluster-Level Evaluations

We determined the number of runs needed to detect the anticipated difference in each hospital-level (i.e., cluster-level) performance measure in four calculations. First, we calculated the number of runs needed to detect a difference in the average weekly number of patients waiting for appointments during weeks when no appointments were available. According to provisional runs of the simulation model, the hypothesized value of this average was 25.4 patients (SD = 1.7) among hospitals using the pooled-list method. We estimated the number of simulation runs needed to detect a reduction in this average of eight patients with the individual-lists or shortest-list method. From the previous experiment, we anticipated a small number of hospitals per group. Instead of using the formula based on the normal distribution, which assumes a large number of runs, we used the calculation based on the t distribution. The number of simulation runs needed was about three per experimental group.

Second, we estimated the number of runs needed to detect a difference in the average weekly clearance time for appointment lists. The provisional runs showed that the hypothesized average weekly clearance time for appointments was 3.7 weeks (SD = 0.25) among hospitals using the pooled-list method. The number of simulation runs needed to detect a reduction of one week in this average clearance time in the individual-lists or shortest-list group was estimated. Again, from the previous experiment, we anticipated a small number of hospitals per group. Instead of using the formula based on the normal distribution, which assumes a large number of runs, we used the calculation based on the t distribution. The estimated number of simulation runs was three runs per experimental group.

Third, we estimated the number of runs needed to detect a difference in the proportion of hospitals with delay of any high-priority elective procedures. According to the provisional runs, the hypothesized proportion of hospitals with delay of any high-priority elective procedures was 0.53 among hospitals using the reference booking method (i.e., pooled-list method). The number of simulation runs needed to detect a decrease of 0.20 in this proportion in the individual-lists or shortest-list group was estimated. Using (8.8), we calculated the number of simulation runs needed (rounding up to the nearest integer) as follows:

$$\begin{aligned} k &= \left[\frac{1.96\sqrt{2(0.43)(1-0.43)} + 1.28\sqrt{0.53(1-0.53)+0.33(1-0.33)}}{0.33-0.53} \right]^2 \\ &\approx 127. \end{aligned}$$

Finally, for the purpose of regression analysis, we determined the number of runs to generate an adequate number of observations per regression variable. Our primary experimental factor was represented by two variables for methods of booking surgical consultation appointments. In addition, we used two variables for clearance times for appointment lists at the start of simulation, three variables for clearance times for surgical wait lists at the start of simulation, two variables for clearance times for inpatient surgical queues at the start of simulation, one variable for methods of booking surgery, and one variable for allocation of operating room slots. Therefore, with a total of 11 variables, we estimated that 37 ($\approx 11 \times 10/3$) observed events per booking method would be needed, allowing for 10 events per regression variable. From provisional runs of the model, the event of a hospital having a delay for any high-priority procedures occurred about 43% of the time. Therefore, we calculated that we would need at least 86 runs ($\approx 37/0.43$) per method of booking surgical consultation appointments.

Number of Runs for Individual-Level Evaluations

Similarly, we calculated the number of runs needed to detect the anticipated difference in each patient-level performance measure in four calculations. For analyses at the patient level, the dependence between experimental responses within each hospital necessitated adjustment for within-hospital correlation.

First, we estimated the number of runs needed to detect a difference in appointment rates among referrals. Given the results of provisional runs of the simulation model, we assumed an average of 3,132 patient-weeks per simulation run and a coefficient of variation of 0.03. The hypothesized weekly rate of appointments was 33 per 100 patient-weeks among hospitals using the pooled-list booking method. We estimated that six runs per booking method would allow us to detect a 10% increase in the weekly appointment rate between the pooled-list group and either the individual-lists or shortest-list group. [49]. It may be undesirable to assume an equal number of patient-weeks across hospitals and identical coefficients of variation between experimental groups. We therefore used (9.24) (Hayes method) to estimate the number of runs. We determined that for comparisons between the pooled-list and shortest-list methods, we would need five runs per method (rounding up to the nearest integer):

$$\begin{aligned} k &= 1 + \frac{(1.96 + 1.28)^2}{(0.33 - 0.33 \times 1.10)^2} \times \left(\frac{0.33}{2{,}201} + \frac{0.33 \times 1.10}{3{,}643} + 0.0001120 \right) \\ &\approx 5. \end{aligned}$$

Similarly, we determined that for comparisons between the pooled-list and individual-lists methods, we would need six runs per method (rounding up to the nearest integer):

$$\begin{aligned} k &= 1 + \frac{(1.96 + 1.28)^2}{(0.33 - 0.33 \times 1.10)^2} \times \left(\frac{0.33}{2{,}201} + \frac{0.33 \times 1.10}{3{,}513} + 0.0001647 \right) \\ &\approx 6. \end{aligned}$$

Second, we calculated the number of runs required to detect a difference in rates of surgery among registered patients. From the provisional runs, we assumed an average of 1,788 patient-weeks per simulation run and a coefficient of variation of

0.13. The hypothesized weekly rate of surgery was 30 per 100 patient-weeks among hospitals using the pooled-list method. We estimated that 44 runs per booking method would allow us to detect a 10% increase in the weekly surgery rate between groups of patients [49]. Again, it may be undesirable to assume an equal number of patient-weeks across hospitals and identical coefficients of variation between experimental groups. We therefore used the alternative (9.24) (Hayes' method) to estimate the number of runs (rounding up to the nearest integer) as follows:

$$\begin{aligned} k &= 1 + \frac{(1.96 + 1.28)^2}{(0.30 - 0.30 \times 1.10)^2} \times \left(\frac{0.30}{1{,}878} + \frac{0.30 \times 1.10}{1{,}695} + 0.003219 \right) \\ &\approx 43. \end{aligned}$$

Similarly, we estimated the number of runs needed for comparisons between the pooled-list and individual-lists methods:

$$\begin{aligned} k &= 1 + \frac{(1.96 + 1.28)^2}{(0.30 - 0.30 \times 1.10)^2} \times \left(\frac{0.30}{1{,}698} + \frac{0.30 \times 1.10}{1{,}695} + 0.002845 \right) \\ &\approx 39. \end{aligned}$$

Third, we estimated the number of runs required to detect a difference in the proportion of patients undergoing elective procedures after the recommended time. The hypothesized proportion of patients whose surgery was delayed was 0.10 among patients whose surgical consultation appointments were booked with the pooled-list method. We estimated that seven runs per booking method would yield 90% power to detect a 0.05 decrease in this proportion between groups of patients [49]. We used (9.9) to calculate the intracluster correlation coefficient, ρ, which is the ratio of the between-cluster and within-cluster variation, as follows:

$$\hat{\rho} = \frac{0.08434 - 0.01009}{0.08434 + (702.3 - 1)(0.01009)} \approx 0.01049.$$

Then, using (9.14), we estimated the inflation factor:

$$\text{IF} = 1 + (702 - 1)(0.01049) \approx 8.4.$$

Therefore, because of the clustered nature of the experimental design, we determined that we would need almost nine times as many patients in our experiment with randomization at the level of runs than in an experiment with randomization at the level of individual patients. We then computed the number of runs per experimental group using (9.13) (rounding up to the nearest integer):

$$k = \frac{(1.96 + 1.28)^2[0.10(1 - 0.10) + 0.05(1 - 0.05)]}{707(0.05 - 0.10)^2} 8.4 \approx 7.$$

Table 14.17 Number of simulation runs required to compare three methods of booking surgical consultation appointments with 0.05 significance level and 90% power, per experimental group

Performance measure	Reference value	Effect size	No. of runs
Hospital level			
Average weekly number of patients waiting for appointments during weeks when no appointments available (standard deviation)	25.4 (1.7)	8-patient decrease	3
Average clearance time for appointments in weeks (standard deviation)	3.7 (0.25)	1-week decrease	3
Proportion of hospitals with delay of any high-priority procedures	0.53	0.20 decrease	127*
Patient level			
Appointment rate per 100 patient-weeks	33	10% increase	6
Surgery rate per 100 patient-weeks	30	10% increase	43
Proportion of patients with surgery after recommended time	0.10	0.05 decrease	7

*86 runs required to allow 10 events per regression variable in cluster-level evaluation

Finally, for the purpose of the regression analyses, we determined the number of runs needed to generate an adequate number of observations per regression variable. Our primary study factor was represented by two variables for methods of booking surgical consultation appointments. In addition, we used two variables for clearance times for appointment lists at the start of simulation, three variables for clearance times for surgical wait lists at the start of simulation, two variables for clearance times for inpatient surgical queues at the start of simulation, one variable for methods of booking surgery, and one variable for allocation of operating room slots. The patient-level variables included one variable for sex, four variables for age groups, two variables for categories of coronary anatomy affected, two variables for categories of comorbidity, two variables for priorities at registration, one time-dependent continuous variable for the weekly number of inpatient and emergency procedures, and one time-dependent continuous variable for wait-list clearance time at registration. Therefore, with a total of 24 variables, we estimated that 80 ($=24\times10/3$) observed events per booking method would be needed, allowing for 10 events per regression variable [73]. From provisional runs of the model, the event of a patient's surgery being delayed after the recommended time occurred about 1.0% of the time, and there were about 707 patients per hospital. Therefore, we calculated that at least 11 runs ($\approx 80/(0.0103\times 707)$) per method would be needed.

The estimates of the number of simulation runs required for each performance measure are summarized in Table 14.17. To ensure adequate power to detect clinically significant differences between the experimental groups in each performance measure, the minimum number of simulation runs per experimental group had to meet the requirements for the performance measure with the largest number of simulation runs required. Therefore, the minimum number of simulation runs was

Table 14.18 Coding for a set of two indicator variables representing three methods of booking surgical consultation appointments

Method	Variable I_1	Variable I_2
Pooled list	0	0
Individual lists	1	0
Shortest list	0	1

127 per experimental group. In our simulation experiment, we actually allocated 128 runs per group. Because 128 is divisible by two and four, the number of runs with each value of a hospital-level factor with two or four categories could then be equally distributed.

14.5.9 Evaluation of Experiment

We compared the three methods of booking surgical consultation appointments using the same performance measures and statistical instruments as were used to compare two booking methods (see Sect. 14.4). In the regression analyses, we used a set of two indicator variables to represent the three methods of booking appointments, with the pooled-list method as the reference group. For regression analyses at the hospital level, the linear regression coefficients for the indicator variables, I_1 and I_2, measured the effects of using the individual-lists method and the shortest-list method, respectively, relative to the pooled-list method, on the average weekly number of patients waiting for appointments during weeks when no appointments were available and the average clearance times for appointment lists (Table 14.18). The odds ratios derived from logistic regressions measured the effects of using the individual-lists and shortest-list methods on the probability that any high-priority elective procedures would be delayed, relative to using the pooled-list method.

For regression analyses at the patient level, the odds ratios derived from discrete-time survival regressions measured the effects of using the individual-lists and shortest-list methods on the weekly proportion of patients on the appointment lists who received their appointments and who underwent the operation, relative to using the pooled-list method [139]. The odds ratios derived from logistic regressions measured the effects of using the individual-lists and shortest-list methods on the odds that a patient's access to surgery would be delayed, relative to the pooled-list method.

Hospital and Patient Characteristics

The 384 simulation runs generated a total of 289,989 referrals for elective procedures, 285,486 urgent cases, and 20,557 emergency cases over six 18-week cycles starting on the arbitrarily chosen date of September 1, 2008. On average, the simulation model generated 364 elective referrals, 358 urgent cases, and 26 emergency arrivals per modeled hospital in one year. The modeled surgical services performed 660 procedures per year on average.

Table 14.19 Characteristics of simulated hospitals for three methods of booking surgical consultation appointments

	Booking method; no. (%) of hospitals		
Characteristic	Pooled list (n = 128)	Individual lists (n = 128)	Shortest list (n = 128)
Method of booking surgery			
Wait-list booking	64 (50.0)	64 (50.0)	64 (50.0)
Advance booking	64 (50.0)	64 (50.0)	64 (50.0)
Allocation of OR slots between elective and urgent procedures			
Weekly split	64 (50.0)	64 (50.0)	64 (50.0)
Daily split	64 (50.0)	64 (50.0)	64 (50.0)
Clearance time for appointment lists at start of simulation (weeks)			
1	42 (32.8)	43 (33.6)	43 (33.6)
2	43 (33.6)	42 (32.8)	43 (33.6)
3	43 (33.6)	43 (33.6)	42 (32.8)
Clearance time for surgical wait lists at start of simulation (weeks)			
3	32 (25.0)	32 (25.0)	32 (25.0)
4	32 (25.0)	32 (25.0)	32 (25.0)
5	32 (25.0)	32 (25.0)	32 (25.0)
6	32 (25.0)	32 (25.0)	32 (25.0)
Clearance time for inpatient surgical queues at start of simulation (weeks)			
0	43 (33.6)	43 (33.6)	42 (32.8)
1	42 (32.8)	43 (33.6)	43 (33.6)
2	43 (33.6)	42 (32.8)	43 (33.6)

Abbreviation: OR = operating room

By design, the distribution of hospitals by hospital-level factors was uniform across booking methods (Table 14.19). The distribution of referrals by patient-level factors was also similar across booking methods (Table 14.20). The majority of referrals were for men (83.7%), and 37.8% of the patients were 60–69 years old. Most patients had multivessel disease (73.6%) and either major or minor concurrent conditions (49.3%).

At the time of referral, 92.9% of the patients had low priority for the consultation. Regardless of the method of booking surgical consultation appointments, most of the referred patients had a consultation by the end of the simulation (95.7% for the pooled-list method, 93.9% for the individual-lists method, and 93.8% for the shortest-list method). The rest of the patients were still waiting for an appointment because their referral times were close to the end of the simulation period.

At the time of registration on a surgical wait list, 7.2% of the patients had high priority of the operation, 70.5% had medium priority, and 22.3% had low priority. The waiting time for elective surgery was less than half a week for 69.4% of the patients booked through the individual-lists method and for 65.7% of those booked

Table 14.20 Characteristics of simulated patients for three methods of booking surgical consultation appointments

	Booking method; no. (%) of referrals		
Characteristic	Pooled list ($n = 96,037$)	Individual lists ($n = 96,570$)	Shortest list ($n = 97,382$)
Age group (years)			
<50	6,926 (7.2)	6,801 (7.0)	6,851 (7.0)
50–59	21,841 (22.7)	22,115 (22.9)	22,154 (22.7)
60–69	36,166 (37.7)	36,422 (37.7)	37,125 (38.1)
70–79	28,155 (29.3)	28,207 (29.2)	28,167 (28.9)
≥80	2,949 (3.1)	3,025 (3.1)	3,085 (3.2)
Sex			
Male	80,165 (83.5)	80,949 (83.8)	81,531 (83.7)
Female	15,872 (16.5)	15,621 (16.2)	15,851 (16.3)
Coronary anatomy affected			
Left main	16,238 (16.9)	16,158 (16.7)	16,481 (16.9)
Multivessel*	70,406 (73.3)	71,346 (73.9)	71,719 (73.6)
Limited†	9,393 (9.8)	9,066 (9.4)	9,182 (9.4)
Comorbidity			
Major conditions‡	21,529 (22.4)	21,377 (22.1)	21,824 (22.4)
Other conditions§	26,153 (27.2)	26,119 (27.0)	26,442 (27.2)
None	48,355 (50.4)	49,074 (50.8)	49,116 (50.4)
Priority of elective referral			
High	6,911 (7.2)	6,909 (7.2)	6,880 (7.1)
Low	89,126 (92.8)	89,661 (92.8)	90,502 (92.9)
Method of booking surgery			
Wait-list booking	47,878 (49.9)	48,317 (50.0)	48,706 (50.0)
Advance booking	48,159 (50.1)	48,253 (50.0)	48,676 (50.0)
Allocation of OR slots between elective and urgent procedures			
Weekly split	48,083 (50.1)	48,092 (49.8)	48,765 (50.1)
Daily split	47,954 (49.9)	48,478 (50.2)	48,617 (49.9)
Clearance time for appointment lists at start of simulation (weeks)			
1	31,654 (33.0)	32,483 (33.6)	32,815 (33.7)
2	32,027 (33.3)	31,745 (32.9)	33,028 (33.9)
3	32,356 (33.7)	32,342 (33.5)	31,539 (32.4)
Clearance time for surgical wait lists at start of simulation (weeks)			
3	24,046 (25.0)	24,109 (25.0)	24,514 (25.2)
4	23,969 (25.0)	24,208 (25.1)	24,156 (24.8)
5	23,986 (25.0)	24,145 (25.0)	24,251 (24.9)
6	24,036 (25.0)	24,108 (25.0)	24,461 (25.1)

(continued)

Table 14.20 (continued)

	Booking method (no. (%) of referrals)		
Characteristic	Pooled list ($n = 96,037$)	Individual lists ($n = 96,570$)	Shortest list ($n = 97,382$)
Clearance time for inpatient surgical queues at start of simulation (weeks)			
0	32,035 (33.4)	32,185 (33.3)	31,936 (32.8)
1	31,426 (32.7)	32,639 (33.8)	32,829 (33.7)
2	32,576 (33.9)	31,746 (32.9)	32,617 (33.5)

Abbreviation: OR = operating room
*Two- or three-vessel disease with proximal left anterior descending (PLAD) artery
†Two-vessel disease with no PLAD or one-vessel disease with PLAD
‡Congestive heart failure, diabetes mellitus, chronic obstructive pulmonary disease, rheumatoid arthritis, cancer
§Peripheral vascular disease, cerebrovascular disease, dementia, peptic ulcer disease, hemiplegia, renal disease, liver disease

through the shortest-list method, but for only 54.4% of those booked with the pooled-list method.

Of all the patients who were registered on a surgical wait list, 78.5% underwent the planned procedure. The reasons for removal from the lists without surgery were similar across booking methods: 8.2% of planned procedures were canceled because no beds were available in the intensive care unit for recovery after surgery, and 8.9% of planned procedures were canceled because an inpatient was admitted for surgery. Another 4.2% of patients were removed from the list for other reasons, or they remained on the wait list at the end of the simulation.

Number of Patients on Appointment Lists

On average, about 37 and 39 patients per week were waiting for surgical consultation appointments during weeks when no appointments were available in hospitals using the individual-lists and shortest-list methods, respectively, whereas about 25 patients were waiting in hospitals using the pooled-list method. After adjustment for hospital-level factors, the average weekly numbers of patients waiting were about 12 and 14 more with the individual-lists and shortest-list methods, respectively, than with the pooled-list method (Table 14.21).

Clearance Times for Appointment Lists

The average clearance time for appointment lists was longer when appointments were booked with the individual-lists method (5.1 weeks) or the shortest-list method (5.4 weeks) rather than the pooled-list method (3.6 weeks). After adjustment for hospital-level factors, the average clearance time was about 1.5 weeks longer for the individual-lists method and 1.8 weeks longer for the shortest-list method than for the pooled-list method (Table 14.22).

Table 14.21 Average weekly number of patients on appointment lists when no appointments were available for three methods of booking surgical consultation appointments

Method	No. of patients waiting (SD)	Crude difference (95% CI)	Adjusted difference∗ (95% CI)
Pooled list	25.0 (1.6)	Reference	Reference
Individual lists	36.9 (3.7)	12.0 (11.3–12.6)	12.0 (11.3–12.6)†
Shortest list	39.0 (2.1)	14.0 (13.4–14.7)	14.0 (13.4–14.7)†

Abbreviations: SD = standard deviation, CI = confidence interval, df = degrees of freedom
∗Adjusted for method of booking surgery, allocation of operating room slots, clearance times for appointment lists, surgical wait lists, and inpatient surgical queues at the start of the simulation
†Difference between individual-lists and shortest-list methods: F statistic = 39.3; df = 1, 372; $p < 0.001$

Table 14.22 Average clearance time for appointment lists for three methods of booking surgical consultation appointments

Method	Clearance time (SD)	Crude difference (95% CI)	Adjusted difference∗ (95% CI)
Pooled list	3.6 (0.2)	Reference	Reference
Individual lists	5.1 (0.5)	1.5 (1.4–1.6)	1.5 (1.4–1.6)†
Shortest list	5.4 (0.3)	1.8 (1.7–1.8)	1.8 (1.7–1.8)†

Abbreviations: SD = standard deviation, CI = confidence interval, df = degrees of freedom
∗Adjusted for method of booking surgery, allocation of operating room slots, clearance times for appointment lists, surgical wait lists, and inpatient surgical queues at the start of the simulation
†Difference between individual-lists and shortest-list methods: F statistic = 33.8; df = 1, 372; $p < 0.001$

Proportion of Hospitals with Delay of Surgery

The proportion of hospitals with delay of any high-priority elective procedures was about 10% lower with the individual-lists method and the shortest-list method (both about 38%) than with the pooled-list method (about 48%). The odds of a hospital having delays for high-priority elective procedures were more than 60% lower with both the individual-lists and shortest-list methods than the pooled-list method, after adjustment for hospital-level factors (Table 14.23).

Weekly Rate of Appointments

In the high-priority group, about 6,500 appointments were received in each experimental group over a varying number of total patient-weeks (6,614 appointments over 15,804 patient-weeks with the pooled-list method, 6,554 appointments over 26,632 patient-weeks with the individual-lists method, and 6,455 appointments over 31,925 patient-weeks with the shortest-list method). The average weekly number of appointments was smaller with the individual-lists method (about 25 per 100 patients remaining on the list) and with the shortest-list method (about 20 per 100 patients

Table 14.23 Proportion of hospitals with delay of any high-priority elective procedures for three methods of booking surgical consultation appointments

Method	% (no. of hospitals with delays/ total no. of hospitals)	Odds ratio (95% CI)∗
Pooled list	47.7 (61/128)	1.00
Individual lists	38.3 (49/128)	0.38 (0.17–0.86)†
Shortest list	36.7 (47/128)	0.36 (0.16–0.79)†

Abbreviations: CI = confidence interval, df = degrees of freedom
∗Adjusted for method of booking surgery, allocation of operating room slots, clearance times for appointment lists, surgical wait lists, and inpatient surgical queues at the start of the simulation
†No difference between individual-lists and shortest-list methods: Wald chi-square statistic = 0.3; df = 1, $p = 0.86$

remaining on the list) than with the pooled-list method (about 42 per 100 patients remaining on the list) (Table 14.24).

High-priority patients whose appointments were booked by the individual-lists and shortest-list methods had longer waiting times (with about half having their appointments within 4 and 5 weeks, respectively) than those booked by the pooled-list method (with about half having their appointments within 2 weeks) (Fig. 14.8). After adjustment for hospital-level and patient-level factors, the weekly odds that a high-priority patient on the wait list would have his or her appointment were about 73% and 82% lower for the individual-lists and shortest-list methods, respectively, relative to the pooled-list method (Table 14.24). The effects of booking patients using the individual-lists or shortest-list method relative to the pooled-list method were similar after additional adjustment for correlation between patients in the same hospital (adjusted odds ratio = 0.27, 95% CI 0.26–0.29 for individual-lists method vs. pooled-list method; adjusted odds ratio = 0.18, 95% CI 0.17–0.19 for shortest-list method vs. pooled-list method).

The method of booking appointments had a similar effect on appointment rates for patients with low priority at referral. In the low-priority group, about 85,000 appointments were received in each experimental group over an average of about 371,000 patient-weeks (85,279 appointments over 252,699 patient-weeks with the pooled-list method, 84,132 appointments over 421,933 patient-weeks with the individual-lists method, and 84,887 appointments over 438,867 patient-weeks with the shortest-list method). The average weekly number of appointments was also smaller with the individual-lists method (about 20 per 100 patients remaining on the list) and the shortest-list method (about 19 per 100 patients remaining on the list) than with the pooled-list method (about 34 per 100 patients remaining on the list) (Table 14.24).

Low-priority patients who were booked in hospitals using the individual-lists or shortest-list method had longer waiting times (with about half having their appointments within 5 weeks) than those booked by the pooled-list method (with about half having their appointments within 3 weeks) (Fig. 14.9). After adjustment for hospital-level and patient-level factors, the weekly odds that a low-priority patient on the wait list would have his or her appointment were about 80% lower

Table 14.24 Weekly rate of surgical consultation appointments for three booking methods, by priority at referral

	High priority		Low priority	
Method	Appointment rate* (95% CI)	Ratio of weekly odds (95% CI)†	Appointment rate* (95% CI)	Ratio of weekly odds (95% CI)†
Pooled list	41.9 (40.8–42.9)	1.00	33.7 (33.5–34.0)	1.00
Individual lists	24.6 (24.0–25.2)	0.27 (0.26–0.28)‡	19.9 (19.8–20.1)	0.22 (0.22–0.22)§
Shortest list	20.2 (19.7–20.7)	0.18 (0.17–0.19)‡	19.3 (19.2–19.5)	0.21 (0.21–0.22)§

Abbreviations: CI = confidence interval, df = degrees of freedom

*Per 100 patient-weeks, calculated as the number of appointments divided by the total time in patient-weeks

†Adjusted for method of booking surgery, allocation of operating room slots, clearance times for appointment lists, surgical wait lists, and inpatient surgical queues at the start of the simulation, age, sex, coronary anatomy affected, comorbidities, and week from referral

‡Difference between individual-lists and shortest-list methods: Wald chi-square statistic = 350.6, df = 1, $p < 0.01$

§Difference between individual-lists and shortest-list methods: Wald chi-square statistic = 27.3, df = 1, $p < 0.01$

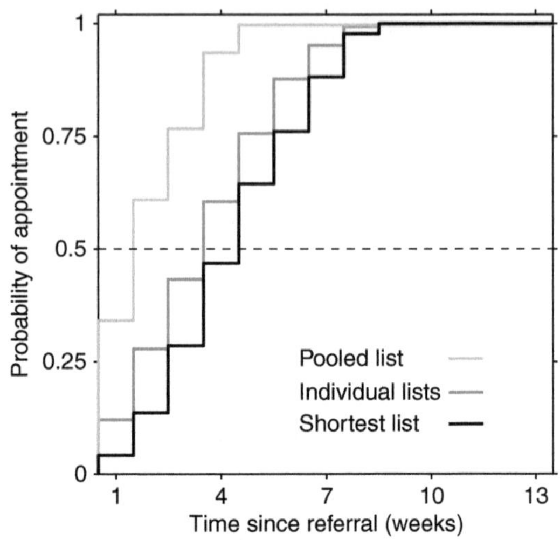

Fig. 14.8 Probability of surgical consultation within a certain time since referral among patients with high priority at referral, in a comparison of three methods of booking appointments

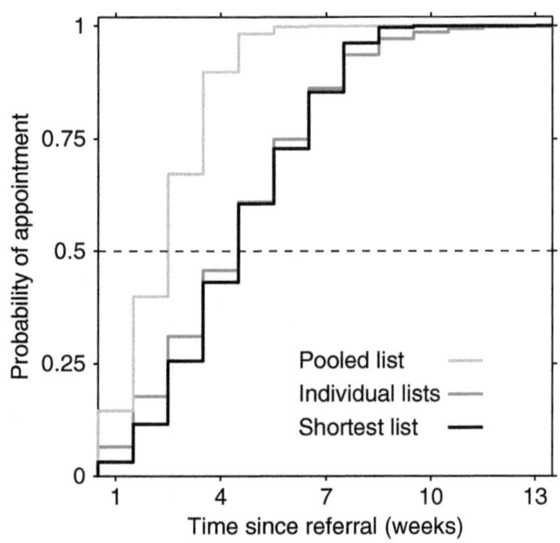

Fig. 14.9 Probability of surgical consultation within a certain time since referral among patients with low priority at referral, in a comparison of three methods of booking appointments

for the individual-lists and shortest-list methods relative to the pooled-list method (Table 14.24).

Weekly Rate of Surgery

We modeled registration on a surgical wait list where patients were assigned to one of three priority groups. In the high-priority group, the average weekly number of operations was similar for the shortest-list and pooled-list methods (about 83 procedures for every 100 patients remaining on the wait list), whereas the rate was slightly higher with the individual-lists method (about 85 procedures for every 100 patients remaining on the wait list) (Table 14.25).

Table 14.25 Weekly rate of elective surgery for three methods of booking surgical consultation appointments, by priority at registration

	High priority		Medium priority		Low priority	
Method	Surgery rate* (95% CI)	Ratio of weekly odds (95% CI)†	Surgery rate* (95% CI)	Ratio of weekly odds (95% CI)†	Surgery rate* (95% CI)	Ratio of weekly odds (95% CI)†
Pooled list	83.4 (81.2–85.7)	1.00	32.3 (32.0–32.6)	1.00	20.2 (19.9–20.6)	1.00
Individual lists	85.4 (83.1–87.6)	1.17 (1.05–1.30)‡	34.7 (34.4–35.0)	1.15 (1.13–1.17)§	22.7 (22.3–23.0)	1.19 (1.16–1.22)‖
Shortest list	83.5 (81.3–85.7)	1.09 (0.98–1.20)‡	34.3 (34.0–34.6)	1.12 (1.10–1.14)§	22.5 (22.2–22.9)	1.18 (1.15–1.22)‖

Abbreviations: CI = confidence interval, df = degrees of freedom

*Per 100 patient-weeks, calculated as the number of procedures divided by the total time in patient-weeks and is reported per 100 patient-weeks

†Adjusted for method of booking surgery, allocation of operating room slots, clearance times appointment lists, surgical wait lists, and inpatient surgical queues, age, sex, coronary anatomy affected, comorbidities, wait-list clearance times at registration, and week from registration

‡No difference between individual-lists and shortest-list methods: Wald chi-square statistic = 1.9, df = 1, $p = 0.17$

§Difference between individual-lists and shortest-list methods: Wald chi-square statistic = 7.6, df = 1, $p < 0.01$

‖No difference between individual-lists and shortest-list methods: Wald chi-square statistic = 0.07, df = 1, $p = 0.70$

Regardless of the method of booking surgical consultation appointments, high-priority patients had similar waiting times (with over half having their operations within 1 week). After adjustment for hospital-level and patient-level factors, the weekly odds that a high-priority patient on the wait list for elective surgery would undergo the operation did not differ between the shortest-list and pooled-list methods, but the likelihood of operation were about 17% higher with the individual-lists method than with the pooled-list method (Table 14.25). The likelihood of operation decreased by 84% for every eight additional procedures performed without registration on a wait list (odds ratio = 0.16, 95% CI 0.14–0.19). After adjustment for correlation between patients within the same hospital, the ratio of weekly odds of surgery did not change (for shortest-list method vs. pooled-list method, odds ratio = 1.08, 95% CI 0.96–1.22; for individual-lists method vs. pooled-list method, odds ratio = 1.17, 95% CI 1.04–1.31).

In the medium-priority group, almost 50,000 operations were performed in each experimental group over about 150,000 patient-weeks (49,719 procedures over 153,772 patient-weeks with the pooled-list method, 49,471 procedures over 142,583 patient-weeks with the individual-lists method, and 49,885 procedures over 145,279 patient-weeks with the shortest-list method). The average weekly number of operations was slightly higher in hospitals using the individual-lists or the shortest-list method than in hospitals using the pooled-list method (Table 14.25). Regardless of the booking method, more than half of the medium-priority elective patients had their operations within 2 weeks. After adjustment for hospital-level and patient-level factors, the weekly odds that a medium-priority patient waiting for elective surgery would undergo the operation were 15% higher in hospitals using the individual-lists method and 12% higher in hospitals using the shortest-list method than in hospitals using the pooled-list method (Table 14.25). The likelihood of operation decreased by 63% for every eight additional procedures performed without registration on a wait list (odds ratio = 0.37, 95% CI 0.36–0.38). After adjustment for correlation between patients within the same hospital, the ratio of weekly odds of surgery did not change (for individual-lists method vs. pooled-list method, adjusted odds ratio = 1.16, 95% CI 1.14–1.19; for shortest-list method vs. pooled-list method, adjusted odds ratio = 1.14, 95% CI 1.11–1.17).

The trends for the low-priority group were similar to those for the medium-priority group. The numbers of procedures performed were 16,806 over 82,993 patient-weeks with the pooled-list method, 16,698 over 73,600 patient-weeks with the individual-lists method, and 16,632 over 73,798 patient-weeks with the shortest-list method. The average weekly number of operations was higher with the individual-lists and shortest-list methods than with the pooled-list method (Table 14.25). Low-priority patients had shorter waiting times with the individual-lists and shortest-list methods (with half having their operations within 3 weeks) than with the pooled-list method (with half having their operations within 4 weeks). The weekly odds of undergoing the operation were 19% higher among patients booked by the individual-lists method and 18% higher among patients booked by the shortest-list method relative to the pooled-list method (Table 14.25). The likelihood of operation decreased by 53% for every eight additional procedures performed without registration on a wait list (odds ratio = 0.47, 95% CI 0.46–0.48). After adjustment for correlation between patients within the same hospital, the weekly odds of surgery were 27% higher with the individual-lists method and 31% higher with the shortest-list method than with the pooled-list method (individual-lists method vs. pooled-list method, adjusted odds ratio = 1.27, 95% CI 1.21–1.34; shortest-list method vs. pooled-list method, adjusted odds ratio = 1.31, 95% CI 1.24–1.38).

Proportion of Surgeries After the Recommended Time

As described above, each simulated patient was assigned to one of three priority groups at the time of registration on the surgical wait list. A patient was classified as having high priority if the recommended time to surgery was within 3 days, medium priority if the suggested time was within 6 weeks, and low priority if the suggested time was within 12 weeks. A patient who waited longer than the recommended time was considered to have delayed access to surgery.

Among high-priority patients, access to surgery was delayed for 348 of 6,614 procedures in the pooled-list group, 256 of 6,554 procedures in the individual-lists group, and 300 of 6,455 procedures in the shortest-list group. Among these high-priority patients, access to surgery was delayed for a higher percentage of those booked in hospitals using the pooled-list method relative to the individual-lists or shortest-list method (Table 14.26). The likelihood of delayed access to surgery was 29% lower with the individual-lists method and 18% lower with the shortest-list method than with the pooled-list method (Table 14.26). There was no difference between the individual-lists and shortest-list methods.

Similar results were observed for both the medium-priority and low-priority patients waiting for elective surgery. Among medium-priority patients, delays occurred for 667 of 64,615 procedures in the pooled-list group, 404 of 63,902 procedures in the individual-lists group, and 453 of 64,602 procedures in the shortest-list group. Relative to the pooled-list method, the odds of delayed access to surgery for these medium-priority patients were 35% lower with the individual-lists method and 29% lower with the shortest-list method (Table 14.26). Among low-priority patients, delays occurred for 178 of 20,664 procedures in the pooled-list group, 63 of 20,230 procedures in the individual-lists group, and 58 of 20,285 procedures in the shortest-list group. Relative to the pooled-list method, the odds of delayed access to surgery for these low-priority patients were about one-third lower with both the individual-lists and shortest-list methods (Table 14.26).

14.5.10 Conclusion

The most common method of booking appointments for surgical consultation is the individual-lists method, where the patient's name is placed on the appointment list of the surgeon specified in the referral. In this chapter, we described the simulation

Table 14.26 Probability of undergoing surgery after the recommended time in comparison of three methods of booking surgical consultation appointments, by priority at registration

	High priority		Medium priority		Low priority	
Method	Procedures with delay, %	Odds ratio (95% CI)*	Procedures with delay, %	Odds ratio (95% CI)*	Procedures with delay, %	Odds ratio (95% CI)*
Pooled list	5.3	1.00	1.0	1.00	0.9	1.00
Individual lists	3.9	0.71 (0.60–0.85)†	0.6	0.65 (0.57–0.74)‡	0.3	0.68 (0.49–0.94)§
Shortest list	4.6	0.82 (0.69–0.97)†	0.7	0.71 (0.63–0.80)‡	0.3	0.66 (0.49–0.91)§

Abbreviations: CI = confidence interval, df = degrees of freedom

*Adjusted for method of booking surgery, allocation of operating room slots, clearance times for appointment lists, surgical wait lists, and inpatient surgical queues at the start of the simulation, age, sex, coronary anatomy affected, comorbidities, and wait-list clearance time at registration

†No difference between individual-lists and shortest-list methods: Wald chi-square statistic = 2.3, df = 1, $p = 0.13$

‡No difference between individual-lists and shortest-list methods: Wald chi-square statistic = 1.6, df = 1, $p = 0.20$

§No difference between individual-lists and shortest-list methods: Wald chi-square statistic = 0.02, df = 1, $p = 0.88$

study of two alternative methods of booking these appointments. In the pooled-list method, appointments are booked by placing all patients' names on one appointment list and booking each appointment with the first available surgeon. In the shortest-list method, appointments are booked by placing patients on the list of the surgeon with the fewest patients waiting. Our results suggest that clearance times will be shorter in hospitals where patients wait for surgical consultation appointments in a single queue and that each week a larger proportion of patients are likely to have an appointment if they are waiting in a single queue.

However, our simulation model had two limitations. First, although we were able to account for the availability of surgeons, we lacked information about shortages of other hospital staff, so our model did not consider fluctuations in their availability. A second limitation is related to the size of the modeled surgical service. Coordinating clinic and operating room schedules for surgeons might have a different effect in a larger service. Whether the effect of the shortest-list system depends on the number of surgeons who share these duties requires further investigation.

The results of our simulation experiments may have implications for policies on managing access to elective surgery in a regional network of hospitals. If the size of the appointment lists and the weekly number of referrals vary significantly from one hospital to another, policy-makers may consider redistributing the cases across surgical services, which would require a centrally managed appointment system. Our findings suggest that compared to other alternatives, pooling referrals will substantially reduce access time for appointment at the expense of a slight delay in the timing of elective operations. Adopting this appointment system in the surgical services setting would present the patient with the choice of waiting to schedule an appointment with the surgeon named in the referral or seeing another surgeon. Further research is required to explore the impact of patient preferences on the performance of various appointment systems.

Chapter 15
Managing Presurgical Screening

In this chapter, we describe a simulation study developed for comparing two methods of presurgical screening of patients in terms of cancellation of elective procedures and time to surgery. We used discrete-event simulation with a cluster randomized design, in which the unit of allocation was the hospital and the units of analysis were both the hospital and the patient. Our results suggest that both the number of surgical cancellations and the likelihood that patients on the wait list would undergo their operations were lower in hospitals that screened all patients before admission for surgery.

15.1 The Simulation Study

15.1.1 Background

Once a surgeon has decided that an operation is indicated and the patient has consented to the procedure, a consultation is sought for the patient to undergo a preoperative assessment. This assessment serves four main purposes: providing education about anesthesia and postoperative care [101, 110, 149]; determining any health problems, surgical factors, and anesthetic factors that might increase the patient's risk of adverse outcomes; modifying surgical risks through further medical tests, medical treatments, or consultations with other health professionals; and identifying medical, nursing, and social issues that may affect planning for discharge from hospital [149]. Depending on hospital policy, preoperative assessment could be required for all patients before admission to hospital for an elective procedure, or some patients may undergo the presurgical screening after admission to hospital [163]. The latter option is expected to reduce the demand on the preadmission clinic, yet could be associated with cancellation of scheduled procedures if a patient admitted to hospital is unfit for the operation.

B. Sobolev et al., *Health Care Evaluation Using Computer Simulation: Concepts, Methods, and Applications*, DOI 10.1007/978-1-4614-2233-4_15,

Box 15.1 What is already known and what this study adds on managing screening

What is already known

- When possible, all patients booked for an elective procedure undergo preoperative assessment before admission for surgery [163].
- Alternatively, these patients could undergo preoperative assessment after admission to hospital, if attempts to book a visit to the preadmission clinic before the planned date of elective surgery are unsuccessful.
- Some evidence suggests that preoperative assessment before admission for surgery reduces the frequency of cancellation of surgery relative to assessment on the day of surgery [21, 121].
- However, the effects of these methods are not well understood, in particular, in terms of the number of cancellations due to the patient being unfit for surgery and the time to surgery.

What this study adds

- This simulation study shows the effects of two methods of arranging presurgical screening on the number of cancellations because the patient was unfit for surgery and the time to surgery in the context of cardiac surgical services.

15.1.2 The Study Rationale

The purpose of this simulation study was to estimate the effects of various methods of managing presurgical screening on the number of cancellations of elective procedures in the context of cardiac surgical services. We compared two methods—the all-screened method and the some-screened method—in terms of the following performance measures: the proportion of hospitals with the rate of cancellation because the patient was unfit for surgery meeting a specific benchmark, the weekly rate of elective surgery among patients registered for operations, the proportion of patients with surgery after the recommended time, and the proportion of procedures canceled from the final operating room list. In particular, we were interested in whether the all-screened method would reduce the rate of cancellations due to the patient's being unfit for surgery, increase the weekly rate of elective surgery among patients registered for an operation, decrease the proportion of registered patients undergoing surgery after the recommended time, and decrease the proportion of patients whose surgery was canceled from the final operating room list. Box 15.1 summarizes the study rationale.

15.1.3 The Management Alternatives

We studied two methods of managing presurgical screening of patients undergoing elective surgery: the all-screened method and the some-screened method. With the all-screened method, all patients who have been booked for elective surgery are required to undergo preoperative assessment before the planned date of surgery to ensure that they are ready for the procedure. With the some-screened method, an attempt is made to book an appointment at the preadmission clinic within the three-week period before the planned date of each patient's surgery, but if this is not possible, patients may be admitted for surgery without having had a consultation at the preadmission clinic, in which case they are assessed in hospital [163].

15.1.4 Study Questions

This simulation study was designed to address the following questions:

- Does the all-screened method of presurgical screening result in fewer surgical cancellations than the some-screened method?
- Is the time to surgery shorter with the all-screened method than with the some-screened method?

15.2 The Simulation Model

We developed a discrete-event simulation model of patient flow representing the process of cardiac surgical care, as described in detail in Chap. 13. As before, we modeled three care paths that patients are likely to experience: the elective path, which applies to patients for whom surgical consultation and subsequent operation can be safely delayed; the inpatient path, which applies to patients admitted to hospital directly from the catheterization laboratory when urgent surgical assessment is necessary; and the emergency path, which applies to patients requiring immediate surgical intervention.

15.2.1 Modeling Requirements

Patients for whom an elective procedure is planned are assigned a date for a preoperative assessment at the preadmission clinic at the same time as the projected date for the operation is determined. With the all-screened method, all patients who are to undergo an elective procedure are assessed at the preadmission clinic within the three-week period before the projected date of the operation. If no slots are available at the preadmission clinic within that period, the operation is canceled from the projected operating room list and rescheduled; a new date for the surgical consultation is then determined. With the some-screened method, an attempt is made to book each patient for a consultation at the preadmission clinic within the three-week period before the projected date of the operation. If no slots are available at the preadmission clinic within that period, the patient is admitted to hospital one day before the projected date of the operation for an in-hospital preoperative assessment. It is expected that some of these patients will require further tests after the in-hospital assessment. In this situation, the operation is canceled from the current operating room list and rescheduled so that a new date for consultation at the preadmission clinic can be determined.

With both methods of managing presurgical screening, and in addition to the types of cancellations described above, some patients may be deemed unsuitable for the operation after their initial preoperative assessment at the preadmission clinic, and these patients may require additional assessment. In this situation, the operation is canceled on the projected operating room list and is rescheduled so that a date for the additional assessment at can be determined. These additional assessments are booked differently for the two methods. With the all-screened method, if no slots are available for the additional assessment at the preadmission clinic within the three-week period before the projected date of the operation, the operation is canceled from the projected operating room list and is rescheduled so that a date for the additional assessment can be determined. With the some-screened method, if no slots are available for the additional assessment at the preadmission clinic within the three-week period before the projected date of the operation, the patient is admitted to hospital one day before the projected date of operation for an in-hospital assessment.

15.2.2 Modeling Assumptions

The complete list of assumptions of the discrete-event simulation model appears in Sect. 13.3. For the reader's convenience, the modeling assumptions related to the management of preoperative assessments are repeated here.

Preoperative Assessment

1. Twenty appointments for preoperative assessments are available at the preadmission clinic each week, and all patients attend their appointments.
2. Inpatients and previous inpatients who were discharged with a promise to readmit are assessed in hospital on the day of the operation.
3. By definition, emergency patients are deemed suitable for the operation and do not require a preoperative assessment.

15.2.3 Configurations of the Model

We developed six configurations of the discrete-event simulation model to implement the two methods of managing presurgical screening with variation in the method of booking surgical consultation appointments (Table 15.1). The method

Table 15.1 Configurations of the discrete-event simulation model for comparing two methods of managing presurgical screening (based on the configurations outlined in Tables 14.1 and 14.16)

Configuration	Appointments	Presurgical screening
B1	Individual lists	All screened
B2	Individual lists	Some screened
D1	Pooled list	All screened
D2	Pooled list	Some screened
F1	Shortest list	All screened
F2	Shortest list	Some screened

Table 15.2 Values of input parameters for capacity for comparing two methods of managing presurgical screening

Capacity	Values
No. of surgeons	3
Weekly no. of slots for elective operations	7
Weekly no. of slots for urgent operations	8
Weekly no. of consultations in preadmission clinic	20
Horizon for advance booking (weeks)	36

of booking surgery—advance booking—was the same for all simulation runs. In configurations B1, D1, and F1, the all-screened method was implemented as an extension of configurations B, D, and F, respectively (Tables 14.1 and 14.16). In configurations B2, D2, and F2, the some-screened method was also implemented as an extension of configurations B, D, and F, respectively.

15.2.4 Input Parameters

The input parameters for the model correspond to the workload and capacities of a typical cardiac surgery service. The full list of input parameters is provided in Table 13.5. For the reader's convenience, the input parameters related to the management of presurgical screening are repeated in Table 15.2.

15.2.5 Output Data

During each simulation run, patient records were stored in internal queues, whereas the occurrence and timing of simulation events, such as cancellations, were stored in external data stores. After a simulation run, we re-created individual patient paths by importing records from the data stores into a relational database and then linking the data stores by the combination of run and patient identification numbers that uniquely specified all rows in each data store. We then used the re-created paths for individual patients to construct the output data according to our predetermined data dictionaries. We used data dictionaries that were similar to those for the studies described in Chap. 14. The data dictionaries for the analytical data set are shown in Tables D.1 and D.2 of Appendix D. The data set for the elective pathway contained information on our study population, including hospital characteristics, patient attributes, and outcomes. In particular, this data set had a variable `meth_pac` for the method of managing presurgical screening. The data set for the inpatient pathway was used to compute the weekly number of inpatient or emergency procedures, which was used for adjustment in the regression analysis.

15.3 Plan of Experiment

15.3.1 Primary Study Factor

The primary study factor for this experiment, the method of managing presurgical screening, had two categories: some screened and all screened. This study factor was represented by one indicator variable, where we defined the some-screened method as the reference group. This indicator variable was calculated from the variable `meth_pac`.

15.3.2 Performance Measures

We studied performance at the level of both the hospital and the patient. In particular, we considered the following hospital-level performance measure:

- Proportion of hospitals with a rate of cancellation from the final operating room list because the patient was unfit for surgery of less than 3.2% of high-priority elective and urgent procedures.

We also considered the following patient-level performance measures:

- Weekly rate of surgery among patients remaining on wait lists.
- Proportion of wait-listed patients undergoing surgery after the recommended time.
- Proportion of elective procedures canceled from the final operating room list.

Here, we provide a brief explanation of our choice of the hospital-level performance measure. The purpose of consultation at the preadmission clinic is to assess whether the patient is fit for surgery before he or she is admitted to hospital for the procedure. For the hospital-level performance measure, we wanted to determine the proportion of hospitals that met a certain benchmark for surgical cancellations caused by the patient being deemed unfit for surgery among patients scheduled for high-priority elective surgery. However, with the all-screened method, there should be no elective procedures cancelled from the final operating room list for this reason, since all patients will have undergone a preadmission assessment before being admitted to hospital. Therefore, we could not choose a benchmark of zero cancellations caused by the patient being deemed unfit for surgery, since all hospitals using the all-screened method would meet this performance criterion. To introduce background variation between hospitals that were using the all-screened method, we modified the performance criterion to a specific benchmark of procedures canceled from the final operating room list among patients with high priority for elective procedures and patients with high or low priority for urgent procedures. Both methods of presurgical screening pertain to patients booked for elective surgery, so cancellations of urgent procedures should be similar with both approaches. The benchmark percentage of cancellations caused by the patient being deemed unfit for surgery (3.2%) was computed from the average observed proportions in preliminary runs of the reference group (the some-screened method).

15.3.3 Experimental Responses

We computed the performance measures from experimental responses (i.e., output data) generated by the simulation runs. The following hospital-level experimental response was generated:

- For each hospital, whether or not the proportion of its cancellations of high-priority elective and urgent procedures from the final operating room list because the patient was deemed unfit for surgery was less than 3.2% (indicator variable).

The following patient-level experimental responses were generated:

- For each patient, whether the patient underwent planned surgery (indicator variable), and the number of weeks from registration to surgery or removal from the list (continuous variable).
- For each patient, whether surgery was performed after the recommended time (indicator variable).
- For each patient, whether the elective procedure was canceled from the final operating room list (indicator variable).

15.3.4 Hospital-Level and Patient-Level Factors

We varied five experimental hospital-level factors that might have affected the experimental responses, namely, method of booking surgical consultation appointments, allocation of operating room slots, and clearance times for appointments, elective surgery, and inpatient surgery at the start of simulation. We also varied seven patient-level factors that might have affected the outcomes, namely, sex, age, coronary anatomy affected, comorbidity, priority of registration on the surgical wait list, clearance time at time of registration on a wait list, and weekly number of inpatient and emergency procedures [141].

15.3.5 Measure of Effect Size

To compare the effects of the methods of managing presurgical screening at the hospital level, we used the following measure of effect size corresponding to the performance measure:

- Odds ratio that a hospital's rate of cancellation of high-priority elective and urgent procedures from the final operating room list because the patient was unfit for surgery was less than 3.2%.

Similarly, we used the following effect-size measures to compare the effects of the methods of managing presurgical screening at the patient level:

- Ratio of weekly odds for undergoing surgery among patients remaining on wait lists.
- Odds ratio for undergoing surgery after the recommended time.
- Odds ratio for cancellation of an elective procedure from the final operating room list.

15.3.6 Design of Experiment

We used a cluster randomized design, in which the unit of allocation was a simulated hospital, as described in Sect. 7.3. A simulated hospital was produced by one run of the simulation model. The number of runs was chosen to detect the anticipated effects of the methods of managing presurgical screening with high probability. We performed provisional runs of the simulation model, with 30 hospitals per experimental group, to estimate the magnitude of each performance measure in the reference group and to estimate the measures of variability and correlation needed for estimating the number of runs. We calculated that 124 simulation runs per experimental group would be needed. This estimate was based on the maximum estimated number of runs across the hospital-level and patient-level performance measures of interest, as described below. All calculations assumed a two-sided test with 0.05 significance level and 90% power. We used the Fedorov algorithm to ensure optimal distribution of the experimental factors across the runs [55]. This algorithm randomly assigned each group of patients from simulation runs with the specified combination of values of the hospital-level factors to an experimental group.

Number of Runs for Cluster-Level Evaluations

First, we determined the number of runs needed to detect the anticipated difference in the proportion of hospitals meeting the specified benchmark for cancellations. We computed the benchmark percentage of cancellations caused by the patient being unfit for surgery, 3.2%, from the average observed proportions during preliminary runs of the some-screened method. According to these preliminary runs, the hypothesized proportion of hospitals was 0.50 among hospitals using the some-screened method. We estimated the number of simulation runs needed to detect a decrease of 0.20 in this proportion. Using (8.8), we calculated the required number of simulation runs (rounding up to the nearest integer) as follows:

$$k = \left[\frac{1.96\sqrt{2(0.40)(1-0.40)} + 1.28\sqrt{0.50(1-0.50)+0.30(1-0.30)}}{0.30-0.50}\right]^2$$
$$\approx 124.$$

Next, for the purpose of the regression analysis, we determined the number of runs to generate an adequate number of observations per regression variable. Our primary experimental factor was represented by one variable for methods of managing presurgical screening. In addition, we used two variables for clearance times for appointment lists at the start of simulation, three variables for clearance times for surgical wait lists at the start of simulation, two variables for clearance times for inpatient surgical queues at the start of simulation, two variables for methods of booking surgical consultation appointments, and one variable for allocation of operating room slots. Therefore, with a total of 11 variables, we estimated that 55 ($=11 \times 10/2$) observed events per booking method would be needed, allowing for 10 events per regression variable [73]. From provisional runs of the model, the event of a hospital having cancellation of any high-priority elective or urgent procedure occurred about 70% of the time. Therefore, we calculated that at least 79 runs ($\approx$55/0.70) per method would be needed.

Number of Runs for Individual-Level Evaluations

We then calculated the number of runs needed to detect the anticipated difference in each patient-level performance measure. For analyses at the patient level, the dependence between experimental responses within each hospital necessitated adjustment for within-hospital correlation [140]. First, we estimated the number of runs to detect a difference in rates of surgery among registered patients. Given the results of provisional runs of the simulation model, we assumed an average of 2,248 patient-weeks per simulation run and a coefficient of variation of 0.04 [74]. The hypothesized weekly rate of surgery was 33 per 100 patient-weeks among hospitals using the some-screened method of managing presurgical screening. We estimated that 11 runs per method would allow us to detect a 10% increase in the weekly surgery rate between groups of patients [49]. It may be undesirable to assume an equal number of patient-weeks across hospitals and identical coefficients of variation between experimental groups. We therefore used the Hayes method in (9.24) to estimate the number of runs (rounding up to the nearest integer) as follows:

$$k = 1 + \frac{(1.96 + 1.28)^2}{(0.33 - 0.33 \times 1.10)^2} \times \left(\frac{0.33}{1{,}709} + \frac{0.33 \times 1.10}{2{,}726} + 0.0006897 \right) \approx 11.$$

Second, we calculated the number of runs required to detect a difference in the proportion of patients whose surgery was delayed after the recommended time. The hypothesized proportion of patients with surgical delay was 0.10 among patients at hospitals that used the some-screened method of managing presurgical screening. We estimated that 11 runs per method would allow us to detect a 0.05 decrease in this proportion between groups of patients [49]. We used (9.9) to calculate the intracluster correlation coefficient

$$\hat{\rho} = \frac{0.5968 - 0.04339}{0.5968 + (717 - 1)(0.04339)} \approx 0.01748.$$

Then, using (9.14), we estimated the inflation factor

$$\text{IF} = 1 + (717 - 1) \times 0.01748 \approx 13.5.$$

Therefore, we would need about 13.5 times more runs in our experiment with randomization at the level of runs than in an experiment with randomization at the level of individual patients. We then computed the number of runs per experimental group (rounding up to the nearest integer) using the estimated IF and (9.13):

$$k = \frac{(1.96 + 1.28)^2[0.10(1 - 0.10) + 0.05(1 - 0.05)]}{717(0.05 - 0.10)^2} 13.5 \approx 11.$$

Third, we determined the number of runs needed to detect a difference in the proportion of patients whose surgery was canceled from the final operating room list. Preliminary runs indicated that the hypothesized proportion of patients with such cancellations was 0.22 for hospitals using the some-screened method of managing presurgical screening. We estimated that three runs per method would allow us to detect a 0.05 decrease in this proportion between groups of patients [49]. We used (9.9) to calculate the intracluster correlation coefficient

$$\hat{\rho} \approx \frac{0.2054 - 0.1491}{0.2054 + (717 - 1)(0.1491)} \approx 0.0005264.$$

Then, using (9.14), we estimated the inflation factor

$$\text{IF} = 1 + (717 - 1) \times (0.0005264) \approx 1.4.$$

Therefore, we would need about 1.4 times more runs in our experiment with randomization at the level of runs than in an experiment with randomization at the level of individual patients. We then computed the number of runs per group (rounding up to the nearest integer) using IF in (9.13):

$$k = \frac{(1.96 + 1.28)^2[0.22(1-0.22) + 0.17(1-0.17)]}{717(0.17-0.22)^2} 1.4 \approx 3.$$

Finally, for the purpose of the regression analysis, we determined the number of runs needed to generate an adequate number of observations per regression variable. As described above, the primary experimental factor was represented by one variable for methods of managing presurgical screening. In addition, we used two variables for clearance times for appointment lists at the start of simulation, three variables for clearance times for surgical wait lists at the start of simulation, two variables for clearance times for inpatient surgical queues at the start of simulation, two variables for methods of booking surgical consultation appointments, and one variable for allocation of operating room slots. The patient-level variables included one variable for sex, four variables for age groups, two variables for categories of coronary anatomy affected, two variables for categories of comorbidity, two variables for priorities at registration, one continuous variable for the weekly number of inpatient and emergency procedures, and one time-dependent continuous variable for wait-list clearance time at registration. Therefore, with a total of 24 variables, we estimated that 120 ($=24 \times 10/2$) observed events per method would be needed, allowing for 10 events per regression variable [73]. Provisional runs of the model indicated that the event of surgery after the recommended time occurred about 4.8% of the time, and there were about 717 patients per hospital. Therefore, we estimated that we would need at least four runs ($\approx 120/(0.048 \times 717)$) per method.

The estimates of the number of simulation runs required for each performance measure are summarized in Table 15.3. To ensure adequate power to detect clinically significant differences between the two experimental groups in each performance measure, the minimum number of simulation runs per experimental group had to meet the requirements for the performance measure with the largest number of simulation runs required. Therefore, the minimum number of simulation runs was 124.

15.4 Evaluation of Experiment

Analyses were conducted at the level of both the hospital and the patient. For analyses at the hospital level, we report differences between the two methods of managing presurgical screening in terms of the odds that cancellation of high-priority elective and urgent procedures would be below a certain benchmark (3.2%). For analyses at the patient level, we report differences between these two methods

Table 15.3 Number of simulation runs required to compare methods of managing presurgical screening with 0.05 significance level and 90% power, per experimental group

Performance measure	Reference value	Effect size	No. of runs
Hospital level			
Proportion of hospitals with frequency of cancellation of high-priority elective or urgent procedures <3.2%*	0.50	0.20 decrease	124†
Patient level			
Surgery rate per 100 patient-weeks	33	10% increase	11
Proportion of patients with delay of surgery after recommended time	0.10	0.05 decrease	11
Proportion of patients with cancellation from final OR list	0.22	0.05 decrease	3

Abbreviation: OR = operating room
*For cancellations caused by the patient being unfit for surgery
†79 runs required to allow 10 events per regression variable in cluster-level evaluation

in terms of the weekly odds that a patient would undergo planned surgery, the odds that surgery would occur after the recommended time, and the odds of cancellation from the final operating room list.

15.4.1 Statistical Instruments

We used logistic regression methods to model the probability of falling below the benchmark for cancellations of high-priority procedures in relation to the method of managing presurgical screening, with adjustment for hospital-level factors (see Table D.1 in Appendix D). In the hospital-level regression analyses, we adjusted for hospital-level factors by including sets of indicator variables, as described in the previous section. The odds ratios derived from these logistic regressions measured the effect of using the all-screened method of managing presurgical screening on the odds that a hospital would have a rate of cancellation of high-priority elective or urgent procedures below 3.2% relative to the some-screened method [139].

To assess performance at the patient level, we plotted the access curves from registration to surgery by method of managing presurgical screening and by priority group. We used discrete-time survival regression to model the relation between time to elective surgery and method of screening, with adjustment for hospital-level and patient-level factors (see Table D.1 in Appendix D). We used logistic regression to model the relation between the method of presurgical screening and the odds of an event, in particular, delay or cancellation of surgery, with adjustment for other factors and for correlation between patients in the same hospital. In these regression models, we adjusted for hospital-level and patient-level variables by including sets of indicator variables, as described in the previous section. The odds ratios derived from discrete-time survival regressions measured the effects of using the all-screened method of managing presurgical screening on the weekly proportion of patients who underwent the operation, relative to the some-screened method [139]. The odds ratios derived from logistic regressions measured the effects of using the all-screened method on the odds that surgery would be after the recommended time and on the odds of cancellation, relative to the some-screened method.

15.4.2 Hospital and Patient Characteristics

The 248 simulation runs generated a total of 187,403 referrals for elective procedures, 181,059 urgent cases, and 13,547 emergency cases over six 18-week cycles of assignment of clinic and operating time starting on the arbitrarily chosen date of September 1, 2008. On average, the simulation model generated 364 elective referrals, 352 urgent cases, and 26 emergency arrivals per modeled hospital in one year. The modeled surgical services performed 655 procedures per year on average.

The distribution of referrals by patient-level factors was also similar across methods of managing presurgical screening. The majority of referrals were for men (83.6%), and 37.7% of the patients were 60–69 years old. Most patients had multivessel disease (73.5%) and either major or minor concurrent conditions (49.6%).

At the time of referral, 92.9% of the patients had low priority for surgical consultation. Regardless of the method of managing presurgical screening, most of the referred patients had a surgical consultation by the end of the simulation (94.5% for the some-screened method and 94.4% for the all-screened method). The rest of the patients were still waiting for an appointment because their referral times were close to the end of the simulation period.

At the time of registration on a surgical wait list, 70.6% of the patients had medium priority for the operation. The waiting time for elective surgery was less than half a week for 63.0% of the patients with the some-screened method of managing presurgical screening, but only 32.9% with the all-screened method (Table 15.4).

Of all the patients who were registered on a surgical wait list, 78.5% underwent the planned procedure. The reasons for removal from a list without surgery were similar across methods of managing presurgical screening: 8.3% of planned procedures were canceled because no beds were available in the intensive care unit for recovery after surgery, and 7.8% of planned procedures were canceled because an inpatient was admitted for surgery. Another 5.4% of patients were removed from the list for other reasons, or they remained on the wait list at the end of the simulation.

Table 15.4 Characteristics of simulated patients registered for elective surgery, by method of managing presurgical screening

	Method; no. (%) of patients			
	Some screened		All screened	
Characteristic	(n = 88,655)		(n = 88,363)	
Age group (years)				
<50	6,260	(7.1)	6,327	(7.2)
50–59	20,178	(22.8)	20,214	(22.9)
60–69	33,417	(37.7)	33,430	(37.8)
70–79	25,956	(29.3)	25,572	(28.9)
≥80	2,844	(3.2)	2,820	(3.2)
Sex				
Male	74,071	(83.5)	73,946	(83.7)
Female	14,584	(16.5)	14,417	(16.3)
Coronary anatomy affected				
Left main	14,748	(16.6)	14,731	(16.7)
Multivessel*	65,297	(73.7)	64,974	(73.5)
Limited†	8,610	(9.7)	8,658	(9.8)
Comorbidity				
Major conditions‡	19,714	(22.2)	19,622	(22.2)
Other conditions§	23,975	(27.0)	24,150	(27.3)
None	44,966	(50.7)	44,591	(50.5)
Priority at time of registration				
High	6,362	(7.2)	6,351	(7.2)
Medium	62,610	(70.6)	62,434	(70.7)
Low	19,683	(22.2)	19,578	(22.2)
Clearance time at registration				
Less than half week	55,823	(63.0)	29,103	(32.9)
Less than half month	30,189	(34.1)	35,524	(40.2)
More than half month	2,643	(3.0)	23,736	(26.9)

*Two- or three-vessel disease with proximal left anterior descending (PLAD) artery
†Two-vessel disease with no PLAD or one-vessel disease with PLAD
‡Congestive heart failure, diabetes mellitus, chronic obstructive pulmonary disease, rheumatoid arthritis, cancer
§Peripheral vascular disease, cerebrovascular disease, dementia, peptic ulcer disease, hemiplegia, renal disease, liver disease

15.4.3 Proportion of Hospitals Meeting Cancellation Benchmark

The proportion of hospitals with cancellation of less than 3.2% of high-priority elective and urgent procedures because patients were unfit for surgery was higher with the all-screened method than with the some-screened method (80.6% vs. 65.3%) (Table 15.5). The odds of a hospital meeting this performance

Table 15.5 Proportion of hospitals canceling less than 3.2% of high-priority procedures because patients are unfit for surgery, in relation to method of managing presurgical screening

Method	% (no. of hospitals with <3.2% cancellations/total no. of hospitals)	Odds ratio (95% CI)*
Some screened	65.3 (81/124)	1.00
All screened	80.6 (100/124)	2.32 (1.28–4.22)

Abbreviation: CI = confidence interval

*Adjusted for method of booking surgical consultation, method of booking surgery, allocation of operating room slots, clearance times for appointment lists, surgical wait lists, and inpatient surgical queues at the start of simulation

criterion were more than two times higher if the hospital screened all patients before admission than if the hospital screened only some patients (Table 15.5).

15.4.4 Weekly Rate of Surgery

Each patient recommended for elective surgery was registered on a surgical wait list and assigned to one of three priority groups. If a patient was found to be unfit for surgery in the preadmission clinic or in the hospital, the patient's surgery was canceled, and he or she was registered on the surgical wait list again. We compared methods of managing presurgical screening in terms of the total waiting time from the first time the patient was registered on the wait list until removal from the wait list because the surgery was performed or for some reason other than being unfit for surgery.

In the high-priority group, 4,820 procedures were performed over 12,659 patient-weeks in hospitals using the all-screened method, and 5,367 procedures were performed over 6,470 patient-weeks in hospitals using the some-screened method. At 38.1 procedures per 100 patient-weeks (95% CI 37.0–39.2), the average weekly rate of surgery was lower among hospitals using the all-screened method than among those using the some-screened method (83.0 procedures per 100 patient-weeks, 95% CI 80.7–85.2) (Table 15.6). More than half of the high-priority patients had their operations within two weeks in hospitals using the all-screened method, whereas more than half had their operations within one week in hospitals using the some-screened method (Fig. 15.1). After adjustment for hospital-level and patient-level factors, the weekly odds that a patient waiting for high-priority elective surgery would undergo the operation were 87% lower among patients registered at hospitals using the all-screened method relative to patients registered at hospitals using the some-screened method (Table 15.6). After adjustment for correlation between patients within the same hospital, the ratio of weekly odds did not change

Table 15.6 Weekly rate of elective surgery in relation to method of managing presurgical screening, by priority at time of registration

	High priority		Medium priority		Low priority	
Method	Surgery rate* (95% CI)	Ratio of weekly odds (95% CI)†	Surgery rate* (95% CI)	Ratio of weekly odds (95% CI)†	Surgery rate* (95% CI)	Ratio of weekly odds (95% CI)†
Some screened	83.0 (80.7–85.2)	1.00	33.9 (33.6–34.2)	1.00	26.8 (26.4–27.2)	1.00
All screened	38.1 (37.0–39.2)	0.13 (0.12–0.14)	19.9 (19.8–20.1)	0.59 (0.58–0.60)	18.3 (18.0–18.6)	0.56 (0.54–0.57)

Abbreviation: CI = confidence interval

*Per 100 patient-weeks, calculated as the number of procedures divided by the total time in patient-weeks

†Adjusted for method of booking surgical consultation appointments, method of booking surgery, allocation of operating room slots, clearance times for appointment lists, surgical wait lists, and inpatient surgical queues at the start of the simulation, age, sex, coronary anatomy affected, comorbidities, wait-list clearance times at registration, and week from registration

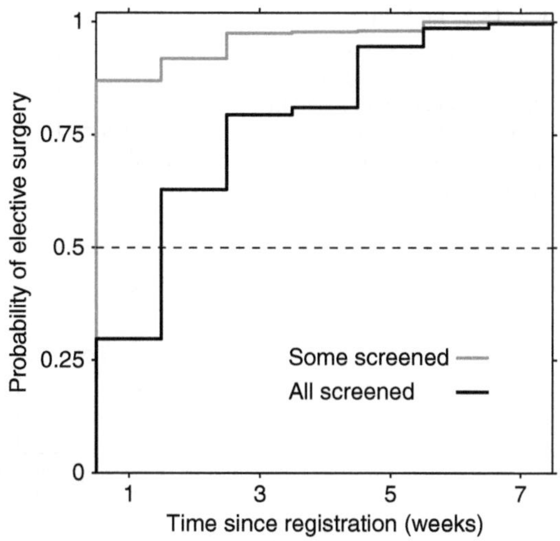

Fig. 15.1 Probability of undergoing surgery within a certain time since registration among patients with high priority at registration, by method of managing presurgical screening

(odds ratio = 0.12, 95% CI 0.11–0.14). The likelihood of operation decreased by 50% for every eight additional procedures performed without registration on a wait list (odds ratio = 0.50, 95% CI 0.46–0.55).

In contrast, in the medium-priority group, a similar number of procedures were performed in each experimental group (48,158 procedures in hospitals using the some-screened method of managing presurgical screening and 47,456 procedures in hospitals using the all-screened method), but the period of time that patients waited was almost double in hospitals that screened all patients (238,023 patient-weeks vs. 142,095 patient-weeks in hospitals using the some-screened method). The weekly rate of elective surgery was lower in hospitals using the all-screened method. More than half of patients waiting for medium-priority elective surgery at hospitals using the some-screened method had their operations within two weeks, but among those waiting for surgery at hospitals using the all-screened method, about half had their surgery within four weeks (Fig. 15.2). After adjustment for hospital-level and patient-level factors, the weekly odds that a patient waiting for medium-priority elective surgery would undergo the operation were 41% lower for hospitals using the all-screened method than for hospitals using the some-screened method (Table 15.6). The likelihood of operation decreased by 68% for every eight additional procedures performed without registration on a wait list (odds ratio = 0.32, 95% CI 0.31–0.33).

In the low-priority group, a similar number of procedures were performed in each experimental group (16,884 in hospitals using the some-screened method and 16,329 in hospitals using the all-screened method), but the total time that patients waited was longer when all patients were screened before admission (62,953 patient-weeks vs. 89,139 patient-weeks, respectively). These patients had longer individual waiting times with the all-screened method (with half having their operations within four weeks) than with the some-screened

Fig. 15.2 Probability of undergoing surgery within a certain time since registration among patients with medium priority at registration, by method of managing presurgical screening

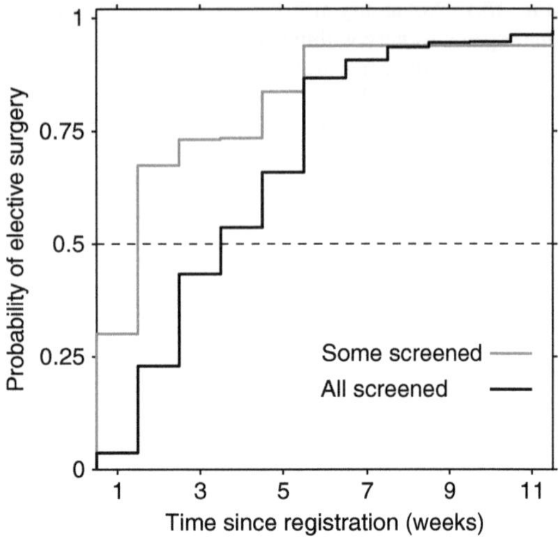

Fig. 15.3 Probability of undergoing surgery within a certain time since registration among patients with low priority at registration, by method of managing presurgical screening

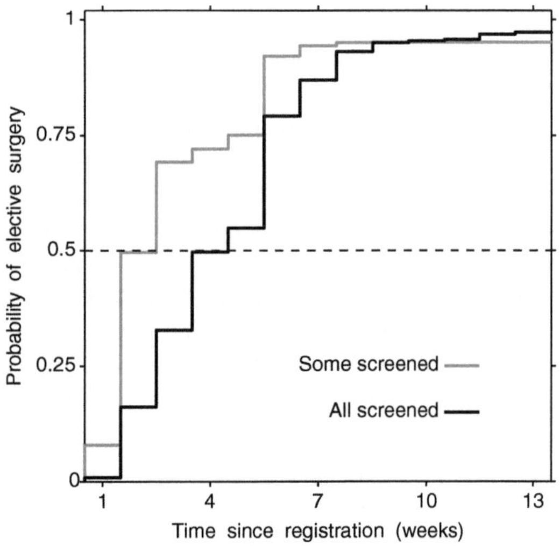

method (with half having their operations within two weeks) (Fig. 15.3). The weekly odds of undergoing the operation were 44% lower among patients whose presurgical screening was booked by the all-screened method (Table 15.6). After adjustment for correlation between patients within the same hospital, the ratio of weekly odds of operation did not change dramatically (odds ratio = 0.58, 95% CI 0.56–0.60). The likelihood of operation decreased by 58% for every eight additional procedures performed without registration on a wait list (odds ratio = 0.42, 95% CI 0.41–0.44).

15.4.5 *Proportion of Surgeries After the Recommended Time*

As described above, each patient was assigned to one of three priority groups at the time of registration on a surgical wait list. A patient was classified as having high priority if the suggested time to surgery was within three days, medium priority if the suggested time was within six weeks, and low priority if the suggested time was within 12 weeks. A patient who waited longer than the suggested time was considered to have delayed access to surgery. Among high-priority patients waiting for elective surgery, there was a large difference between methods of managing presurgical screening in the proportion of patients whose surgery was delayed: 5.2% (329 of 6,362 patients) in the some-screened group and 55.0% (3,491 of 6,351 patients) in the all-screened group. In this patient group, the odds of delayed access to surgery were higher in hospitals using the all-screened method than in those using the some-screened method (Table 15.7). After adjustment for correlation within hospitals, the effect was similar (odds ratio = 23.18, 95% CI 20.43–26.30).

Similarly, in the medium-priority group, a higher proportion of patients had surgery after the recommended time with the all-screened method: 6.3% (3,911 of 62,434 patients) vs. 1.1% (700 of 62,610) with the some-screened method. Relative to hospitals using the some-screened method, the odds of delayed access to surgery were almost two times higher in hospitals using the all-screened method (Table 15.7). After adjustment for correlation within hospitals, the odds were over two times higher (odds ratio = 2.47, 95% CI 2.17–2.81).

Among patients in the low-priority group, less than 1% had surgery after the recommended time, regardless of the method of managing presurgical screening. After adjustment for hospital-level and patient-level factors, the odds of delayed access to surgery were 52% lower with the all-screened method than with the some-screened method (Table 15.7). After adjustment for correlation within hospitals, the effect was similar (odds ratio = 0.52, 95% CI 0.36–0.77).

15.4.6 *Proportion of Patients with Cancellation of Surgery*

The effect of the method of managing presurgical screening on cancellation of elective procedures differed across priority. The proportion of high-priority patients whose procedures were canceled from the final operating room list was lower in hospitals using the all-screened method than in hospitals using the some-screened method: 4.7% (299 of 6,351 patients) vs. 10.9% (693 of 6,362 patients). The odds of cancellation of a high-priority elective procedure were 60% lower in the all-screened group (Table 15.8). The effect remained similar after accounting for correlation between patients in the same hospital (odds ratio = 0.40, 95% CI 0.35–0.46).

Among medium-priority patients, the all-screened method also yielded better performance, but the effect size was smaller than for high-priority patients. Almost one-quarter of medium-priority patients (15,508 of 62,610 patients) in

Table 15.7 Probability of undergoing surgery after the recommended time in relation to method of managing presurgical screening, by priority at registration

	High priority		Medium priority		Low priority	
Method	Procedures with delay, %	Odds ratio (95% CI)*	Procedures with delay, %	Odds ratio (95% CI)*	Procedures with delay, %	Odds ratio (95% CI)*
Some screened	5.2	1.00	1.1	1.00	0.5	1.00
All screened	55.0	23.15 (20.48–26.16)	6.3	1.87 (1.70–2.05)	0.5	0.48 (0.35–0.67)

Abbreviation: CI = confidence interval
*Adjusted for method of booking surgical consultation appointments, allocation of operating room slots, clearance times for appointment lists, surgical wait lists, and inpatient surgical queues at the start of the simulation, age, sex, coronary anatomy affected, comorbidities, and wait-list clearance times at time of registration

Table 15.8 Probability of cancellation from the final operating room list in relation to method of managing presurgical screening, by priority at registration

	High priority		Medium priority		Low priority	
Method	Cancellations, %	Odds ratio (95% CI)*	Cancellations, %	Odds ratio (95% CI)*	Cancellations, %	Odds ratio (95% CI)*
Some screened	10.9	1.00	24.8	1.00	12.1	1.00
All screened	4.7	0.40 (0.35–0.47)	17.6	0.61 (0.59–0.63)	11.1	0.87 (0.83–0.95)

Abbreviation: CI = confidence interval

*Adjusted for method of booking surgical consultation appointments, allocation of operating room slots, clearance times for appointment lists, surgical wait lists, and inpatient surgical queues at the start of the simulation, age, sex, coronary anatomy affected, comorbidities, and wait-list clearance times at time of registration

the some-screened group experienced cancellation from the final operating room list, whereas the proportion was less than one-fifth for the all-screened group (10,977 of 62,434 patients). The odds of cancellation of a medium-priority elective procedure were about 39% lower with the all-screened method (Table 15.8). The effect remained the same after adjustment for correlation within hospitals (odds ratio = 0.61, 95% CI 0.59–0.63).

The effect of the method of managing presurgical screening was less pronounced for low-priority elective procedures: 12.1% (2,383 of 19,683 patients) in hospitals using the some-screened method and 11.1% (2,180 of 19,578 patients) in hospitals using the all-screened method. The odds of cancellation of a low-priority elective procedure were about 13% lower with the all-screened method (Table 15.8). The effect remained similar after accounting for correlation between patients in the same hospital (odds ratio = 0.89, 95% CI 0.83–0.95).

15.4.7 Conclusion

When possible, all patients who have been booked for elective surgery undergo preoperative assessment before the planned date of surgery. If an appointment at the preadmission clinic cannot be booked within that period, the operation is canceled and rescheduled, and a new date for the preoperative assessment is then determined. Alternatively, if a visit to the preadmission clinic cannot be booked within that period, the patient is admitted to hospital one day before surgery for an in-hospital assessment. Our results suggest that even though the number of surgical cancellations was lower in hospitals that screened all patients before admission for surgery, these hospitals also had a lower weekly likelihood that patients remaining on the wait list would have their operations within the recommended time.

As discussed in Chap. 14, our simulation model had some limitations. For example, our model did not account for variations in the availability of staff in the preadmission clinics or hospital staff needed for in-hospital assessment. In addition, we did not control the distribution of patient-level factors through the design of experiment but instead assigned these factors randomly according to their frequency in the patient population from one jurisdiction. The case mix of patients needing elective operations could be different in other regions of the world. For example, women consistently accounted for 20% of patients undergoing isolated coronary artery bypass surgery in the United Kingdom, Norway, France, Italy, and Japan in the period 2000–2005 [86, 112]. Conversely, patients who undergo this procedure in the United States are slightly older, with greater proportions of women, diabetic patients, smokers, and patients with lung disease. Reasons offered for the lower rates of coronary artery bypass grafting among women include greater comorbidity, which augments the operative risk, and smaller size of the coronary arteries, which presents greater technical challenges and increases the potential for incomplete revascularization [65]. Determining whether the effect of the appointment system is independent of the case mix requires further investigation.

Chapter 16
Booking Elective Surgery

In this chapter, we describe a simulation study developed for comparing two methods of booking elective surgery in terms of cancellation of elective procedures and time to surgery. We used discrete-event simulation with a cluster randomized design, in which the unit of allocation was the hospital and the units of analysis were both the hospital and the patient. Our results suggest that hospitals with advance booking of surgery dates had fewer surgical cancellations and a higher weekly likelihood that a medium-priority patient would actually undergo the operation.

16.1 The Simulation Study

16.1.1 Background

After deciding that an operation is indicated, and after the patient has consented to the procedure, the surgeon sends a request to the hospital booking office to book an operating room. The process of booking surgery determines the dates of admission to hospital and of the operation itself and also reserves hospital resources to ensure appropriate patient care during and after the operation [67]. The booking process takes into account the urgency of treatment, the availability of postoperative resources, the specialists' schedules, and the number of slots available for booked (elective) and emergency cases. Booking patients for elective surgery involves three activities: allocating operating room time to various surgical services [17], assigning blocks of operating time to surgeons [18], and booking patients into the operating room slots of their respective surgeons [47].

The most common method of booking elective procedures, the wait-list booking method, is to schedule surgery when a slot in the operating room becomes available. Advance booking has been suggested as an alternative method for booking elective surgery [66]. Instead of keeping patients on wait lists until an operating room slot becomes available, the consulting surgeon prebooks the operation date at the time

B. Sobolev et al., *Health Care Evaluation Using Computer Simulation: Concepts, Methods, and Applications*, DOI 10.1007/978-1-4614-2233-4_16,

of the decision to operate [103]. However, the effects of these methods on surgical cancellations and time to surgery are not well understood, especially considering that surgeons perform various other activities within their respective practices, such as examining patients in their offices, teaching, administrative duties, and performing operations in other hospitals where they have admitting privileges, and therefore may not be available to perform operations on certain days.

16.1.2 The Study Rationale

The purpose of this simulation study was to estimate the effects of two methods of booking elective surgery on the number of surgical cancellations and on the time to surgery in the context of cardiac surgical services. We compared two booking methods—wait-list booking and advance booking—in terms of the following performance measures: the proportion of hospitals with delay of any high-priority elective procedures, the proportion of hospitals with no cancellations of high-priority elective procedures, the weekly rate of elective surgery among patients registered for operations, the proportion of patients undergoing surgery after the recommended time, and the proportion of procedures canceled from the final operating room list. In particular, we were interested in whether advance booking would reduce the proportion of hospitals with delay of any high-priority elective procedures, increase the proportion of hospitals with no cancellations of high-priority elective procedures, increase the weekly rate of elective surgery among patients registered for operations, decrease the registered proportion of patients undergoing planned surgery after the recommended time, and decrease the proportion of patients whose surgery was canceled from the final operating room list. Box 16.1 summarizes the study rationale.

16.1.3 The Management Alternatives

We considered two methods of booking elective surgery: wait-list booking and advance booking. With wait-list booking, the patient's name is placed on a wait list without a projected date of operation, and attempts to book the operation are made periodically until an appropriate operating room slot becomes available. With advance booking, the date of surgery is booked at the time of the decision to operate.

16.1.4 Study Questions

This simulation study was designed to address the following study questions:

Box 16.1 What is already known and what this study adds on booking surgery

What is already known

- Booking surgery determines the day of the operation and reserves resources to ensure appropriate patient care during and after the operation [67].
- The most common method of booking operations is the wait-list booking method in which surgery for a wait-listed patient is booked when a slot in the operating room becomes available.
- Booking the date of the operation at the time of the decision to operate has been suggested as an alternative to the wait-list booking method [66].
- However, the effects of these methods are not well understood, in particular, in terms of the number of cancellations originating with the hospital and the time to surgery.

What this study adds

- The simulation study shows the effects of using the advance booking method, compared to the wait-list booking method, on the number of surgical cancellations and the time to surgery in the context of cardiac surgical services.

- Does booking surgery in advance result in fewer surgical cancellations than booking from wait lists?
- Is the time to surgery shorter with advance booking of surgery than with wait-list booking?

16.2 The Simulation Model

We developed a discrete-event simulation model of patient flow representing the process of cardiac surgical care, as described in detail in Chap. 13. As before, we modeled three care paths that patients are likely to experience: the elective path, which applies to patients for whom surgical consultation and subsequent operation can be safely delayed; the inpatient path, which applies to patients admitted to hospital directly from the catheterization laboratory when urgent surgical assessment is necessary; and the emergency path, which applies to patients requiring immediate surgical intervention.

16.2.1 Modeling Requirements

With wait-list booking, patients for whom an elective procedure is planned are registered on the wait list of the consulting surgeon without a projected date of operation. A surgical priority (high, medium, or low) is assigned to each patient according to the urgency of the operation. The patient remains on the wait list until the operation can be scheduled. Attempts to book each patient for the operation are made periodically until an appropriate operating room slot becomes available. A draft operating room list for the following week is generated every Friday. This list contains the scheduled elective operations of patients selected from wait lists, low-priority inpatients staying in hospital, and patients whose previously booked surgery was canceled with a promise to readmit. On Mondays, the draft operating room list, containing the operations that have been booked for the current week, becomes the current list.

With advance booking, elective patients are registered on a wait list with a projected date of operation. This projected date is the date of the next available operating room slot assigned to the consulting surgeon on the projected list of the 36-week period after the patient's outpatient surgical consultation. Similar to the process for wait-list booking, a draft operating room list, generated every Friday is the basis for the next week's list generated the following Monday. The draft operating room list contains the operations of patients booked for elective surgery in the coming week, the operations of inpatients waiting in hospital, and the operations of patients whose surgery was previously canceled with a promise to readmit.

With both methods of booking operations, the current operating room list may be modified unexpectedly by the arrival of patients requiring emergency surgery and by inpatients, who are given preferential access to operating room slots, which in turn causes cancellation of previously booked operations.

16.2.2 Modeling Assumptions

The complete list of assumptions of the discrete-event simulation model appears in Sect. 13.3. For the reader's convenience, the modeling assumptions related to the booking of operations are repeated here.

Booking of operations

1. With wait-list booking, elective patients with high priority for their operations are booked before those with low priority, and patients with the same priority are booked by their respective dates of registration.
2. With wait-list booking, patients with any priority may be booked into any urgent slots available to the consulting surgeon, so long as no inpatients are waiting in hospital.
3. With advance booking, patients with high and medium priority are eligible for booking into both elective and urgent slots available to the consulting surgeon, whereas those with low priority may be booked only into elective slots available to the consulting surgeon.
4. Each week, seven operating room slots are available for elective surgery and eight for urgent procedures. Two methods for allocating operating room slots over weekdays are modeled: a weekly or a daily split between elective and urgent procedures.

5. Emergency patients and high-priority inpatients are booked on the current operating room list immediately. They are booked into urgent slots, if such are available; otherwise, previously booked operations may be canceled to accommodate these cases.
6. Low-priority inpatients are booked for surgery on the current operating room list if urgent slots are available; otherwise, they are booked into available urgent slots the following week.

Cancellation of scheduled operations

1. The scheduled operation of an elective patient may be canceled by the arrival of an emergency patient or a high-priority inpatient.
2. The scheduled operation of a high-priority inpatient may be canceled by the arrival of an emergency patient.
3. The scheduled operation of a low-priority inpatient may be canceled by the arrival of an emergency patient or a high-priority inpatient.
4. The scheduled operation of a patient whose surgery was previously canceled with a promise to readmit may be canceled by the arrival of an emergency patient or a high-priority inpatient.
5. The scheduled operation of an emergency patient cannot be canceled.
6. Canceled high- and medium-priority elective operations are rebooked as inpatient operations after the operations of all previously registered inpatients have been booked.
7. Canceled low-priority elective operations are rebooked as "promise-to-readmit" operations after the operations of all previously registered "promise-to-readmit" patients have been booked.
8. Canceled high-priority inpatient operations are rebooked as high-priority inpatient operations ahead of the operations for any previously registered high-priority inpatients.
9. Canceled low-priority inpatient operations are rebooked as low-priority inpatient operations ahead of the operations for any previously registered low-priority inpatients.
10. Canceled "promise-to-readmit" operations are rebooked as "promise-to-readmit" operations ahead of the operations for any previously registered "promise-to-readmit" patients.

16.2.3 Configurations of the Model

We developed six configurations of the discrete-event simulation model to implement all possible combinations of the two methods of booking elective operations and three methods of booking surgical consultation appointments (Table 16.1). Configurations A, C, and E implemented the wait-list booking method, and configurations B, D, and F implemented the advance booking method. We studied

Table 16.1 Configurations of the discrete-event simulation model for comparing two methods of booking elective surgery

Configuration	Appointments	Elective operations
A	Individual lists	Wait-list booking
B	Individual lists	Advance booking
C	Pooled list	Wait-list booking
D	Pooled list	Advance booking
E	Shortest list	Wait-list booking
F	Shortest list	Advance booking

Table 16.2 Values of input parameters for comparing two methods of booking surgery

Input parameter	Values
Priority group	
Operation	High, medium, low
Probability of progression (elective operation)	
High priority for consultation to high priority for operation	1
Low priority for consultation to medium priority for operation	0.76
Low priority for consultation to low priority for operation	0.24
Probability of progression (urgent operation)	
High priority for assessment to high priority for operation	1
Low priority for assessment to low priority for operation	0.5
Low priority for assessment to promise-to-readmit status	0.5
Capacity	
No. of surgeons	3
Weekly no. of slots for elective operations	7
Weekly no. of slots for urgent operations	8
No. of beds in CS-ICU	4
Horizon for advance booking (weeks)	36

Abbreviation: CS-ICU = cardiac surgery intensive care unit

the methods of booking surgery while varying the method of booking surgical consultation appointments to evaluate the net effect of choosing an alternative method of booking elective surgery. The independent effects of different methods of booking surgical consultation appointments are described in detail in Chap. 14.

16.2.4 Input Parameters

The input parameters for the model correspond to the workload and capacities of a typical cardiac surgical service. The full list of input parameters is provided in Table 13.5. For the reader's convenience, the input parameters related to the booking of operations are repeated in Table 16.2.

16.2.5 Output Data

During each simulation run, patient records were stored in internal queues, whereas the occurrence and timing of simulation events, such as cancellations, were stored in external data stores. After a simulation run, we re-created individual patient paths by importing records from the data stores into a relational database and then linking the data stores by the combination of run and patient identification numbers that uniquely specified all rows in each data store. We then used the re-created paths for individual patients to construct the output data. We used data dictionaries that were similar to those for the studies described in Chaps. 14 and 15. The data dictionaries for the analytical data set for elective patients and for inpatients are shown in Tables D.1 and D.2 of Appendix D, respectively. The data set for elective cases contained information on our study population, including hospital characteristics, patient attributes, and outcomes. In particular, this data set had a variable `meth_sx` for the method of booking surgery. The data set for inpatient cases was used to compute the weekly number of inpatient or emergency procedures, which was used for adjustment in the regression analysis.

16.3 Plan of Experiment

16.3.1 Primary Study Factor

Our primary study factor for this experiment, the method of booking surgery, had two categories: wait-list booking and advance booking. This study factor was represented by one indicator variable, where we defined the wait-list booking method as the reference group. This indicator variable was calculated from the variable `meth_sx`.

16.3.2 Performance Measures

We were interested in performance measures at the level of both the hospital and the patient. We considered the following hospital-level performance measures:

- Proportion of hospitals with delay of any high-priority elective procedures.
- Proportion of hospitals with no cancellations of high-priority elective procedures.

We also considered the following patient-level performance measures:

- Weekly rate of surgery among patients remaining on wait lists.
- Proportion of wait-listed patients undergoing surgery after the recommended time.
- Proportion of elective procedures canceled from the final operating room list.

16.3.3 Experimental Responses

The following hospital-level experimental responses were generated by the simulation runs:

- For each hospital, whether any high-priority elective procedures were delayed (indicator variable).
- For each hospital, whether the number of high-priority elective procedures canceled was zero (indicator variable).

The patient-level experimental responses were:

- For each patient, whether the patient underwent planned surgery (indicator variable) and the number of weeks from registration to surgery or removal from the list (continuous variable).
- For each patient, whether surgery was performed after the recommended time (indicator variable).
- For each patient, whether the elective procedure was canceled from the final operating room list (indicator variable).

16.3.4 Hospital-Level and Patient-Level Experimental Factors

We identified several experimental hospital-level factors that might have affected the experimental responses: method of booking surgical consultation appointments, allocation of operating room slots, and clearance times for appointment lists, surgical wait lists, and inpatient surgical queues at the start of simulation. We also identified seven patient-level factors that might have affected the outcomes, namely, sex, age group, coronary anatomy affected, comorbidity, priority at the time of registration on the surgical wait list, clearance time at time of registration on the wait list, and weekly number of inpatient and emergency procedures [141].

16.3.5 Measure of Effect Size

To compare the effects of the methods of booking surgery on the performance measures of interest at the hospital level, we used the following measures of effect size corresponding to those performance measures:

- Odds ratio for delay of any high-priority elective procedures.
- Odds ratio for a hospital having no cancellations of high-priority elective procedures.

Similarly, we used the following measures of effect size to compare the effects of the methods of booking surgery on the performance measures of interest at the patient level:

- Ratio of weekly odds for undergoing surgery among patients remaining on wait lists.
- Odds ratio for undergoing surgery after the recommended time.
- Odds ratio for cancellation of an elective procedure from the final operating room list.

16.3.6 Design of Experiment

Similar to the study designs in Chaps. 14 and 15, we used a cluster randomized design, in which the unit of allocation was a simulated hospital, as described in Sect. 7.3. We calculated that 144 simulation runs per experimental group would be needed to detect the anticipated effects of the methods of booking surgery with high probability. All calculations assumed a two-sided test with 0.05 significance level and 90% power. The estimated 144 runs were based on the maximum number of runs across the hospital-level and patient-level performance measures of interest, as described below. We used the Fedorov algorithm to ensure optimal distribution of the experimental factors across the runs [55]. This algorithm randomly assigned each group of patients from simulation runs with the specified combination of values of the hospital-level factors to an experimental group. These combinations of values for each run were specified by a design matrix (see Sect. 7.3).

Number of Runs for Cluster-Level Evaluations

We determined the number of runs needed to detect the anticipated difference in each hospital-level performance measure. First, we calculated the number of runs needed to detect a difference in the proportion of hospitals with delay of any high-priority elective procedures. According to provisional runs of the simulation model, the hypothesized proportion of hospitals with delay of any high-priority elective procedures was 0.67 among hospitals using the wait-list method of booking surgery. We estimated the number of simulation runs needed to detect a decrease of 0.20 in this proportion. Using (8.8), the required number of simulation runs (rounding up to the nearest integer) is as follows:

$$\begin{aligned} k &= \left[\frac{1.96\sqrt{2(0.57)(1-0.57)} + 1.28\sqrt{0.67(1-0.67)+0.47(1-0.47)}}{0.47-0.67}\right]^2 \\ &\approx 127. \end{aligned}$$

Second, according to provisional runs of the simulation model, the hypothesized proportion of hospitals with no cancellations of high-priority elective procedures from the final operating room list was 0.07 among hospitals using the wait-list booking method. We estimated the number of simulation runs needed to detect an increase of 0.20 in this proportion. Using (8.8), the required number of simulation runs (rounding up to the nearest integer) is as follows:

$$k = \left[\frac{1.96\sqrt{2(0.17)(1-0.17)} + 1.28\sqrt{0.07(1-0.07)+0.27(1-0.27)}}{0.27-0.07}\right]^2$$
$$\approx 73.$$

For the purpose of the multivariable regression analysis, we determined the number of runs to generate an adequate number of observations per regression variable. Our primary experimental factor required one variable for the method of booking surgery. In addition, we used two variables for clearance times for appointment lists at the start of simulation, three variables for clearance times for surgical wait lists at the start of simulation, two variables for clearance times for inpatient surgical queues at the start of simulation, two variables for methods of booking surgical consultation appointments, and one variable for allocation of operating room slots. Therefore, with a total of 11 variables, we estimated that 55 ($= 11 \times 10/2$) observed events per booking method would be needed, allowing for 10 events per regression variable [73]. From provisional runs of the model, the event of a hospital having delay of any high-priority elective procedures occurred about 38.5% of the time. Therefore, we calculated that at least 143 runs ($\approx$55/0.385) per method would be needed.

Number of Runs for Individual-Level Evaluations

We then calculated the number of runs needed to detect the anticipated difference in each patient-level performance measure. For analyses at the patient level, the dependence between experimental responses within each hospital necessitated adjustment for within-hospital correlation [140]. First, we estimated the number of runs to detect a difference in rates of surgery among registered patients. Given the results of provisional runs of the simulation model, we assumed an average of 1,791 patient-weeks per simulation run and a coefficient of variation of 0.06 [74]. The hypothesized weekly rate of surgery was 28 per 100 patient-weeks among hospitals using the wait-list booking method. We estimated that 14 runs per booking method would allow us to detect a 10% increase in the weekly surgery rate between groups of patients [49]. Using the Hayes method in (9.24), the required number of simulation runs (rounding up to the nearest integer) is as follows:

$$k = 1 + \frac{(1.96+1.28)^2}{(0.28-0.28\times 1.10)^2} \times \left(\frac{0.28}{1{,}980} + \frac{0.28\times 1.10}{1{,}578} + 0.0005595\right)$$
$$\approx 14.$$

Second, we calculated the number of runs required to detect a difference in the proportion of patients whose surgery was delayed after the recommended time.

The hypothesized proportion of patients with surgical delay was 0.10 among hospitals that used the wait-list booking method. We estimated that five runs per booking method would allow us to detect a 0.05 decrease in this proportion between groups of patients [49]. We used (9.9) to calculate the intracluster correlation coefficient, ρ, which is the ratio of the between-cluster and within-cluster variation, as follows:

$$\hat{\rho} = \frac{0.05062 - 0.00878}{0.05062 + (716.7 - 1)(0.00878)} \approx 0.006605.$$

Then, using (9.14), we estimated the inflation factor, IF, as follows:

$$\mathrm{IF} = 1 + (717 - 1) \times 0.006605 \approx 5.7.$$

Therefore, because of the clustered nature of the experimental design, we determined that we would need almost six times more runs in our experiment with randomization at the level of runs than in an experiment with randomization at the level of individual patients. We then computed the number of runs per booking method using (9.13) (rounding up to the nearest integer):

$$k = \frac{(1.96 + 1.28)^2[0.10(1 - 0.10) + 0.05(1 - 0.05)]}{717(0.05 - 0.10)^2}5.7 \approx 5.$$

Third, we determined the number of runs needed to detect a difference in the proportion of patients whose surgery was canceled from the final operating room list. Preliminary runs indicated that the hypothesized proportion of patients with cancellations was 0.17 for hospitals using the wait-list booking method. Using (9.9), (9.13), and (9.14), we estimated that one run per booking method would allow us to detect a 0.10 decrease in this proportion between groups of patients [49].

Finally, for the purpose of the multivariable regression analysis, we determined the number of runs needed to generate an adequate number of observations per regression variable. As described above, the primary experimental factor was represented by one variable for methods of booking surgery. In addition, we used two variables for clearance times for appointment lists at the start of simulation, three variables for clearance times for surgical wait lists at the start of simulation, two variables for clearance times for inpatient surgical queues at the start of simulation, two variables for methods of booking surgical consultation appointments, and one variable for allocation of operating room slots. The patient-level variables included one variable for sex, four variables for age groups, two variables for categories of coronary anatomy affected, two variables for categories of comorbidity, two variables for priorities at registration, one continuous variable for the weekly number of inpatient and emergency procedures, and one time-dependent continuous variable for wait-list clearance time at registration. Therefore, with a total of 24 variables, we estimated that 120 ($= 24 \times 10/2$) observed events per booking method would be needed, allowing for 10 events per regression variable

Table 16.3 Number of simulation runs required to compare methods of booking surgery with 0.05 significance level and 90% power per experimental group

Performance measure	Reference value	Effect size	No. of runs
Hospital level			
Proportion of hospitals with delay of any high-priority elective procedures	0.67	0.20 decrease	127*
Proportion of hospitals with no cancellations of high-priority elective procedures	0.07	0.20 increase	73
Patient level			
Surgery rate per 100 patient-weeks	28	10% increase	14
Proportion of patients with surgical delay after recommended time	0.10	0.05 decrease	5
Proportion of patients with cancellation from final OR list	0.17	0.10 decrease	1

Abbreviation: OR = operating room
*143 runs required to allow 10 events per regression variable in cluster-level evaluation

[73]. Provisional runs of the model indicated that the event of surgery performed after the recommended time occurred about 0.9% of the time, and there were about 717 patients per hospital. Therefore, we estimated that we would need at least 19 runs ($\approx 120/[0.009 \times 717]$) per method.

The estimates of the number of simulation runs required for each performance measure are summarized in Table 16.3. To ensure adequate power to detect clinically significant differences between the two experimental groups in each performance measure, the minimum number of simulation runs per experimental group had to meet the requirements for the performance measure with the largest number of simulation runs. Therefore, the minimum number of simulation runs was 143 per method. We included 144 runs per method in our experiment to allow for an equal number of runs across hospital-level variables with two categories.

16.4 Evaluation of Experiment

Analyses were conducted at the level of both the hospital and the patient. For analyses at the hospital level, we report differences between the two methods of booking surgery in terms of the odds of delay of any high-priority elective procedures and the odds of a hospital having no cancellations of high-priority elective procedures. For analyses at the patient level, we report differences between the two booking methods in terms of the weekly odds that a patient would undergo elective surgery, the odds that a surgery would occur after recommended time, and the odds of cancellation from the final operating room list.

16.4.1 Statistical Instruments

We used logistic regression methods to model the relation between method of booking surgery and delay of any high-priority elective procedures or no cancellations of high-priority elective procedures. In multivariable regression analyses, we adjusted the difference between the two booking methods for hospital-level factors by including sets of indicator variables, as described in the previous section. The odds ratios derived from these logistic regressions measured the effect of advance booking on the odds that a hospital would delay any high-priority elective procedures and on the odds that a hospital would have no cancellations of high-priority elective procedures, relative to hospitals using wait-list booking (see Table D.1 in Appendix D).

To assess performance at the patient-level, we plotted the access curves from registration to surgery by method of booking surgery and by priority group. We used discrete-time survival regression to model the relation between booking method and time to elective surgery, with adjustment for hospital-level and patient-level factors (see Table D.1 in Appendix D). We used logistic regression, with adjustment for correlation between patients in the same hospital, to model the relation between the booking method and undergoing surgery after the recommended time or cancellation from the final operating room list. In these regression models, we adjusted for hospital-level and patient-level variables by including sets of indicator variables, as described in the previous section.

The odds ratios derived from discrete-time survival regressions measured the effects of advance booking of surgery on the weekly proportion of patients undergoing the operation, relative to what occurred with wait-list booking [139]. The odds ratios derived from logistic regressions measured the effects of advance booking, relative to wait-list booking, on the odds of surgery after the recommended time and on the odds of cancellation.

16.4.2 Hospital and Patient Characteristics

The 288 simulation runs generated a total of 218,310 referrals for elective procedures, 214,664 urgent cases, and 15,480 emergency cases over six 18-week cycles of assignment of clinic and operating time starting on the arbitrarily chosen date of September 1, 2008. On average, the simulation model generated 365 elective referrals, 359 urgent cases, and 26 emergency arrivals per modeled hospital in one year. The modeled surgical services performed 662 procedures per year on average.

The distribution of referrals by patient-level factors was also similar across methods of booking surgery. The majority of referrals were for men (83.6%), and 37.9% of patients were 60–69 years old. Most patients had multivessel disease (73.5%) and either major or minor concurrent conditions (49.5%).

Table 16.4 Characteristics of simulated patients registered for elective surgery by method of booking surgery

	Booking method; no. (%) of patients			
	Wait-list booking		Advance booking	
Characteristic	(n = 102,696)		(n = 103,681)	
Age group (years)				
<50	7,263	(7.1)	7,407	(7.1)
50–59	23,444	(22.8)	23,429	(22.6)
60–69	38,930	(37.9)	39,224	(37.8)
70–79	29,890	(29.1)	30,468	(29.4)
≥80	3,169	(3.1)	3,153	(3.0)
Sex				
Male	86,065	(83.8)	86,790	(83.7)
Female	16,631	(16.2)	16,891	(16.3)
Coronary anatomy affected				
Left main	16,968	(16.5)	17,319	(16.7)
Multivessel*	75,568	(73.6)	76,386	(73.7)
Limited†	10,160	(9.9)	9,976	(9.6)
Comorbidity				
Major conditions‡	22,794	(22.2)	23,018	(22.2)
Other conditions§	27,916	(27.2)	27,913	(26.9)
None	51,986	(50.6)	52,750	(50.9)
Priority at time of registration				
High	7,421	(7.2)	7,444	(7.2)
Medium	72,181	(70.3)	73,195	(70.6)
Low	23,094	(22.5)	23,042	(22.2)
Clearance time at registration				
Less than half week	59,024	(57.5)	70,044	(67.6)
Less than half month	34,144	(33.2)	31,877	(30.7)
More than half month	9,528	(9.3)	1,760	(1.7)

*Two- or three-vessel disease with proximal left anterior descending (PLAD) artery
†Two-vessel disease with no PLAD or one-vessel disease with PLAD
‡Congestive heart failure, diabetes mellitus, chronic obstructive pulmonary disease, rheumatoid arthritis, cancer
§Peripheral vascular disease, cerebrovascular disease, dementia, peptic ulcer disease, hemiplegia, renal disease, liver disease

At the time of referral, 92.8% of the patients had low priority for surgical consultation. Regardless of the method of booking surgery, most of the referred patients had a surgical consultation by the end of the simulation (94.4% for those booked from a wait list and 94.6% for those booked in advance). The rest of the patients were still waiting for an appointment because their referral times were close to the end of the simulation period.

At the time of registration on a surgical wait list, 70.4% of the patients had medium priority for the operation and 22.4% had low priority (Table 16.4). The

Table 16.5 Proportion of hospitals with delay of high-priority elective procedures in relation to method of booking surgery

Method	% (no. of hospitals with delay/ total no. of hospitals)	Odds ratio (95% CI)*
Wait-list booking	73.6 (106/144)	1.00
Advance booking	6.9 (10/144)	0.01 (0.00–0.01)

Abbreviation: CI = confidence interval
*Adjusted for method of booking surgical consultation appointments, allocation of operating room slots, clearance times for appointment lists, surgical wait lists, and inpatient surgical queues at the start of the simulation

waiting time for elective surgery was less than half a week for 57.5% of the patients booked from wait lists and for 67.6% of those with advance booking.

Of all the patients who were registered on a surgical wait list, 78.6% underwent the planned procedure. The reasons for removal from the list without surgery were similar across methods of booking surgery: 8.3% of planned procedures were canceled because no beds were available in the intensive care unit for recovery after surgery, and 8.7% of planned procedures were canceled because an inpatient was admitted for surgery. Another 4.3% of patients were removed from the list for other reasons, or they remained on the wait list at the end of the simulation.

16.4.3 Proportion of Hospitals with Surgical Delay

The proportion of hospitals with delay of any high-priority elective procedures was substantially lower among hospitals using the advance booking method than among those with wait-list booking (6.9% vs. 73.6%) (Table 16.5). The odds of a hospital delaying surgery for high-priority elective procedures were much lower with advance booking than with wait-list booking, after adjustment for hospital-level factors (Table 16.5).

16.4.4 Proportion of Hospitals with no Cancellations

The proportion of hospitals with no cancellations of any high-priority elective procedures was lower among hospitals using the advance booking method than among those using wait-list booking (2.8% vs. 5.6%) (Table 16.6). After adjustment for hospital-level factors, the odds of a hospital having no cancellations of high-priority elective procedures were not significantly different between the two booking methods (Table 16.6).

Table 16.6 Proportion of hospitals with no cancellation of high-priority elective procedures in relation to method of booking surgery

Method	% (no. of hospitals with no cancellations/total no. of hospitals)	Odds ratio (95% CI)*
Wait-list booking	5.6 (8/144)	1.00
Advance booking	2.8 (4/144)	0.44 (0.13–1.57)

Abbreviation: CI = confidence interval
*Adjusted for method of booking surgical consultation appointments, allocation of operating room slots, clearance times for appointment lists, surgical wait lists, and inpatient surgical queues at the start of the simulation

Table 16.7 Weekly rate of elective surgery among patients with high priority at registration, in relation to method of booking surgery

Factor	No. of procedures	No. of patient-weeks	Surgery rate* (95% CI)	Ratio of weekly odds (95% CI)†
Booking method				
Wait-list booking	5,987	7,898	75.8 (73.9–77.7)	1.00
Advance booking	6,278	6,788	92.5 (90.2–94.8)	2.30 (2.05–2.58)
Nonelective procedures‡				0.15 (0.13–0.18)

Abbreviation: CI = confidence interval
*Per 100 patient-weeks, calculated as the number of procedures divided by the total time in patient-weeks
†Adjusted for method of booking clinic appointments, allocation of operating room slots, clearance times for appointment lists, surgical wait lists, and inpatient surgical queues at the start of the simulation, age, sex, coronary anatomy affected, comorbidities, wait-list clearance times at registration, and week from registration
‡Associated with eight additional procedures performed without wait-list registration (the average weekly number)

16.4.5 Weekly Rate of Surgery

Each patient registered on a surgical wait list was assigned to one of three priority groups. In the high-priority group, the average weekly number of operations was higher with advance booking than with wait-list booking (92.5 vs. 75.8 procedures per 100 patient-weeks) (Table 16.7). Regardless of the booking method, more than half of high-priority patients had their operations within one week (Fig. 16.1). After adjustment for hospital-level and patient-level factors, the weekly odds that a high-priority patient waiting for elective surgery would undergo the operation were over two times higher among patients booked in advance than among those booked from a wait list (Table 16.7). After adjustment for correlation between patients within the same hospital, the ratio of weekly odds did not change (odds ratio = 2.46, 95% CI 2.13–2.84).

In the medium-priority group, the weekly rate of elective surgery was slightly higher in hospitals with advance booking than in those that used wait-list booking (36.2 vs. 31.2 per 100 patient-weeks) (Table 16.8). In both experimental groups,

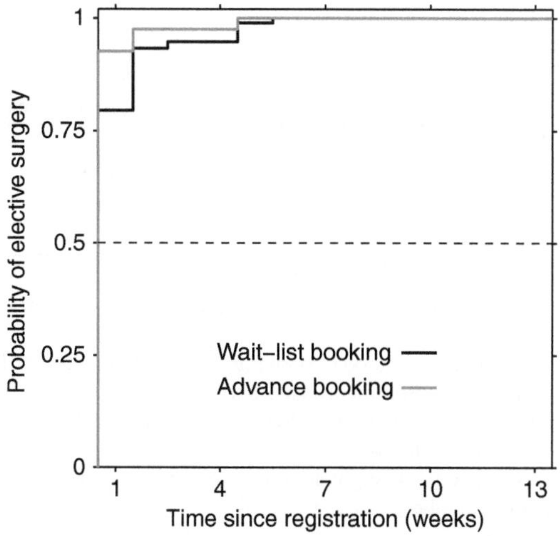

Fig. 16.1 Probability of undergoing surgery within a certain time since registration among patients with high priority at registration by method of booking surgery

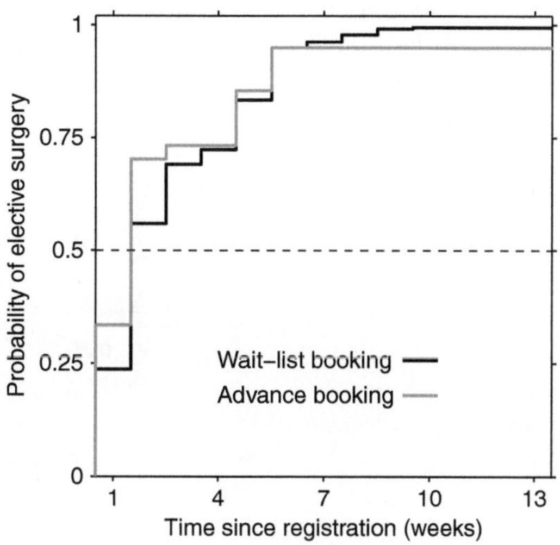

Fig. 16.2 Probability of undergoing surgery within a certain time since registration among patients with medium priority at registration by method of booking surgery

more than half of the medium-priority patients waiting for an elective procedure had their operations within two weeks (Fig. 16.2). After adjustment for hospital-level and patient-level factors, the weekly odds that a medium-priority patient would undergo the operation were just 3% higher among patients in hospitals with advance booking than in hospitals with wait-list booking. After adjustment for correlation between patients within the same hospital, the ratio of weekly odds of operation were similar (odds ratio = 1.11, 95% CI 1.08–1.14).

Low-priority patients had longer waiting times in hospitals that used wait-list booking (with half of these patients having their operations within four weeks) than in hospitals that used advance booking (with half having their operations within three weeks) (Fig. 16.3). The weekly odds of undergoing the operation were more

Table 16.8 Weekly rate of elective surgery among patients with medium priority at registration in relation to method of booking surgery

Factor	No. of procedures	No. of patient-weeks	Surgery rate* (95% CI)	Ratio of weekly odds (95% CI)†
Booking method				
Wait-list booking	56,099	179,543	31.2 (31.0–31.5)	1.00
Advance booking	55,922	154,479	36.2 (35.9–36.5)	1.03 (1.01–1.04)
Nonelective procedures‡				0.36 (0.36–0.37)

Abbreviation: CI = confidence interval

*Per 100 patient-weeks, calculated as the number of procedures divided by the total time in patient-weeks

†Adjusted for method of booking clinic appointments, allocation of operating room slots, clearance times for appointment lists, surgical wait lists, and inpatient surgical queues at the start of the simulation, age, sex, coronary anatomy affected, comorbidities, wait-list clearance times at registration, and week from registration

‡Associated with eight additional procedures performed without wait-list registration (the average weekly number)

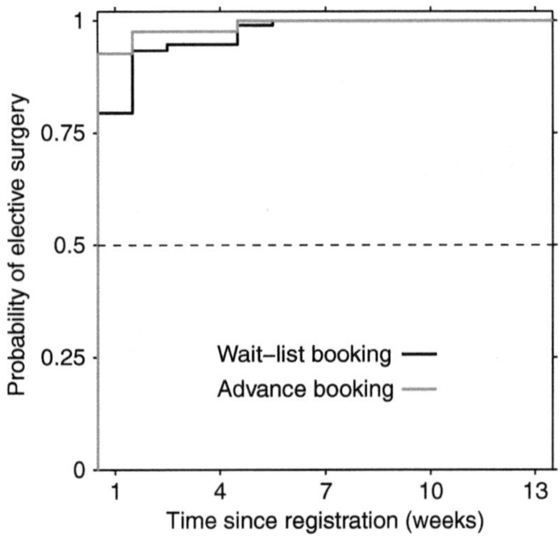

Fig. 16.3 Probability of undergoing surgery within a certain time since registration among patients with low priority at registration by method of booking surgery

than two times higher among patients booked in advance than among those booked from wait lists (Table 16.9). After adjustment for correlation between patients within the same hospital, the ratio of weekly odds of undergoing the operation did not change dramatically (odds ratio = 2.08, 95% CI 2.00–2.18).

16.4.6 Proportion of Surgeries After the Recommended Time

As described above, each patient was assigned to one of three priority groups at the time of registration on a surgical wait list. A patient was classified as having high priority if the suggested time to surgery was within three days, medium priority if

Table 16.9 Weekly rate of elective surgery among patients with low priority at registration in relation to method of booking surgery

Factor	No. of procedures	No. of patient-weeks	Surgery rate∗ (95% CI)	Ratio of weekly odds (95% CI)†
Booking method				
Wait-list booking	18,278	104,043	17.6 (17.3–17.8)	1.00
Advance booking	19,577	70,973	27.6 (27.2–28.0)	2.17 (2.11–2.23)
Nonelective procedures‡				0.46 (0.47–0.49)

Abbreviation: CI = confidence interval

∗Per 100 patient-weeks, calculated as the number of procedures divided by the total waiting time in patient-weeks

†Adjusted for method of booking clinic appointments, allocation of operating room slots, clearance times for appointment lists, surgical wait lists, and inpatient surgical queues at the start of the simulation, age, sex, coronary anatomy affected, comorbidities, wait-list clearance times at registration, and week from registration

‡Associated with eight additional procedures performed without wait-list registration (the average weekly number)

Table 16.10 Probability of undergoing surgery after the recommended time among patients with high priority at registration in relation to method of booking surgery

Method	% (no. of procedures with delay/ total no. of procedures)	Odds ratio (95% CI)∗
Wait-list booking	9.6 (716/7,421)	1.00
Advance booking	0.2 (15/7,444)	0.03 (0.01–0.03)

Abbreviation: CI = confidence interval

∗Adjusted for method of booking clinic appointments, allocation of operating room slots, clearance times for appointment lists, surgical wait lists, and inpatient surgical queues at the start of the simulation, age, sex, coronary anatomy affected, comorbidities

the suggested time was within six weeks, and low priority if the suggested time was within 12 weeks. A patient who waited longer than the suggested time was considered to have delayed access to surgery. Regardless of the priority group, surgery was delayed for less than 1% of patients scheduled for elective surgery at hospitals using the advance booking method. For patients booked at hospitals using the wait-list booking method, almost 10% of those with high-priority had delayed access to surgery (Table 16.10). For high-priority patients, the odds of a delay were substantially lower with advance booking than with wait-list booking (Table 16.10).

Among medium-priority patients, the proportion with delayed access to surgery in the advance booking group was about half the proportion in the wait-list booking group, and the odds of a delay were 51% lower with advance booking than with wait-list booking (Table 16.11). Among low-priority patients, almost all those whose procedures were scheduled at hospitals using advance booking underwent surgery within the specified timeframe of 12 weeks, and the odds of a delay were 87% lower with advance booking than with wait-list booking (Table 16.12).

Table 16.11 Probability of undergoing surgery after the recommended time among patients with medium priority at registration in relation to method of booking surgery

Method	% (no. of procedures with delay/ total no. of procedures)	Odds ratio (95% CI)*
Wait-list booking	1.1 (806/72,181)	1.00
Advance booking	0.5 (392/73,195)	0.49 (0.44–0.56)

Abbreviation: CI = confidence interval
*Adjusted for method of booking clinic appointments, allocation of operating room slots, clearance times for appointment lists, surgical wait lists, and inpatient surgical queues at the start of the simulation, age, sex, coronary anatomy affected, comorbidities

Table 16.12 Probability of undergoing surgery after the recommended time among patients with low priority at registration in relation to method of booking surgery

Method	% (no. of procedures with delay/ total no. of procedures)	Odds ratio (95% CI)*
Wait-list booking	1.0 (231/23,094)	1.00
Advance booking	<0.1 (11/23,042)	0.13 (0.07–0.24)

Abbreviation: CI = confidence interval
*Adjusted for method of booking clinic appointments, allocation of operating room slots, clearance times for appointment lists, surgical wait lists, and inpatient surgical queues at the start of the simulation, age, sex, coronary anatomy affected, comorbidities

16.4.7 Proportion of Patients with Cancellation of Surgery

The effect of the method of booking surgery differed across priority groups. The proportion of high-priority patients whose procedures were canceled from the final operating room list was lower in hospitals that used advance booking than in hospitals that used wait-list booking (5.3% vs. 7.4%) (Table 16.13). The odds of cancellation of a high-priority elective procedure were about 29% lower with advance booking than with wait-list booking (Table 16.13).

In contrast, among medium-priority patients, the proportion of cancellations from the final operating room list seemed higher with advance booking than with wait-list booking (20.5% vs. 18.3%) (Table 16.14). The odds of cancellation of a medium-priority elective procedure were about 15% higher with advance booking than with wait-list booking (Table 16.14).

The situation for low-priority patients was similar to that for high-priority patients, and their operations seemed to be canceled less often in hospitals that used advance booking (11.5% vs. 15.5%) (Table 16.15). The odds of cancellation of a low-priority elective procedure were about 29% lower with advance booking than with wait-list booking (Table 16.15).

Table 16.13 Probability of cancellation from the final operating room list among patients with high priority at registration in relation to method of booking surgery

Method	% (no. of procedures canceled/ total no. of patients)	Odds ratio (95% CI)*
Wait-list booking	7.4 (547/7,421)	1.00
Advance booking	5.3 (394/7,444)	0.71 (0.62–0.81)

Abbreviation: CI = confidence interval
*Adjusted for method of booking clinic appointments, allocation of operating room slots, clearance times for appointment lists, surgical wait lists, and inpatient surgical queues at the start of the simulation, age, sex, coronary anatomy affected, comorbidities, and wait-list clearance times at registration

Table 16.14 Probability of cancellation from the final operating room list among patients with medium priority at registration in relation to method of booking surgery

Method	% (no. of procedures canceled/ total no. of patients)	Odds ratio (95% CI)*
Wait-list booking	18.3 (13,215/72,181)	1.00
Advance booking	20.5 (14,991/73,195)	1.15 (1.12–1.18)

Abbreviation: CI = confidence interval
*Adjusted for method of booking clinic appointments, allocation of operating room slots, clearance times for appointment lists, surgical wait lists, and inpatient surgical queues at the start of the simulation, age, sex, coronary anatomy affected, comorbidities, and wait-list clearance times at registration

Table 16.15 Probability of cancellation from the final operating room list among patients with low priority at registration in relation to method of booking surgery

Method	% (no. of procedures canceled/ total no. of patients)	Odds ratio (95% CI)*
Wait-list booking	15.5 (3,590/23,094)	1.00
Advance booking	11.5 (2,650/23,042)	0.71 (0.67–0.75)

Abbreviation: CI = confidence interval
*Adjusted for method of booking clinic appointments, allocation of operating room slots, clearance times for appointment lists, surgical wait lists, and inpatient surgical queues at the start of the simulation, age, sex, coronary anatomy affected, comorbidities, and wait-list clearance times at registration

16.4.8 Conclusion

The most common method of booking elective surgery is the wait-list booking method, whereby the patients name is placed on a wait list without a projected date of operation, and attempts to book the operation are made periodically until an appropriate operating room slot becomes available. With the advance booking method, the consulting surgeon prebooks the date of the procedure at the time of the decision to operate, instead of keeping patients on wait lists until an operating room slot becomes available.

Our results suggest that cancellations of high-priority elective procedures were less likely in hospitals that booked surgery dates in advance and that a larger proportion of both high-priority and low-priority patients waiting for elective surgery were likely to undergo their operations each week with advance booking. Given that the weekly proportion of operations in relation to the size of the wait lists estimates the conditional probability of the operation taking place while waiting, the latter observation means shorter times to elective surgery [139]. Higher cancellation rates after wait-list booking may be attributable to a higher proportion of patients who need elective surgery being scheduled in the on-call slot with this method of booking. Therefore, these patients are at higher risk of cancellation caused by the arrival of emergency patients or inpatients. Shorter time to surgery after advance booking may be a result of scheduling cases in the order of booking requests; in contrast, with wait-list booking, newly registered cases with higher priority delay scheduling of cases with lower priority already on the lists.

In this study, we evaluated two methods of booking elective surgery using specifications of perioperative activities that constitute the process of cardiac surgical care. Because these managerial and clinical activities are generic across surgical services, the results of our evaluation may be applicable to other settings in which wait lists are used to manage access to surgical procedures in hospital. Indeed, by varying other factors that are likely to influence service performance, such as allocation of operating room slots and method of booking surgical consultation appointments, we were able to delineate the independent effect of booking methods. However, some limitations of our model should be recognized in assessing our results. For example, although we were able to account for availability of surgeons for operations, fluctuations in availability of intensive care beds due to staff shortage and bed blockage were not considered in the model. The results may not be applicable to a network of hospitals where surgeons have admitting rights to multiple hospitals. Although the schedules of three surgeons with operating room, office, and on-call duties were modeled in one hospital, these schedules, and hence the model, would be different in a network of hospitals.

Further research is required to explore the implications of booking systems on patient flow, specifically, the impact of the ratio of slots allocated for urgent and elective procedures on time to surgery for patients needing procedures urgently; the implications of policies for postponement or cancellation of elective procedures and rescheduling canceled surgeries in relation to time to surgery; and the effects of the order of elective procedures on a given day, patient segmentation, the partitioning of inpatient and outpatient facilities, and dedicated operating rooms. Other remaining questions include whether successful management solutions developed in one hospital can be transferred to other institutions.

Chapter 17
Booking Anesthesiology Consultations

In this chapter, we describe our plans for a simulation study to investigate the management of anesthesiology consultations in the context of cardiac surgical care. This chapter differs from Chaps. 14–16 in that here, we focus on the planning of a simulation study rather than evaluating the results of such a study. In particular, we describe our plans for extending our simulation model, for designing the simulation experiment, and for evaluating the effect of adopting a pooled-list method for booking anesthesiology consultations. These plans are discussed using our analytical framework of a simulation experiment, as described in Chap. 7. Specifically, we discuss the modeling requirements, study and experimental factors, and patient attributes for such a study. We also discuss the information that will be reported to help the reader understand the objectives and hypotheses of the study (see item 5 of Table 10.1).

17.1 Background

In the process of surgical care, patients for whom an operation is deemed necessary and who consent to the procedure undergo a preoperative assessment. During this assessment, the anesthesiologist determines factors that may increase the risk of adverse outcomes and provides education about anesthesia and postoperative care (Fig. 3.1). A consultation with an anesthesiologist is a part of presurgical screening, discussed in Chap. 15. For a patient who undergos elective surgery, the anesthesiology consultation is booked after registration on a surgical wait list. A commonly used model for booking anesthesiology consultations is to refer patients to a clinic run by anesthesiologists with subsequent referrals to internists or other medical subspecialists if needed. Pooling anesthesiology referrals on a single list may reduce the chances that consultations cannot be scheduled due to unavailability of a particular anesthesiologist, relative to booking consultations with a preferred anesthesiologist. Few studies have assessed the effect of booking practices for

B. Sobolev et al., *Health Care Evaluation Using Computer Simulation: Concepts, Methods, and Applications*, DOI 10.1007/978-1-4614-2233-4_17,

Box 17.1 What is already known about booking anesthesiology consultations

- Several approaches to preoperative assessment have been used in the real world, including referral of patients to a preoperative assessment clinic run by anesthesiologists [25].
- Any approach to managing these preoperative assessments entails some amount of waiting, which could lead to inconvenience for the patient and potential postponement of the scheduled operation.
- Few studies have assessed the effect of the various approaches to preoperative assessment on patient or treatment outcomes [21, 121, 134, 154].

anesthesiology consultations on time to surgery. The study question of interest for this simulation study is *Does use of a pooled referral list for booking anesthesiology consultations affect the time to surgery?*

17.2 The Management Alternatives

In this planned simulation study, we will compare two methods of booking anesthesiology consultations: individual consultation lists and pooled consultation list. In the case of individual lists, each consultation is booked with the surgeon's preferred anesthesiologist. This method ensures that each patient is assessed by the anesthesiologist chosen by the referring surgeon. In the case of a pooled list, each consultation is booked with the first available anesthesiologist. Box 17.1 summarizes what is already known about this topic.

17.3 The Simulation Model

17.3.1 Modeling Requirements

This simulation experiment will be based on discrete-event simulation of patient flow, described in detail in Chap. 13. The simulation model for this particular study will be based on the model specifications developed for the analysis presented in Chap. 15, with the addition of two alternative methods of booking anesthesiology consultations: individual consultation lists and pooled consultation list. We will consider a setting in which four anesthesiologists are available for assessments every weekday, with each anesthesiologist available for one assessment per weekday.

Patients requiring further medical tests after the initial anesthesiology consultation are booked for an additional consultation with the anesthesiologist, which may delay the operation. Under the individual consultation lists method, patients are offered the possibility of booking the additional anesthesiology consultation through the pooled-list method. Conversely, under the pooled consultation list

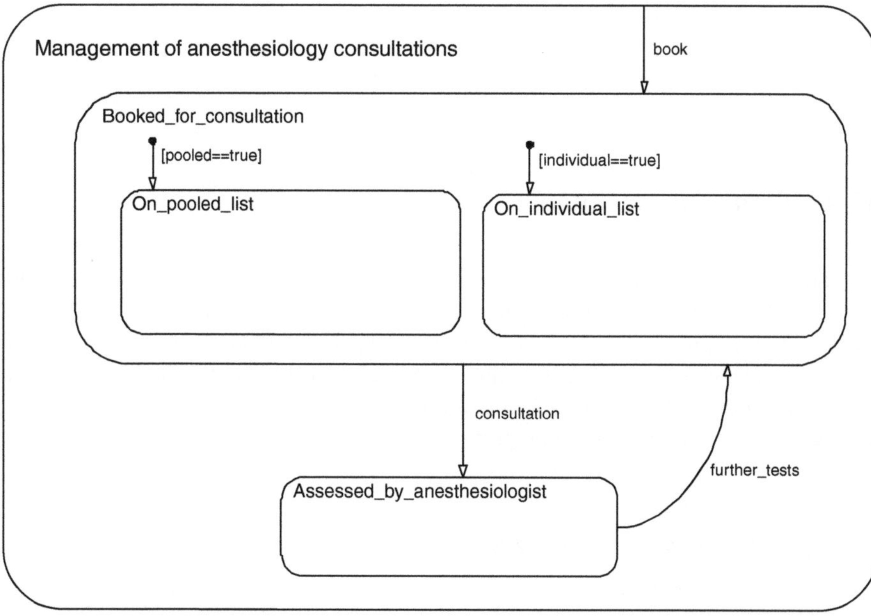

Fig. 17.1 Statechart for two methods of booking anesthesiology consultations: individual consultation lists and pooled consultations list

method, patients are offered the possibility of booking the additional anesthesiology consultation with the anesthesiologist who performed the initial assessment.

Figure 17.1 depicts the Statechart for the two alternative methods of booking anesthesiology consultations. Triggering of the event `book` causes a transition to the state `Booked_for_consultation`. In this state, the patient is in the substate `On_individual_list`, if the booking method is individual consultation lists, or the state `On_pooled_list`, if the booking method is pooled consultation list. Triggering of the event `consultations` causes a transition to the state `Assessed_by_anesthesiologist`. If the event `further tests` is triggered in this state, the patient moves back to the state `Booked_for_consultation`.

17.3.2 Modeling Assumptions

The modeling assumptions particular to this simulation study are in addition to the ones listed in Chaps. 13 and 15. These additional assumptions are as follows:

1. Four anesthesiologists are available for consultations, and each is available for one assessment per weekday.
2. Twenty anesthesiology consultations are available each week.

3. All patients attend their appointments.
4. The progress of patients requiring additional anesthesiology consultations is governed by binomial probability distributions.

17.4 Plan of Experiment

We will use elements from our analytical framework (Sect. 7.2) and experimental design (Sect. 7.3) to plan our simulation experiment. Our analytical framework operationalizes the hypothesis by identifying the primary study factor, experimental outcomes, performance measures, and measures of effect size. The experimental design determines the unit of randomization, the number of simulation runs, and the allocation of runs to experimental groups.

17.4.1 Primary Study Factor

Our primary study factor will be the method of booking anesthesiology consultations, and this factor will have two categories: individual consultation lists and pooled consultation list. This primary study factor will be represented by one indicator variable, with the individual-lists method defined as the reference group.

17.4.2 Experimental Responses and Performance Measures

We are interested in measuring system performance at the levels of both the hospital and the patient. We anticipate that the methods of booking anesthesiology consultations may have different effects on the overall performance of a hospital and on the timing of surgery for individual patients, so we will study more than one performance measure to understand these different perspectives. These performance measures will allow a decision-maker to evaluate the effects of the booking methods on times to surgery.

The hospital-level response is a system-related outcome reflecting the effect, an intervention on the simulated health care system (see Sect. 2.4). During the simulation experiment, the following hospital-level experimental response will be generated:

- For each hospital, whether any high-priority elective procedures are delayed (indicator variable).

The following hospital-level performance measure will be used to summarize the results of the experiment:

- Proportion of hospitals with delay of any high-priority elective procedures.

The patient-level responses are patient-related outcomes reflecting the effect of an intervention on patients who are treated in the simulated health care system (see Sect. 2.4). During the simulation experiment, the following patient-level experimental responses will be generated:

- For each patient, whether surgery is performed (indicator variable) and the number of weeks from registration to surgery or removal from the list (continuous variable).
- For each patient, whether surgery is after the recommended time (indicator variable).

The following patient-level performance measures will be of interest:

- Weekly rate of surgery among patients remaining on wait lists.
- Proportion of wait-listed patients undergoing surgery after the recommended time.

17.4.3 Hospital-Level and Patient-Level Experimental Factors

For our planned simulation experiment, we will identify hospital-level and patient-level factors that may impede or enhance occurrence of the outcomes (see Sect. 2.3). We will use these factors in regression analyses to adjust for differences in distributions between the experimental groups. We will then attribute to the method of booking anesthesiology consultations any differences between experimental groups that cannot be explained by the hospital-level and patient-level factors.

We anticipate that six hospital-level factors might affect the experimental responses: method of booking surgical consultation appointments, method of managing presurgical screening, allocation of operating room slots, the clearance times for appointment lists, surgical wait lists, and inpatient surgical queues at the start of simulation. A variety of patient-level factors, such as sex, age group, coronary anatomy affected, comorbidity, priority of registration on the surgical wait list, clearance time at time of registration on a wait list, and weekly numbers of inpatient and emergency procedures, may all affect the time to elective surgery, as well as the chance that a procedure will be delayed [141].

17.4.4 Measure of Effect Size

To compare the effects of the methods of booking anesthesiology consultations on the hospital-level performance measure of interest, we will use the following measure of effect size:

- Odds ratio for delay of any high-priority elective procedures.

Similarly, to compare the effects of the booking methods on the patient-level performance measures of interest, we will use the following two measures of effect size:

- Ratio of weekly odds for undergoing surgery among patients remaining on wait lists.
- Odds ratio for undergoing surgery after the recommended time.

17.4.5 Allocation of Runs

In this experiment, each run will generate a cluster of simulated patients served in a simulated hospital. As such, the study will be a cluster randomized trial, with the unit of allocation being a simulated hospital. A full factorial design for this type of simulation experiment will have one run for every possible combination of values of the seven cluster-level experimental factors (see Sect. 7.3). More specifically, there will be two categories for the method of booking anesthesiology consultations, three categories for the method of booking surgical consultation appointment, two categories for the method of managing presurgical screening, two categories for the allocation of operating room slots, three categories for clearance time for appointment lists, four categories for clearance time for surgical wait lists, and three categories for clearance time for inpatient surgical queues. Therefore, the number of combinations (i.e., design points) for this simulation experiment will be 864 $(=2 \times 3 \times 2 \times 2 \times 3 \times 4 \times 3)$.

The design matrix corresponding to this full factorial design will have 864 rows (representing the 864 design points) and 12 $(=1+2+1+1+2+3+2)$ columns (representing the indicator variables for the cluster-level experimental factors):

$$
\begin{array}{c}
\\ 1 \\ 2 \\ 3 \\ 4 \\ 5 \\ 6 \\ \vdots \\ 862 \\ 863 \\ 864
\end{array}
\begin{array}{c}
\begin{array}{cccccccccccc} I_1 & I_2 & I_3 & I_4 & I_5 & I_6 & I_7 & I_8 & I_9 & I_{10} & I_{11} & I_{12} \end{array} \\
\begin{pmatrix}
0 & 0 & 0 & 0 & 0 & 0 & 0 & 0 & 0 & 0 & 0 & 0 \\
0 & 0 & 0 & 0 & 0 & 0 & 0 & 0 & 0 & 0 & 1 & 0 \\
0 & 0 & 0 & 0 & 0 & 0 & 0 & 0 & 0 & 0 & 0 & 1 \\
0 & 0 & 0 & 0 & 0 & 0 & 0 & 1 & 0 & 0 & 0 & 0 \\
0 & 0 & 0 & 0 & 0 & 0 & 0 & 1 & 0 & 0 & 1 & 0 \\
0 & 0 & 0 & 0 & 0 & 0 & 0 & 1 & 0 & 0 & 0 & 1 \\
\vdots & \vdots & \vdots & \vdots & \vdots & \vdots & \vdots & \vdots & \vdots & \vdots & \vdots & \vdots \\
1 & 0 & 1 & 1 & 1 & 0 & 1 & 0 & 0 & 1 & 0 & 0 \\
1 & 0 & 1 & 1 & 1 & 0 & 1 & 0 & 0 & 1 & 1 & 0 \\
1 & 0 & 1 & 1 & 1 & 0 & 1 & 0 & 0 & 1 & 0 & 1
\end{pmatrix}
\end{array}
$$

In this design matrix, an experimental factor with two categories are represented by one indicator variable. For example, indicator variable I_1 represents the two methods of booking anesthesiology consultations by taking the value 1 for pooled consultation list method and the value 0 for individual consultation lists method. Factors with two or more categories are represented by sets of indicator variables. The number of variables in each set is one less than the number of categories. For example, the set of two indicator variables I_2 and I_3 represents the three methods of booking surgical consultation appointment. In this set, the values $I_2 = 1$ and $I_3 = 0$ correspond to the individual-lists method, the values $I_2 = 0$ and $I_3 = 1$ correspond to the shortest-list method, and the values $I_2 = 0$ and $I_3 = 0$ correspond to the pooled-list method. Each row of the design matrix will specify the values of cluster-level experimental factors for one simulation run (i.e., one modeled hospital).

As noted above, we plan to use a cluster randomized design, in which the unit of allocation is the simulation run. This number of runs that will actually be executed may be less than the number in the full factorial design. The number of runs should ensure that we detect, with high probability, the anticipated effects of the methods of booking anesthesiology consultations, as described in Sect. 7.3. After determining the number of runs, we will apply the Fedorov algorithm to ensure an optimal distribution of experimental factors across the runs [55]. If the number of runs is less than 864, then the optimal design matrix will contain a subset of the rows from the full design matrix. Pilot data will be needed to estimate the magnitude of the performance measures in the reference group, as well as to estimate the measures of variability and correlation needed for estimating the number of runs (see Chaps. 8 and 9). These pilot data will be generated by performing provisional runs of the simulation model, with 30 hospitals per experimental group.

17.5 Plan of Evaluation

We will use our analytical framework of a simulation study for identifying elements for the analysis of the simulated data (see Sect. 7.4). These elements include identifying the unit of analysis and appropriate regression methods for estimating the effect of the intervention. For this simulation study, we will have two units of analysis, the hospital and the patient. At the hospital level, we will report differences between the methods of booking anesthesiology consultations in terms of the odds of delay for any high-priority elective procedures. At the patient level, we will report differences between the two methods in terms of the weekly odds of undergoing surgery and the odds of delay of high-priority elective procedures.

17.5.1 Statistical Instruments

We plan to use multivariable logistic regressions to model the relation between the method of booking anesthesiology consultations and delay of any high-priority procedures, with adjustment for hospital-level factors. The regression model will have an indicator variable, I_1, to represent the pooled-list booking method (Table 17.1).

Table 17.1 Regression model for estimating effect of method of booking anesthesiology consultations on proportion of hospitals with delay of procedures

Question:	Does use of a pooled-list booking method for anesthesiology consultations affect the proportion of hospitals with delay of any high-priority elective procedures?
Model:	$\log\left(\frac{p^c}{1-p^c}\right) = \beta_0 + \beta_1 I_1 + \beta_2 I_2 + \beta_3 I_3 + \beta_4 I_4 + \beta_5 I_5 + \beta_6 I_6 + \beta_7 I_7 + \beta_8 I_8 + \beta_9 I_9 + \beta_{10} I_{10} + \beta_{11} I_{11} + \beta_{12} I_{12}$
p^c	Proportion of hospitals with delay of any high-priority elective procedures
I_1	Indicator for pooled-list vs. individual-lists booking of anesthesiology consultations
I_2, I_3	Indicators for individual-lists or shortest-list vs. pooled-list booking of surgical consultation appointments
I_4	Indicator for some-screened vs. all-screened management of presurgical screening
I_5	Indicator for daily vs. weekly split of operating room slots between elective and urgent procedures
I_6, I_7	Indicators for 2 or 3 vs. 1 week of clearance time for appointment lists at start of simulation
I_8, I_9, I_{10}	Indicators for 4, 5, or 6 vs. 3 weeks of clearance time for surgical wait lists at start of simulation
I_{11}, I_{12}	Indicators for 1 or 2 vs. 0 weeks of clearance time for inpatient surgical queues at start of simulation

The odds ratio derived from the estimated regression coefficient for this indicator variable (i.e., $\exp[\hat{\beta}_1]$) will measure the effect of using the pooled-list method on the probability of a hospital having delay of any high-priority procedures, relative to using the individual-lists method.

To assess patient-level performance, we will plot access curves from the time of registration to surgery, by method of booking anesthesiology consultations and priority group. We will then use discrete-time survival regression to model time to elective surgery in relation to the booking method, with adjustment for hospital-level and patient-level factors. The odds ratio derived from the estimated regression coefficient for an indicator variable representing the pooled-list method, see Table 17.2, will measure the effects of using the pooled-list method on the weekly proportion of wait-listed patients who undergo the operation, relative to what occurs with the individual-lists method of booking anesthesiology consultations.

We will also use multivariable logistic regressions to model the relation between the method of booking anesthesiology consultations and the odds of undergoing surgery after the recommended time, while adjusting for other hospital-level and patient-level factors and accounting for correlation between patients in the same hospital. This regression model will have an indicator variable I_1 for the pooled-list method of booking anesthesiology consultations (Table 17.3). We will use the odds ratios derived from the logistic regressions to measure the effect of the pooled-list method on the proportion of surgeries performed after the recommended time, relative to the individual-lists method.

Table 17.2 Regression model for estimating effect of method of booking anesthesiology consultations on weekly rate of surgery

Question:	Does use of a pooled-list booking method for anesthesiology consultations affect the weekly proportion of patients who receive access to elective surgery?
Model:	$\log\left(\frac{p_t}{1-p_t}\right) = \beta_{0t} + \beta_1 I_1 + \beta_2 I_2 + \beta_3 I_3 + \beta_4 I_4 + \beta_5 I_5 + \beta_6 I_6 + \beta_7 I_7 + \beta_8 I_8 + \beta_9 I_9 + \beta_{10} I_{10} + \beta_{11} I_{11} + \beta_{12} I_{12} + \beta_{13} I_{13} + \beta_{14} I_{14} + \beta_{15} I_{15} + \beta_{16} I_{16} + \beta_{17} I_{17} + \beta_{18} I_{18} + \beta_{19} I_{19} + \beta_{20} I_{20} + \beta_{21} I_{21} + \beta_{22} x_{22} + \beta_{23} X_{23} + \beta_{24} X_{24} + \beta_{25} X_{25}$
p_t	Proportion of patients who underwent elective surgery at week t
I_1	Indicator for pooled-list vs. individual-lists booking of anesthesiology consultations
I_2, I_3	Indicators for individual-lists or shortest-list vs. pooled-list booking of surgical consultation appointments
I_4	Indicator for some-screened vs. all-screened management of presurgical screening
I_5	Indicator for daily vs. weekly split of operating room slots between elective and urgent procedures
I_6, I_7	Indicators for 2 or 3 vs. 1 week of clearance time for appointment lists at start of simulation
I_8, I_9, I_{10}	Indicators for 4, 5, or 6 vs. 3 weeks of clearance time for surgical wait lists at start of simulation
I_{11}, I_{12}	Indicators for 1 or 2 vs. 0 weeks of clearance time for inpatient surgical queues at start of simulation
I_{13}	Indicator for female sex of patient
$I_{14}, I_{15}, I_{16}, I_{17}$	Indicators for <50, 50–59, 70–79 or ≥80 vs. 60–69 years age group
I_{18}, I_{19}	Indicators for high or low vs. medium priority at time of registration on surgical wait list
I_{20}, I_{21}	Indicators for multivessel or limited vs. left main coronary anatomy affected
I_{22}, I_{23}	Indicators for major conditions or other conditions vs. none
X_{24}	Clearance time for elective surgery at time of registration on the surgical wait list (weeks)
X_{25}	No. of additional surgeries performed without wait-list registration

17.5.2 *Information to Be Reported*

Complete and transparent reporting of information from a computer simulation study helps the reader to reflect on the conceptual challenges posed by modeling operations within a health care system (Sect. 2.5). In Chap. 10, we suggested the items that should be reported from a simulation study on health care evaluation, based on the CONSORT extension statement for cluster randomized trials. In particular, we described the importance of reporting items related to the study question, the methods, and the results. Here, we outline the information that will be reported from this simulation study to help readers understand the study rationale (Sect. 10.2). Specifically, we plan to report details allowing the reader to understand the specific objectives and hypotheses of the study (see item 5 of Table 10.1).

Table 17.3 Regression model for estimating effect of method of booking anesthesiology consultations on proportion of patients undergoing surgery after the recommended time

Question:	Does use of a pooled-list booking method for anesthesiology consultations affect the proportion of patients whose high-priority elective procedures are delayed after the recommended time?
Model:	$\log\left(\frac{p}{1-p}\right) = \beta_0 + \beta_1 I_1 + \beta_2 I_2 + \beta_3 I_3 + \beta_4 I_4 + \beta_5 I_5 + \beta_6 I_6 + \beta_7 I_7 + \beta_8 I_8 + \beta_9 I_9 + \beta_{10} I_{10} + \beta_{11} I_{11} + \beta_{12} I_{12} + \beta_{13} I_{13} + \beta_{14} I_{14} + \beta_{15} I_{15} + \beta_{16} I_{16} + \beta_{17} I_{17} + \beta_{18} I_{18} + \beta_{19} I_{19} + \beta_{20} I_{20} + \beta_{21} I_{21} + \beta_{22} I_{22} + \beta_{23} I_{23} + \beta_{24} X_{24}$
p	Proportion of patients whose high-priority elective surgery was delayed after the recommended time frame
I_1	Indicator for pooled-list vs. individual-lists booking of anesthesiology consultations
I_2, I_3	Indicators for individual-lists or shortest-list vs. pooled-list booking of surgical consultation appointments
I_4	Indicator for some-screened vs. all-screened management of presurgical screening
I_5	Indicator for daily vs. weekly split of operating room slots between elective and urgent procedures
I_6, I_7	Indicators for 2 or 3 vs. 1 week of clearance time for appointment lists at start of simulation
I_8, I_9, I_{10}	Indicators for 4, 5, or 6 vs. 3 weeks of clearance time for surgical wait lists at start of simulation
I_{11}, I_{12}	Indicators for 1 or 2 vs. 0 weeks of clearance time for inpatient surgical queues at start of simulation
I_{13}	Indicator for female sex of patient
I_{14}, I_{15}, I_{16}, I_{17}	Indicators <50, 50–59, 70–79, or ≥80 vs. 60–69 years age group
I_{18}, I_{19}	Indicators for high or low vs. medium priority at time of registration on surgical wait list
I_{20}, I_{21}	Indicators for multivessel or limited vs. left main coronary anatomy affected
I_{22}, I_{23}	Indicators for major conditions or other conditions vs. none
X_{24}	Clearance time for elective surgery at time of registration on the surgical wait list (weeks)

We will describe the statistical hypothesis through operationalizing the study hypothesis. Operationalizing involves determining whether the hypothesis pertains to the individual (patient) level or the cluster (hospital) level, identifying the performance measure of interest, and deciding whether to use one-sided or two-sided hypothesis testing (see Sect. 7.2). Our study question—*Does use of a pooled referral list for booking anesthesiology consultations affect the time to surgery?*—links the method of booking anesthesiology consultations (the primary study factor) and the time to surgery (an experimental outcome). One performance measure that will be of interest in this study is the proportion of hospitals with delay of any high-priority elective procedures. This measure quantifies system performance at the cluster level by summarizing the fraction of hospitals meeting a specific criterion (see Chap. 8). Therefore, a two-sided statistical hypothesis at the cluster level would be appropriate, and such a hypothesis could be formulated as follows:

H_0: There is no difference in the proportion of hospitals with delay of any high-priority elective procedures between hospitals using the individual-lists method of booking anesthesiology consultations and those using the pooled-list method.

H_A: There is a difference in the proportion of hospitals with delay of any high-priority elective procedures between hospitals using the individual-lists method of booking anesthesiology consultations and those using the pooled-list method.

Another performance measure that will be of interest in this study is the weekly rate of elective surgery among patients registered on a wait list. This measure quantifies system performance at the individual level by summarizing how many patients experience the event of surgery over a specified time interval (see Chap. 9). Therefore, a two-sided statistical hypothesis at the individual level would be appropriate, and such a hypothesis could be formulated as follows:

H_0: There is no difference in the weekly rate of elective surgery for registered patients between the individual-lists and pooled-list methods of booking anesthesiology consultations.

H_A: There is a difference in the weekly rate of elective surgery for registered patients between the individual-lists and pooled-list methods of booking anesthesiology consultations.

Reporting the objective of the simulation study will help readers to assess the appropriateness of the statistical methods and will also help them to interpret the results (see Chap. 10). For example, a reader can assess whether hypotheses formulated at the hospital level were evaluated using methods for which the hospital was the unit of analysis (see Chap. 11) and whether hypotheses formulated at the patient level were evaluated using methods for which the patient was the unit of analysis, with adjustment for correlation between patients in the same hospital (see Chap. 12). Whether the hypothesis pertains to the hospital level or the patient level will also help the reader to understand whether the results should be interpreted from the perspective of the hospital or the patient.

Chapter 18
Managing Postoperative Care

In this chapter, we describe our plans for a simulation study to investigate the management of postoperative care in the intensive care unit in the context of cardiac surgical care. This chapter differs from Chaps. 14–16 but is similar to Chaps. 17 and 19 in that here, we focus on the planning of a simulation study rather than evaluating the results of such a study. In particular, we will describe the design of a simulation study and the plan of analysis for comparing methods of managing postoperative care. Specifically, we use the framework for the design of a simulation study, described in Chap. 7, to discuss the modeling requirements, study and experimental factors, and patient attributes for such an experiment. We also discuss the information that will be reported, to help the reader understand how the total number of simulation runs should be determined (item 7 of Table 10.1).

18.1 Background

As presented in the taxonomy of the perioperative processes in Chap. 3, patients recover after surgery in the intensive care unit, where they are monitored and treated for any adverse effects of anesthesia (Fig. 3.1). Following recovery, patients are discharged to the hospital ward. The management of postoperative care in the intensive care unit has a direct impact on access to elective surgery. For example, when the number of beds available in the intensive care unit is insufficient to accept new patients after their surgery, scheduled operations may be postponed or canceled, and then rescheduled. There are no evidence-based guidelines regarding the optimal size of an intensive care unit to ensure access for all patients who need this type of care, including postoperative patients. However, some data suggest that small intensive care units are not cost-effective [15] and that high occupancy within an intensive care unit (i.e., high percentage of beds being occupied) is associated with high mortality [79]. Analytical models have been developed to plan for critical care capacity [38], but these have not been tested in a complex system of surgical care.

B. Sobolev et al., *Health Care Evaluation Using Computer Simulation: Concepts, Methods, and Applications*, DOI 10.1007/978-1-4614-2233-4_18,

Box 18.1 What is already known about the management of postoperative care

- The availability of intensive care beds directly affects access to elective surgery.
- There are no evidence-based guidelines for the optimal size of an intensive care unit to ensure access to postoperative treatment for surgical patients admitting to hospital for elective procedures.
- Small intensive care units are not cost-effective [15], and high occupancy within an intensive care unit is associated with high mortality [79].
- Few studies have assessed the effect of various approaches to managing postoperative care on patient and system outcomes.

The study question of interest for this planned simulation study will be, *Does the method of managing postoperative care in the intensive care unit affect the number of cancellations of elective procedures?*

18.2 The Management Alternatives

In this planned simulation study, we will consider two alternatives for managing postoperative care when no beds are available in the intensive care unit: diverting elective patients to different hospitals before their surgery and rescheduling elective operations. Box 18.1 summarizes what is already known about this issue.

18.3 The Simulation Model

18.3.1 Modeling Requirements

This simulation experiment will be based on discrete-event simulation of patient flow, described in detail in Chap. 13. The simulation model for this particular study will be based on the model specifications developed for the analysis presented in Chap. 16, with the addition of two alternatives for the management of postoperative care in the intensive care unit: diversion of patients and rescheduling of operations. We will consider a setting in which four beds are available for treatment in the cardiac surgery intensive care unit, with recovering patients spending an average of one day in the unit after their surgery. Two additional beds from the hospital's main intensive care unit may be used for emergency patients if no cardiac surgery intensive care beds are available.

Under the management alternative involving diversion of patients, if no beds are available in the cardiac surgery intensive care unit for recovery after a planned operation, the patient is diverted to another hospital; in this case, the operation is

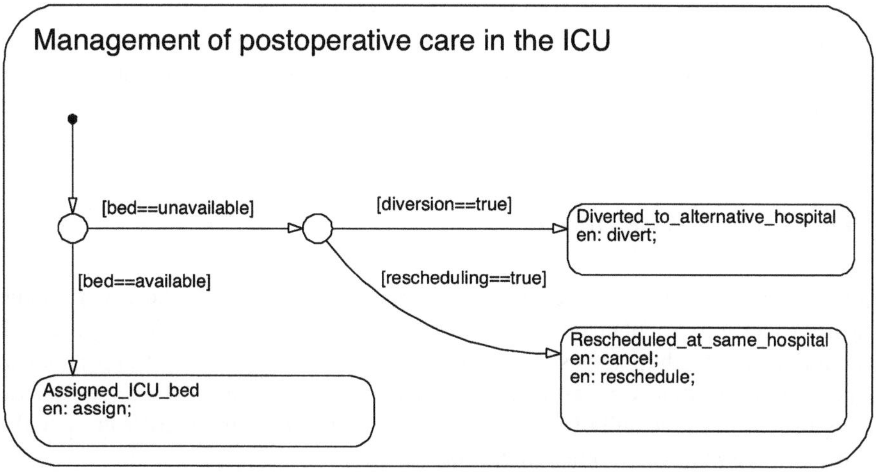

Fig. 18.1 Statechart for two methods of managing postoperative care in the intensive care unit (ICU): diversion of patients and rescheduling of operations

canceled and rebooked at the other hospital. Under the management alternative involving rescheduling of operations, if no beds are available in the cardiac surgery intensive care unit for recovery from a planned operation, the operation is canceled and rescheduled at the same hospital.

Figure 18.1 depicts the Statechart for the two alternatives for managing postoperative care in the intensive care unit. Patients entering the Statechart `Management of postoperative care in the ICU` may reside in one of three states, according to the availability of beds and the management alternative applied. If at least one bed is available, the patient enters the state `Assigned_ICU_bed`, at which point a bed is assigned by triggering of the event `assign`. If no beds are available and the management alternative is the one involving diversion of patients, the patient enters the state `Diverted_to_alternative_hospital`, which triggers the event `divert`. If no beds are available and the management alternative is the one involving rescheduling of operations, the patient enters the state `Rescheduled_at_same_hospital`, at which point the operation is canceled and rescheduled at the same hospital by triggering of the events `cancel` and `reschedule`.

18.3.2 Modeling Assumptions

The following modeling assumptions particular to this simulation study are additional to those listed in Chaps. 13 and 16:

1. Patients recover in the cardiac surgery intensive care unit for an average of one day.

2. Four beds are available in the cardiac surgery intensive care unit.
3. Two additional beds from the hospital's main intensive care unit may be used for emergency patients if no beds are available in the cardiac surgery intensive care unit.

18.4 Plan of Experiment

We will use elements from our analytical framework (Sect. 7.2) and experimental design (Sect. 7.3) to plan our simulation experiment. Our analytical framework operationalizes the hypothesis by identifying the primary study factor, experimental outcomes, performance measures, and measures of effect size. The experimental design determines the unit of randomization, the number of simulation runs, and the allocation of runs to experimental groups.

18.4.1 Primary Study Factor

The primary study factor will be the method of managing postoperative care in the intensive care unit, and this factor will have two categories: diversion of patients and rescheduling of operations. This primary study factor will be represented by one indicator variable, with hospitals using the rescheduling-of-operations method defined as the reference group.

18.4.2 Experimental Responses and Performance Measures

We are interested in measuring system outcomes at the levels of both the hospital and the patient. We anticipate that the method of managing postoperative care may have different effects on the overall performance of a hospital and on the cancellation of elective surgery for individual patients, so we will study more than one performance measure to understand these different perspectives. The performance measures of interest for this study will inform policy on the most efficient method of managing access to postoperative care in the intensive care unit in terms of cancellations of elective procedures.

The hospital-level response is a system-related outcome reflecting the effect of an intervention on the system of delivering care to a group of patients (see Sect. 2.4). During the simulation experiment, the following hospital-level experimental response will be generated:

- For each hospital, whether the number of high-priority elective procedures canceled was zero (indicator variable).

The following hospital-level performance measure will be used to summarize the results of this experiment:

- Proportion of hospitals with no cancellations of high-priority elective procedures.

The patient-level responses are patient-related outcomes reflecting the effect of an intervention on patients who are undergoing treatment in the health care system (see Sect. 2.4). During the simulation experiment, the following patient-level experimental response will be generated:

- For each patient, whether the patient's elective procedure was canceled from the final operating room list (indicator variable).

The following patient-level performance measure will be of interest:

- Proportion of elective procedures canceled from the final operating room list.

18.4.3 Hospital-Level and Patient-Level Experimental Factors

For this planned simulation experiment, we will identify hospital-level and patient-level factors that may impede or enhance occurrence of the experimental outcomes (see Sect. 2.3). Varying these factors in a simulation experiment would be necessary for estimating the independent effect of the method of managing postoperative treatment. We will also use these factors in regression analyses to adjust for differences in distributions between the experimental groups. We will then attribute to the management method any differences between experimental groups that cannot be explained by the hospital-level and patient-level factors.

The hospital-level factors that we anticipate might influence the experimental responses in this simulation study are the method of booking surgical consultation appointments, the method of booking elective surgery, the allocation of operating room slots, and the clearance times for appointment lists, surgical wait lists, and inpatient surgical queues at the start of simulation. A number of patient-level factors, such as sex, age group, coronary anatomy affected, comorbidity, priority of registration on the surgical wait list, clearance time at registration on the wait list, and weekly numbers of inpatient and emergency procedures, may also affect the chances of cancellation.

18.4.4 Measures of Effect Size

To compare the effects of the methods of managing postoperative care in the intensive care unit on the hospital-level performance measure of interest, we will use the following measure of effect size:

- Odds ratio for a hospital having no cancellations of high-priority elective procedures.

Similarly, to compare the effects of the management methods on the patient-level performance measures of interest, we will use the following measure of effect size:

- Odds ratio for cancellation of elective procedures from the final operating room list.

18.4.5 Allocation of Runs

In this planned study, each run will generate a cluster of simulated patients served in a modeled hospital. As such, the study will be a cluster randomized experiment, with the unit of allocation being a hospital. A full factorial design for this type of simulation experiment will have one run for every possible combination of values of the seven cluster-level experimental factors (see Sect. 7.3). More specifically, there will be two categories for the method of managing postoperative care, three categories for the method of booking surgical consultation appointment, two categories for the method of booking surgery, two categories for the allocation of operating room slots, three categories for clearance time for appointment lists, four categories for clearance time for surgical wait lists, and three categories for clearance time for inpatient surgical queues. Therefore, the number of combinations (i.e., design points) for this simulation experiment will be 864 ($=2 \times 3 \times 2 \times 2 \times 3 \times 4 \times 3$).

Similar to the matrix in Chap. 17, the design matrix corresponding to this full factorial design will have 864 rows (representing the 864 design points) and 12 ($=1 + 2 + 1 + 1 + 2 + 3 + 2$) columns (representing the indicator variables for the cluster-level experimental factors). Each row of the design matrix specifies the values of cluster-level experimental factors for one simulation run (i.e., one modeled hospital).

In this design matrix, one indicator variable represents the primary study factor, the method of managing postoperative care, because it has two categories: diverting and rescheduling. Experimental factors that have two or more categories are represented by sets of indicator variables, in which the number of variables is one less than the number of categories. For example, the set of three indicator variables I_8, I_9, and I_{10} represents four clearance times that could be used for surgical wait lists at the start of the simulation. As shown in Table 18.1, the values $I_8 = 1, I_9 = 0$, and $I_{10} = 0$ in this set correspond to the clearance time of 4 weeks, the values $I_8 = 0, I_9 = 1$, and $I_{10} = 0$ correspond to the clearance time of 5 weeks, the values $I_8 = 0, I_9 = 0$, and $I_{10} = 1$ correspond to the clearance time of 6 weeks, and the values $I_8 = 0, I_9 = 0$, and $I_{10} = 0$ correspond to the reference category of, 3 weeks.

We will use a cluster randomized design, in which the unit of allocation is the simulation run and corresponds to a simulated hospital. The number of runs that

Table 18.1 Coding for three indicator variables representing four clearance times for surgical wait lists

Clearance time (weeks)	Variable I_8	Variable I_9	Variable I_{10}
3	0	0	0
4	1	0	0
5	0	1	0
6	0	0	1

will actually be executed may be less than the number of runs in the full factorial design. We will choose the specific number of runs to ensure that we detect, with high probability, the anticipated effects of the methods of managing access to postoperative care in the intensive care unit (see Sect. 7.3). After determining the number of runs needed, we will apply the Fedorov algorithm to ensure an optimal distribution of experimental factors across the runs [55]. If the number of runs is less than 864, then the optimal design matrix will contain a subset of the rows from the full design matrix. Pilot data will be needed to estimate the magnitude of the performance measures in the reference group as well as to estimate the measures of variability and correlation needed for estimating the number of runs (see Chaps. 8 and 9). We will perform provisional runs of the simulation model, with 30 hospitals per experimental group, to generate these pilot data.

18.5 Plan of Evaluation

We will use our framework for the design of a simulation study to identify the required elements for planning our analysis of the simulated data (see Sect. 7.4). For this simulation study, we will have two units of analysis, the hospital and the patient. At the hospital level, we will report differences between the two methods of managing postoperative care in the intensive care unit in terms of the odds of there being no cancellations of high-priority elective procedures. At the patient level, we will report differences between the two management methods in terms of the odds of cancellation of elective procedures from the final operating room list.

18.5.1 Statistical Instruments

We will use multivariable logistic regressions to relate the probability of a hospital having no cancellations of high-priority elective procedures to the method of managing postoperative care, with adjustment for hospital-level factors. An indicator variable, I_1, will be entered into the regression model to represent the diversion method of managing postoperative care vs. the rescheduling method (Table 18.2). The odds ratio, derived from logistic regressions by exponentiating the regression estimate for this variable, will measure the effects of using the diversion method, relative to hospitals using the rescheduling method.

Table 18.2 Regression model for estimating effect of method of managing postoperative care in the ICU on proportion of hospitals with no cancellations of high-priority procedures

Question:	Does use of the diversion-of-patient method of managing postoperative care in the ICU affect the proportion of hospitals with no cancellations of high-priority elective procedures?
Model:	$\log\left(\frac{p^c}{1-p^c}\right) = \beta_0 + \beta_1 I_1 + \beta_2 I_2 + \beta_3 I_3 + \beta_4 I_4 + \beta_5 I_5 + \beta_6 I_6 + \beta_7 I_7 + \beta_8 I_8 + \beta_9 I_9 + \beta_{10} I_{10} + \beta_{11} I_{11} + \beta_{12} I_{12}$
p^c	Proportion of hospitals with no cancellations of any high-priority elective procedures
I_1	Indicator for diversion of patient vs. rescheduling-of-operation method of managing postoperative care
I_2, I_3	Indicators for individual-lists or shortest-list vs. pooled-list booking of surgical consultation appointments
I_4	Indicator for advance vs. wait-list booking of surgery
I_5	Indicator for daily vs. weekly split of operating room slots between elective and urgent procedures
I_6, I_7	Indicators for 2 or 3 vs. 1 week of clearance time for appointment lists at start of simulation
I_8, I_9, I_{10}	Indicators for 4, 5, or 6 vs. 3 weeks of clearance time for surgical wait lists at start of simulation
I_{11}, I_{12}	Indicators for 1 or 2 vs. 0 weeks of clearance time for inpatient surgical queues at start of simulation

Abbreviation: ICU = intensive care unit

We will also use logistic regression to model the relation between the method of managing postoperative care and the odds of cancellation of elective procedures from the final operating room list, with adjustment for other hospital-level and patient-level factors and accounting for correlation between patients in the same hospital. The regression model will have an indicator variable, I_1, for the diversion-of-patient method (Table 18.3). The odds ratios derived from these logistic regressions will measure the effect of diverting patients to another hospital on the odds of cancellation of elective procedures, relative to canceling the operations and rebooking in the same hospital.

18.5.2 Information To Be Reported

Complete and transparent reporting of information from a computer simulation study helps the reader to reflect on the conceptual challenges posed by modeling operations within a health care system (see Sect. 2.5). In Chap. 10, we recommended the items that should be reported from a simulation study on health care evaluation, based on the CONSORT extension statement for cluster randomized trials. In particular, we described the importance of reporting items related to the study question, the methods, and the results. Here, we emphasize what we plan to report from this simulation study of managing postoperative care in the intensive care unit,

Table 18.3 Regression model for estimating effect of method of managing postoperative care in the ICU on proportion of patients whose elective procedure was canceled

Question:	Does use of the diversion-of-patient method of managing postoperative care in the ICU affect the proportion of patients whose elective procedures are canceled?
Model:	$\log\left(\frac{p}{1-p}\right) = \beta_0 + \beta_1 I_1 + \beta_2 I_2 + \beta_3 I_3 + \beta_4 I_4 + \beta_5 I_5 + \beta_6 I_6 + \beta_7 I_7 + \beta_8 I_8 + \beta_9 I_9 + \beta_{10} I_{10} + \beta_{11} I_{11} + \beta_{12} I_{12} + \beta_{13} I_{13} + \beta_{14} I_{14} + \beta_{15} I_{15} + \beta_{16} I_{16} + \beta_{17} I_{17} + \beta_{18} I_{18} + \beta_{19} I_{19} + \beta_{20} I_{20} + \beta_{21} I_{21} + \beta_{22} I_{22} + \beta_{23} I_{23} + \beta_{24} X_{24} + \beta_{25} X_{25}$
p	Proportion of patients whose elective procedure is canceled
I_1	Indicator for diversion-of-patients vs. rescheduling-of-operations method of managing postoperative care
I_2, I_3	Indicators for individual-lists or shortest-list vs. pooled-list booking of surgical consultation appointments
I_4	Indicator for advance vs. wait-list booking of surgery
I_5	Indicator for daily vs. weekly split of operating room slots between elective and urgent procedures
I_6, I_7	Indicators for 2 or 3 vs. 1 week of clearance time for appointment lists at start of simulation
I_8, I_9, I_{10}	Indicators for 4, 5, or 6 vs. 3 weeks of clearance time for surgical wait lists at start of simulation
I_{11}, I_{12}	Indicators for 1 or 2 vs. 0 weeks of clearance time for inpatient surgical queues at start of simulation
I_{13}	Indicator for female sex of patient
I_{14}, I_{15}, I_{16}, I_{17}	Indicators for <50, 50–59, 70–79, or ≥80 vs. 60–69 years age group
I_{18}, I_{19}	Indicators for high or low vs. medium priority at time of registration on surgical wait list
I_{20}, I_{21}	Indicators for multivessel or limited vs. left main coronary anatomy affected
I_{22}, I_{23}	Indicators for major conditions or other conditions vs. none
X_{24}	Clearance time for elective surgery at time of registration on the surgical wait list (weeks)
X_{25}	No. of additional surgeries performed without wait-list registration

Abbreviation: ICU = intensive care unit

to help the reader to understand the methods (Sect. 10.3). Specifically, we will report details, allowing the reader to get a better view of how the total number of simulation runs was determined (see item 7 of Table 10.1).

In determining the appropriate number of runs, we will ensure a sufficient number of runs to detect, with high probability, the anticipated effect of the method of managing postoperative care in the intensive care unit (see Sect. 7.3). In particular, we will follow the steps for estimating the number of simulation runs for each performance measure of interest (see Appendix B). In performing the simulation experiment, we will use the largest of these estimates. First, we will determine the number of runs needed to detect an important difference in the hospital-level performance (see Chap. 8), following the steps outlined in Appendix B. In this experiment, the cluster is a simulated hospital. Second, we will determine the number of runs needed to detect an important difference in the patient-level performance measure (see Chap. 9), following the steps outlined in Appendix B.

18.5.3 Number of Runs for Cluster-Level Evaluations

Step 1: Determine the Statistical Hypothesis

At the cluster (hospital) level, the study question of interest will be, *Does managing postoperative care in the intensive care unit by diverting patients to another hospital when no recovery beds are available affect the proportion of hospitals with no cancellations of high-priority elective procedures?* We can operationalize this study question as a statistical hypothesis by identifying the performance measure of interest and deciding whether to use one-sided or two-sided hypothesis testing.

The performance measure of interest is the proportion of hospitals with no cancellations of high-priority elective procedures, and we will use a two-sided hypothesis test because we are interested in detecting if the diversion-of-patient method performs better or worse than the rescheduling-of-operation method. Therefore, the two-sided hypothesis at the cluster level will be formulated as follows:

H_0: There is no difference in the proportion of hospitals with no cancellations of high-priority elective procedures between those that divert patients to another hospital and those that cancel operations when no beds are available in the intensive care unit for postoperative recovery.

H_A: There is a difference in the proportion of hospitals with no cancellations of high-priority elective procedures between those that divert patients to another hospital and those that cancel operations when no beds are available in the intensive care unit for postoperative recovery.

Step 2: Choose the Significance Level

For this simulation experiment, we will be comfortable with incorrectly concluding that there is a difference between the two methods of managing postoperative care in the intensive care unit about 1 of every 20 times. Therefore, we will choose a 5% significance level.

Step 3: Choose the Desired Statistical Power of the Test

We would like to correctly claim that there is a difference between the methods of managing postoperative care in the intensive care unit about 9 times out of 10. Therefore, we will set the desired statistical power of the test to 90%.

Step 4: Determine the Anticipated Effect Size

We will use pilot data to estimate the proportion of hospitals with no cancellations of high-priority elective procedures (i.e., the cluster-level performance measure) in the rescheduling-of-operations group. We are interested in detecting a 20% difference in this proportion. Therefore, the estimated effect size will be a difference of 0.20 in the proportions.

Step 5: Determine the Cluster Characteristics

Because the hypothesis is formulated at the cluster level, we will not need to determine the cluster characteristics for this analysis.

Step 6: Estimate the Number of Simulation Runs

We will use the information from steps 1–4 and (8.8) to estimate the required number of simulation runs.

18.5.4 Number of Runs for Individual-Level Evaluations

Step 1: Determine the Statistical Hypothesis

At the individual level, the study question of interest will be, *Does managing postoperative care in the intensive care unit by diverting patients to another hospital when no recovery beds are available affect the proportion of patients whose elective procedures are canceled?* We can operationalize this study question as a statistical hypothesis by identifying the performance measure of interest and deciding whether to use one-sided or two-sided hypothesis testing.

The performance measure of interest will be the proportion of patients with cancellation of their elective procedures, and we will use a two-sided hypothesis test because we are interested in detecting if the diversion-of-patient method performs better or worse than the rescheduling-of-operation method. Therefore, the two-sided hypothesis at the patient level will be formulated as follows:

H_0: There is no difference in the proportion of patients with cancellation of their elective procedures from the final operating room list between those treated at hospitals that divert patients to another hospital and those treated at hospitals that cancel operations when no beds are available in the intensive care unit for postoperative recovery.

H_A: There is a difference in the proportion of patients with cancellations of their elective procedures from the final operating room list between those treated at hospitals that divert patients to another hospital and those treated at hospitals that cancel operations when no beds are available in the intensive care unit for postoperative recovery.

Step 2: Choose the Significance Level

For this simulation experiment, we will be comfortable with incorrectly concluding that there is a difference between the two methods of managing postoperative care in the intensive care unit about 1 of every 20 times. Therefore, we will choose a 5% significance level.

Step 3: Choose the Desired Statistical Power of the Test

We would like to correctly claim that there is a difference between the methods of managing postoperative care in the intensive care unit about 9 times out of 10. Therefore, we will set the desired statistical power of the test to 90%.

Step 4: Determine the Anticipated Effect Size

We will use the pilot data to estimate the proportion of patients with cancellation of their elective procedures (i.e., the patient-level performance measure) in the rescheduling-of-operation group. We are interested in detecting a 5% difference in this proportion. Therefore, the estimated effect size will be a difference of 0.05 in the proportions.

Step 5: Determine the Cluster Characteristics

We will also use pilot data to estimate the distribution of cluster characteristics, including the intracluster correlation coefficient and the number of simulated patients per modeled hospital.

Step 6: Estimate the Number of Simulation Runs

We will use the information from steps 1–5 and (9.13) to estimate the required number of simulation runs.

Chapter 19
Discharge Planning

In this chapter, we describe plans for a simulation study to investigate the management of discharge planning in the context of cardiac surgical care. This chapter is similar to Chaps. 17 and 18 in focusing on the planning of the study rather than evaluating results. In particular, we will describe the study design and the plan of analysis for comparing two methods of planning discharge from hospital after surgery. We use the analytical framework of a simulation study, as described in Chap. 7, to discuss the modeling requirements, study and experimental factors, and patient attributes for such an experiment. We also discuss the information that will be reported, to help the reader understand the experimental outcomes and methods for estimating the effect size (see item 17 of Table 10.1).

19.1 Background

In the process of surgical care, postoperative discharge of patients involves a series of tasks, including examination by the surgical specialist, patient education, and arrangement of postoperative services such as home care, rehabilitation, or long-term care [163]. A patient who has undergone surgery is discharged from hospital after a period of recovery in the intensive care unit and treatment on the ward (Fig. 3.1). Admissions for future procedures may be delayed by inefficient management of discharges for earlier procedures, and it has been argued that a more predictable discharge schedule could improve overall patient flow through this process [68]. Other researchers have argued that once a discharge schedule is in place, internal transfers of patients, such as from an intensive care unit to a regular patient care ward, should be synchronized to that schedule. Individual units can then begin scheduling the movement of patients at a local level. This synchronization would allow simultaneous unit-level control and system-wide optimization [68].

To better understand the implications of various discharge planning strategies and the effects of the availability of health services beyond the perioperative process, policy-makers and health care administrators need to determine whether arranging

B. Sobolev et al., *Health Care Evaluation Using Computer Simulation: Concepts, Methods, and Applications*, DOI 10.1007/978-1-4614-2233-4_19,

Box 19.1 What is already known about the management of discharge planning

- Postoperative discharge of patients involves a series of tasks, such as examination by the surgical specialist, patient education, and the arrangement of postoperative services such as home care, rehabilitation, or long-term care [163].
- Admissions for future procedures may be delayed by inefficient management of discharges for earlier procedures.
- It has been argued that a more predictable discharge schedule could improve overall patient flow through this process [68].
- Few studies have assessed the effect of various approaches to discharge planning on patient and system outcomes.

postoperative services before the operation will affect the timing of discharge. They must also determine the effects of unavailability of rehabilitation, home care, and long-term care beds on outcomes for both the patient and the system [163]. The study question of interest for this planned simulation study will be *Does discharge planning before a patient is admitted for an operation affect the postoperative length of stay?*

19.2 The Management Alternatives

In this planned simulation study, we will consider two alternatives for the management of discharge planning in cardiac surgical care: performing discharge planning for all elective procedures before patients' admission to hospital for the surgery and performing discharge planning for only some elective procedures before patients' admission to hospital. Box 19.1 summarizes what is already known about this topic.

19.3 The Simulation Model

19.3.1 Modeling Requirements

This simulation study will be based on the model of patient flow developed for the analysis presented in Chap. 16. In addition, the simulation model will include implementation of two alternatives for the management of discharge planning: discharge planning before admission to hospital for all elective procedures and discharge planning before admission to hospital for only some elective procedures. Under the management alternative involving discharge planning for all elective procedures, booking of postoperative services is attempted before the patient's admission to hospital for an elective procedure, but if some or all of these postoperative services are unavailable, the operation is canceled and rebooked when

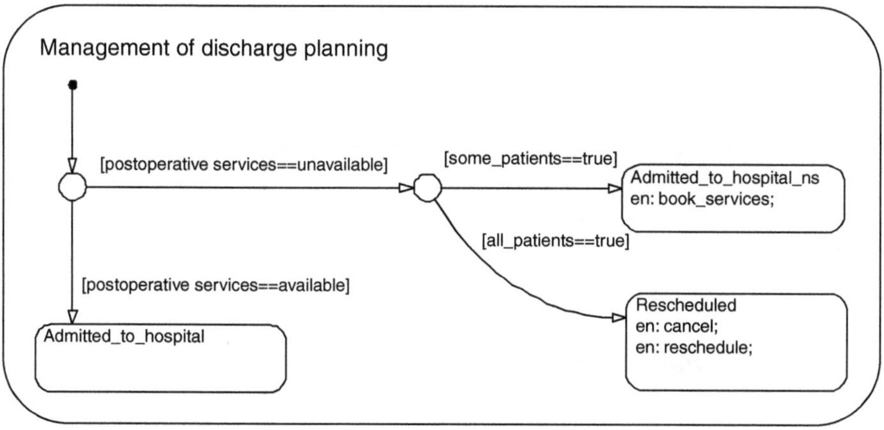

Fig. 19.1 Statechart for two methods of discharge planning: all elective procedures and some elective procedures

availability of all postoperative services can be confirmed. Under the management alternative involving discharge planning for only some elective procedures, booking of all postoperative services is attempted before the patient's admission to hospital for an elective procedure, but if postoperative services are not available, the patient is admitted to hospital anyway, and postoperative services are booked as they become available.

Figure 19.1 depicts the Statechart for the two alternatives for management of discharge planning. Patients entering Statechart `Management of discharge planning` may reside in one of three states, according to the availability of postoperative services and the management alternative applied. If postoperative services are available, the patient enters the state `Admitted_to_hospital`. If postoperative services are unavailable and the management alternative is discharge planning for all elective procedures, the patient enters the state `Rescheduled`, which triggers the events `cancel` and `reschedule`, to cancel and rebook the operation, respectively. If postoperative services are unavailable and the management alternative is discharge planning for only some elective procedures, the patient enters the state `Admitted_to_hospital_ns`, which triggers the event `book_services`, allowing services to be booked as they become available.

19.3.2 Modeling Assumptions

The following modeling assumptions particular to this simulation study are additional to those listed in Chaps. 13 and 16:

1 Before their operations, patients receive education about anesthesia and postoperative care.
2 After undergoing the operation, patient recovers in the cardiac surgery intensive care unit for an average of one day.
3 Four beds are available in the cardiac surgery intensive care unit.
4 Two additional beds from the hospital's main intensive care unit may be used for emergency patients if no beds are available in the cardiac surgery intensive care unit.

19.3.3 Expanding the Model

Our previous modeling requirements were based on the service with three surgeons who closely coordinate their schedules over a 36-week horizon. In this experiment, we will model a surgical service with 10 surgeons, where each surgeon has his or her own combination of duties, which are scheduled at predetermined times. Each surgeon performs operations (operating room duty) and assesses patients in the outpatient clinic (clinic duty); however, only eight surgeons perform emergency operations (on-call duty). Other responsibilities include operating outside the service, monitoring patients in the cardiac intensive care unit (intensive care supervision duty), teaching, conducting research, and performing administrative work. Some surgeons do administrative work concurrently with other responsibilities, and other surgeons have protected time for their administrative work, teaching, and research. When one of the surgeons is on vacation, the other surgeons cover that person's operating room duty, on-call duty, and intensive care supervision duty, if necessary.

Each surgeon will be modeled using a unique Statechart to represent his or her weekly schedule and to model rotation of the responsibilities (see Fig. 19.2). These Statecharts will operate autonomously, with some events being broadcast to individual surgeons on particular days (e.g., to trigger a scheduled research day on the last Monday of the month) and other events being broadcast to all surgeons (to ensure that some duties, such as intensive care supervision, are shared equally among participating surgeons).

19.4 Plan of Experiment

We will use elements from our analytical framework (Sect. 7.2) and experimental design (Sect. 7.3) to plan our simulation experiment. Our analytical framework operationalizes the hypothesis by identifying the primary study factor, experimental outcomes, performance measures, and measures of effect size. The experimental design determines the unit of randomization, the number of simulation runs, and the allocation of runs to experimental groups.

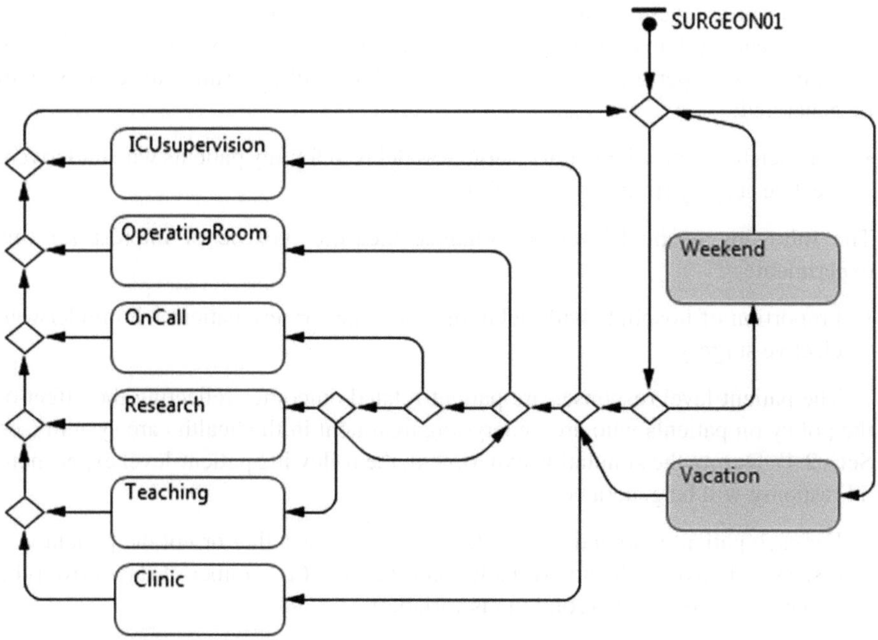

Fig. 19.2 Statechart for duty rotation of a surgeon (ICU = intensive care unit)

19.4.1 Primary Study Factor

The primary study factor will be the method of managing discharge planning, and this factor will have two categories: discharge planning before admission to hospital for all elective procedures and discharge planning for only some elective procedures. This primary study factor will be represented by one indicator variable, with hospitals performing discharge planning for only some elective procedures defined as the reference group.

19.4.2 Experimental Responses and Performance Measures

We are interested in measuring system outcomes at the levels of both the hospital and the patient. We anticipate that the method of managing discharge planning may have different effects on the overall performance of a hospital and on the postoperative length of stay for individual patients undergoing elective surgery, so we will study more than one performance measure to understand these different perspectives. The performance measures of interest for this study will allow a decision-maker to evaluate the effects of the method of managing discharge planning on the postoperative stay following elective procedures.

The hospital-level response is a system-related outcome reflecting the effect on the health care system of delivering care to a group of patients (see Sect. 2.4). During the simulation experiment, the following hospital-level experimental response will be generated:

- For each hospital, whether discharge was delayed for any patients who underwent elective surgery (indicator variable)

The following hospital-level performance measure will be of interest for this experiment:

- Proportion of hospitals with delay of discharge for any patient who underwent elective surgery

The patient-level responses are patient-related outcomes reflecting the effect of the policy on patients who are undergoing treatment in the health care system (see Sect. 2.4). During the simulation experiment, the following patient-level experimental response will be generated:

- For each patient who underwent elective surgery, whether or not the patient was discharged alive (indicator variable) and the time (as number of days) from the procedure to discharge (continuous variable)

The following patient-level performance measure will be of interest:

- Daily discharge rate among those who have undergone surgery

19.4.3 Hospital-Level and Patient-Level Experimental Factors

For our planned simulation experiment, we will identify hospital-level and patient-level factors that may impede or enhance occurrence of the outcomes (see Sect. 2.3). We will use these factors in multivariable regression analyses to adjust for differences in distributions between the experimental groups. We will then attribute to the policy (i.e., the method of managing discharge planning) any differences between experimental groups that cannot be explained by the hospital and patient factors.

The hospital factors that we anticipate might affect the experimental responses in this simulation study are the method of booking surgical consultation appointments, the method of booking elective surgery, the allocation of operating room slots, and the clearance times for appointment lists, surgical wait lists, and inpatient surgical queues at the start of the simulation. A variety of patient-level factors, such as sex, age group, coronary anatomy affected, comorbidity, priority of registration on the surgical wait list, clearance time at registration on the wait list, and weekly numbers of inpatient and emergency procedures, may also affect the chances of discharge.

19.4.4 Measure of Effect Size

To compare the effects of the two methods of managing discharge planning on the hospital-level performance measure of interest, we will use the following measure of effect size:

- Odds ratio for a hospital having any discharges after elective procedures

Similarly, to compare the effects of the two methods of managing discharge planning on the patient-level performance measure, we will use the following measure of effect size:

- Ratio of daily odds of discharge after elective procedure

19.4.5 Allocation of Runs

In this planned simulation study, each run will generate a cluster of simulated patients served in a modeled hospital. As such, the study will be a cluster randomized trial, with the unit of allocation being a hospital (i.e., a simulation run). A full factorial design for this type of simulation experiment will have one run for every possible combination of values of the seven cluster-level experimental factors (see Sect. 7.3). More specifically, there will be two categories for the method of managing discharge planning (the primary study factor), three categories for the method of booking surgical consultation appointment, two categories for the method of booking surgery, two categories for the allocation of operating room slots, three categories for clearance time for appointment lists, four categories for clearance time for surgical wait lists, and three categories for clearance time for inpatient surgical queues. Therefore, the number of combinations (i.e., design points) for this simulation experiment is 864 ($=2 \times 3 \times 2 \times 2 \times 3 \times 4 \times 3$). The design matrix of this full factorial design will have 864 rows, representing the 864 design points, and 12 ($=1+2+1+1+2+3+2$) columns, representing the indicator variables for the experimental factors.

As described in Chap. 17, experimental variables with two categories are represented by one indicator variable in this design matrix, and experimental variables with more than two categories are represented by a corresponding set of indicator variables. For example, the set of two indicator variables, say I_{11} and I_{12} represents three distinct clearances time for inpatient surgical queues that will be used in the simulation experiments. In this set, the values $I_{11} = 1$ and $I_{12} = 0$ correspond to one week, the values $I_{11} = 0$ and $I_{12} = 1$ correspond to two weeks, and the values $I_{11} = 0$ and $I_{12} = 0$ correspond to zero weeks. Because of the full factorial design for the planned simulation experiment, each row of the design matrix specifies a combination of values for the experimental factors for one modeled hospital (i.e., one simulation run).

We will use a cluster randomized design, in which the unit of allocation is the simulation run. As noted above, the number of runs may be less than the number of runs in the full factorial design. We will choose the specific number of runs to ensure that we detect, with high probability, the anticipated effects of the methods of managing discharge planning (see Sect. 7.3). After determining the number of runs needed, we will apply the Fedorov algorithm to ensure an optimal distribution of experimental factors across the runs [55]. If the number of runs is less than 864, then the optimal design matrix will contain a subset of the rows from the full design matrix. Pilot data will be needed to estimate the magnitude of the performance measures in the reference group as well as to estimate the measures of variability and correlation needed for estimating the number of runs (see Chaps. 8 and 9). We will perform provisional runs of the simulation model, with 30 hospitals per experimental group, to generate these pilot data.

19.5 Evaluation of Experiment

We will use our analytical framework of a simulation study to identify the required elements for planning the analysis of the simulated data (see Sect. 7.4). For this simulation study, we will have two units of analysis, the hospital and the patient. At the hospital level, we will report differences between the two methods of managing discharge planning in terms of the odds of delay of discharge. At the patient level, we will report differences between the two methods in terms of the daily odds of discharge for individual patients.

19.5.1 Statistical Instruments

We will use multivariable logistic regressions to model the relation between the methods of managing discharge planning and delay of discharge, with adjustment for hospital-level factors. The regression model will have an indicator variable, I_1, for the method involving discharge planning for all elective procedures (Table 19.1). The odds ratios derived from logistic regressions will measure the effects of using the method of discharge planning for all elective procedures on the probability of a hospital having delays of any discharges, relative to hospitals that perform discharge planning for only some elective procedures.

To assess system performance at the patient level, we will plot access curves from the time of the procedure to discharge, by method of managing discharge planning and priority group. We will then use discrete-time survival regression to model the relation between the method involving discharge planning and time to discharge, with adjustment for hospital-level and patient-level factors. The regression model will have an indicator variable, I_1, for the discharge planning for all elective procedure method of management (Table 19.2). The odds ratio derived from the

Table 19.1 Regression model for estimating effect of method of managing discharge planning on proportion of hospitals with delay of discharge

Question:	Does performing discharge planning for all elective procedures before patients' admission to hospital affect the proportion of hospitals with delay of any discharges?
Model:	$\log\left(\frac{p^c}{1-p^c}\right) = \beta_1 I_1 + \beta_2 I_2 + \beta_3 I_3 + \beta_4 I_4 + \beta_5 I_5 + \beta_6 I_6 + \beta_7 I_7 + \beta_8 I_8 + \beta_9 I_9 + \beta_{10} I_{10} + \beta_{11} I_{11} + \beta_{12} I_{12}$
p^c	Proportion of hospitals with delay of discharge after suregry
I_1	Indicator of discharge planning for all elective procedures vs. some elective procedures
I_2, I_3	Indicators for pooled-list vs. individual-lists or shortest-list booking of appointments
I_4	Indicator for advance vs. wait-list booking of surgery
I_5	Indicator for daily vs. weekly split of operating room slots between elective and urgent procedures
I_6, I_7	Indicators for 2 or 3 vs. 1 week of clearance time for appointment lists at the start of simulation
I_8, I_9, I_{10}	Indicators for 4, 5, or 6 vs. 3 weeks of clearance time for surgical wait lists at the start of simulation
I_{11}, I_{12}	Indicators for 1 or 2 vs. 0 weeks of clearance time for inpatient surgical queues at the start of simulation

estimated regression coefficient of this indicator variable will measure the effects of using the method involving discharge planning for all elective procedures on the daily proportion of patients who are discharged, relative to what occurs when discharge planning is performed for only some elective procedures.

19.5.2 Information To Be Reported

Complete and transparent reporting of information from a computer simulation study helps the reader to reflect on the conceptual challenges posed by modeling operations within the health care system (see Sect. 2.5). In Chap. 10, we recommended the items that should be reported from a simulation study on health care evaluation, based on the CONSORT statement for cluster randomized trials. In particular, we described the importance of reporting items related to the study question, the methods, and the results.

Here, we emphasize what we plan to report from this simulation study of managing discharge planning, to help the reader to understand the results (Sect. 10.4). Specifically, we will report details allowing the reader to understand the outcomes and estimation of effect size (see item 17 of Table 10.1). For each hospital-level and patient-level outcome, we will report a summary of the results for each method of discharge planning, including the estimated effect size and its precision, as measured by a 95% confidence interval. For patient-level measures, we will also report the intracluster correlation coefficient.

Table 19.2 Discrete-time regression for estimating effect of method of managing discharge planning on daily proportion of patients discharged from hospital

Question:	Does performing discharge planning for all elective procedures affect the daily proportion of patients who are discharged?
Model:	$\log\left(\frac{p_t}{1-p_t}\right) = \beta_{0t} + \beta_1 I_1 + \beta_2 I_2 + \beta_3 I_3 + \beta_4 I_4 + \beta_5 I_5 + \beta_6 I_6 + \beta_7 I_7 + \beta_8 I_8 + \beta_9 I_9 + \beta_{10} I_{10} + \beta_{11} I_{11} + \beta_{12} I_{12} + \beta_{13} I_{13} + \beta_{14} I_{14} + \beta_{15} I_{15} + \beta_{16} I_{16} + \beta_{17} I_{17} + \beta_{18} I_{18} + \beta_{19} I_{19} + \beta_{20} I_{20} + \beta_{21} I_{21} + \beta_{22} I_{22} + \beta_{23} I_{23} + \beta_{24} X_{24} + \beta_{25} X_{25}$
p_t	Proportion of patients discharged at day t after surgery
I_1	Indicator of discharge planning for all elective procedures vs. some elective procedures
I_2, I_3	Indicators for individual-lists or shortest-list vs. pooled-list booking of surgical consultation appointments
I_4	Indicator for advance vs. wait-list booking of surgery
I_5	Indicator for daily vs. weekly split of operating room slots between elective and urgent procedures
I_6, I_7	Indicators for 2 or 3 vs. 1 week of clearance time for appointment lists at start of simulation
I_8, I_9, I_{10}	Indicators for 4, 5, or 6 vs. 3 weeks of clearance time for surgical wait lists at start of simulation
I_{11}, I_{12}	Indicators for 1 or 2 vs. 0 weeks of clearance time for inpatient surgical queues at start of simulation
I_{13}	Indicator for female sex of patient
I_{14} to I_{17}	Indicators for <50, 50–59, 70–79, or ≥80 vs. 60–69 years age group
I_{18}, I_{19}	Indicators for high or low vs. medium priority at time of registration on surgical wait list
I_{20}, I_{21}	Indicators for multivessel or limited vs. left main coronary anatomy affected
I_{22}, I_{23}	Indicators for major conditions or other conditions vs. none
X_{24}	Clearance time for elective surgery at time of registration on the surgical wait list (weeks)
X_{25}	No. of additional surgeries performed without wait-list registration

We will summarize the hospital-level outcomes and effects in a table, where we present the results by method of discharge planning (column 1). The performance measure (i.e., the proportion of hospitals with delay of discharges) will be reported as a percentage (column 2), along with the total number of hospitals where discharges were delayed and the total number of hospitals in each experimental group. Reporting these totals will allow the reader to see how the performance measure was estimated. In addition, reporting the total number of hospitals in each group will allow the reader to determine if the hospitals were evenly distributed between the experimental groups and if this number of clusters allowed adequate power to detect the anticipated effect. We will also report the adjusted odds ratio (column 3), along with a measure of precision (the 95% confidence interval). Reporting the estimated size of the effect and its 95% confidence interval will allow

Table 19.3 Template for reporting effect of method of discharge planning on proportion of hospitals with delay of discharge

Method	% (no. of hospitals with delay/ total no. of hospitals)	Odds ratio (95% CI)∗
Some procedures	$a/b \times 100$ (a/b)	1.00
All procedures	$c/d \times 100$ (c/d)	$\exp(\hat{\beta}_1)$†

Abbreviation: CI = confidence interval

∗Adjusted for hospital-level factors

†$\hat{\beta}_1$ is the estimated regression coefficient for the method of managing discharge planning from multivariable logistic regression

Table 19.4 Template for reporting the effect of method of discharge planning on daily proportion of patients discharged from hospital

Method	No. of discharges	No. of patient-days	Discharge rate∗ (95% CI)	Ratio of daily odds (95% CI)†
Some procedures	a	b	$a/b \times 100$	1.00
All procedures	c	d	$c/d \times 100$	$\exp(\hat{\beta}_1)$‡

Abbreviation: CI = confidence interval

∗Per 100 patient-days, calculated as the number of discharges divided by the total time in patient-days

†Adjusted for hospital-level and patient-level factors and for correlation for patients within the same hospital (with specification of estimated measure of similarity)

‡$\hat{\beta}_1$ is the estimated regression coefficient for the experimental group from multivariable discrete-time survival regression

the reader to assess statistical significance and to make decisions about whether the size of effect is large enough to consider applying a particular method of managing discharge planning in a real-world situation. Table 19.3 shows a template table for summarizing these hospital-level results.

Similarly, we will summarize patient-level outcomes and effects in a table and a figure. In the table, we will present the results by method of discharge planning (column 1). The patient-level performance measure (i.e., the daily rate of discharges) will be reported as a rate (per 100 patient-days; column 4), along with the total number of discharges (column 2) and the total number of days that patients in each experimental group spent waiting from the time of the procedure until discharge (column 3). Reporting these totals will allow the reader to see how the performance measure was estimated. We will also report the adjusted ratio of daily odds of discharge (column 5), along with a measure of precision (95% confidence interval). Reporting the estimated size of the effect and its 95% confidence interval will allow the reader to assess the statistical significance and to make decisions about whether the size of the effect is large enough to consider using a particular method of managing discharge planning in a real-world situation. Table 19.4 shows a template table for summarizing these patient-level results. We will also create a figure showing the estimated probability of discharge within a certain time after the procedure, by method of discharge planning. The horizontal axis will display the time since the procedure (in days), and the vertical axis will display the probability of discharge. The body of the figure will show access curves for discharge by method of discharge planning. A higher curve will indicate greater chances of discharge with that method of discharge planning. From this figure, we will estimate the proportion of patients being discharged within a certain number of days since the procedure.

Appendices

Appendix A
Framing the Questions

Table 1.1 in Chap. 1 shows an example of linking a research question with three elements of study design: the hypothesis, the level of analysis, and the summary outcome measure. Table A.1 in this appendix provides more examples for research questions discussed in detail in Chap. 1.

B. Sobolev et al., *Health Care Evaluation Using Computer Simulation: Concepts, Methods, and Applications*, DOI 10.1007/978-1-4614-2233-4,

Table A.1 Research questions linked to hypotheses, level of evaluation, and summary measures of the outcome

Question	Hypothesis	Level	Summary measure
Booking surgical consultation appointments in the outpatient clinic			
Effect of booking method on access to appointments?	Reduced time to appointment	Patient	Proportion of appointments after benchmark time
	More hospitals with improved access to appointments	Hospital	Proportion of hospitals with less than 10% of appointments after benchmark time
Presurgical screening			
Effect of screening method on cancellation of surgery?	Fewer cancellations for patient-related reasons	Patient	Proportion of surgeries canceled because patient is not ready, not educated about procedure, or not medically optimized
	More hospitals with fewer cancellations for patient-related reasons	Hospital	Proportion of hospitals with less than 10% of surgeries canceled because patient is not ready, not educated, not medically optimized
Booking anesthesiology consultations			
Effect of booking method on time to consultation?	Reduced time to anesthesiology consultation	Patient	Proportion of anesthesiology consultations after benchmark time
	More hospitals with improved access to anesthesiology consultations	Hospital	Proportion of hospitals with less than half of anesthesiology consultations delayed
Managing access to elective surgery			
Effect of access-management method?	Reduced time to surgery	Patient	Proportion of admissions within certain times of decision for surgery
	More hospitals with improved access to surgery	Hospital	Proportion of hospitals with less than half of waits for admission longer than benchmark access time

Table A.1 (continued)

Question	Hypothesis	Level	Summary measure
Scheduling patients for surgery			
Effect of booking method on cancellations of surgery for nonclinical reasons?	Increased number of scheduled surgeries done	Patient	Proportion of surgeries canceled on the day of surgery or within 48 h by patient or hospital for nonclinical reasons
	More hospitals with fewer cancellations for nonclinical reasons	Hospital	Proportion of hospitals with less than 10% of surgeries canceled by patient or hospital for nonclinical reasons
Effect of "short-notice pool" method on time to admission?	Reduced time to surgery	Patient	Proportion of admissions within certain times of decision for surgery
	More hospitals with improved access to surgery	Hospital	Proportion of hospitals with less than half of waits for admission longer than benchmark access time
Effect of booking method on cancellations for clinical reasons?	Increased number of scheduled surgeries done	Patient	Proportion of surgeries canceled on the day of surgery or within 48 h by patient or hospital for clinical reasons
	More hospitals with fewer cancellations	Hospital	Proportion of hospitals with less than 10% of surgeries canceled by patient or hospital for clinical reasons
Prioritizing patients for admission to hospital			
Effect of prioritizing interventions on the risk of adverse events?	Fewer adverse events among patients waiting for hospital admission	Patient	Weekly rates of (a) symptom worsening, (b) urgency upgrade, (c) preoperative death, (d) becoming unsuitable for surgery, and (e) unexpected emergency admission before index admission
	More hospitals with reduced risk of adverse events on wait lists	Hospital	Proportion of hospitals with less than 25% of adverse events after benchmark time

(continued)

Table A.1 (continued)

Question	Hypothesis	Level	Summary measure
Rescheduling surgeries that had to be canceled			
Effect of rescheduling interventions on time to admission?	Reduced time to surgery among canceled surgeries	Patient	Proportion of admissions within certain times of decision for surgery
	More hospitals with improved access to surgery	Hospital	Proportion of hospitals with less than half of waits for admission longer than benchmark access time
Effect of increasing priority for canceled surgeries on time to readmission?	Reduced time to readmission after cancellation	Patient	Proportion of readmissions within certain times of surgery being canceled during hospital admission
	More hospitals with improved access to surgery for canceled surgeries	Hospital	Proportion of hospitals with less than half of waits for readmission longer than a week since cancellation
Managing direct admissions			
Effect of direct-admission option on time to surgery?	Reduced time to surgery	Patient	Proportion of surgeries in the week of direct admission to hospital
	More hospitals with improved access to surgery	Hospital	Proportion of hospitals with more than half of surgeries within a week of direct admission
Managing utilization of operating rooms			
Effect of specialty-dedicated operating room?	Increased availability of operating room time	Patient	Proportion of surgeries performed on days that are less than fully booked
	More hospitals with increased availability of operating room time	Hospital	Proportion of hospitals with more than 10% of the time that operating room not fully booked
Effect of emergency-dedicated operating room on cancellation of surgery?	Greater number of scheduled surgeries done	Patient	Proportion of surgeries canceled by hospital on the day of surgery for nonclinical reasons

Table A.1 (continued)

Question	Hypothesis	Level	Summary measure
	More hospitals with fewer cancellations for nonclinical reasons	Hospital	Proportion of hospitals with less than 10% of surgeries canceled by hospital for nonclinical reasons
Sequencing patients for the operating room			
Effect of case-sequencing interventions on cancellations by hospital because of insufficient time?	Greater number of scheduled surgeries done	Patient	Proportion of scheduled surgeries canceled by hospital on the day of surgery because of insufficient time
	More hospitals with fewer cancellations	Hospital	Proportion of hospitals with less than 10% surgeries canceled by hospital because of insufficient time
Managing postanesthesia care			
Effect of holding patients in postanesthesia care unit?	Greater number of scheduled surgeries done	Patient	Proportion of scheduled surgeries canceled by hospital on the day of surgery or within 48 h because no intensive care bed available
	More hospitals with fewer cancellations for nonclinical reasons	Hospital	Proportion of hospitals with less than 10% of surgeries canceled by hospital because no intensive care bed available
Effect of adjusting staffing pattern to fluctuations in case mix?	Greater number of scheduled surgeries done	Patient	Proportion of scheduled surgeries canceled by hospital on the day of surgery because of insufficient nursing and postoperative staff
	More hospitals with fewer cancellations for nonclinical reasons	Hospital	Proportion of hospitals with less than 10% of surgeries canceled by hospital because of insufficient nursing and postoperative staff

(continued)

Table A.1 (continued)

Question	Hypothesis	Level	Summary measure
Planning for discharge before surgery			
Effect of discharge planning on postoperative length of stay?	Reduced time to discharge	Patient	Proportion of patients not discharged in a timely fashion because of no home care arranged, no rehabilitation service available, or no long-term care bed available
	More hospitals with improved access to postoperative care	Hospital	Proportion of hospitals with less than half of patients having an extended postoperative stay
Managing postoperative care			
Effect of diverting surgical surgeries if critical care beds unavailable?	Greater number of scheduled surgeries done	Patient	Proportion of surgeries canceled by hospital on the day of surgery for nonclinical reasons
	More hospitals with fewer cancellations for nonclinical reasons	Hospital	Proportion of hospitals with less than 10% of surgeries canceled by hospital for nonclinical reasons

Appendix B
Determining the Sufficient Number of Simulation Runs

The design of a simulation experiment should ensure a sufficient number of simulation runs to detect the anticipated effect of the intervention as discussed in Chap. 7. In this appendix, we describe the six steps for estimating the required number of runs:

Step 1—Determine the statistical hypothesis.
Step 2—Choose the significance level.
Step 3—Choose the required statistical power of the test.
Step 4—Choose the anticipated effect size.
Step 5—Determine the cluster characteristics.
Step 6—Estimate the number of simulation runs.

Step 1: Determine the Statistical Hypothesis

As described in Sect. 7.2, the statistical hypothesis specifies the experimental groups and indicates how the researcher plans to summarize the outcome of interest into a meaningful quantity or performance measure. The performance measure helps the statistician to determine the corresponding measure of effect size and the appropriate methodology and formulas to estimate the number of simulation runs.

Step 2: Choose the Significance Level

The significance level for simulation experiments, that is, the probability that a result is due to chance, is usually set at 5% ($\alpha = 0.05$). A significance level of 5% means that the researcher will incorrectly conclude that there is a difference between experimental groups when no such difference exists only 1 out of every 20

B. Sobolev et al., *Health Care Evaluation Using Computer Simulation: Concepts, Methods, and Applications*, DOI 10.1007/978-1-4614-2233-4,

times. A researcher with particular concerns about mistakenly claiming that the null hypothesis is untrue can reduce the chances of this type of error by choosing a lower significance level, say 1%, that is, 1 out of 100.

For example, suppose a policy-maker is contemplating replacing the existing method of managing presurgical screening in the preadmission clinic, whereby only some patients are screened before admission, with a new method, whereby all patients are screened before admission, and further suppose the new method will cost millions of dollars more than the existing method. In this scenario, the policy-maker would not want to mistakenly replace the existing system with the much more expensive new system if the two methods perform similarly. To reduce the chances of making such an error, the policy-maker could set the significance level to 1%. At this lower significance level, the policy-maker will incorrectly reject the null hypothesis only about 1 out of 100 times, as opposed to 1 out of 20 times at the 5% level.

In this example, the costs are measured in terms of monetary units, but the concept of costs may also be related to patients' well-being. A policy-maker would not want to mistakenly adopt a new method of presurgical screening in the preadmission clinic if it does not reduce the frequency of cancellations of elective procedures. On the other hand, a policy-maker who would like to decrease the chances of missing a true effect may increase the significance level to 10%. At this higher significance level, the policy-maker will incorrectly reject the null hypothesis about 1 out of 10 times, as opposed to only 1 out of 20 times at the 5% level. A higher significance level is often appropriate for exploratory analysis.

Step 3: Choose the Required Statistical Power of the Test

The power of the statistical test is typically set at 80% (or 90%), to allow the researcher to make a correct claim of a difference between experimental groups 8 (or 9) times out of 10. Consequently, with a power of 80% or 90%, there is an implicit indication that the researcher is comfortable with a 20% or 10% chance, respectively, of mistakenly claiming no effect when an effect does exist. The typical choice for power contrasts with the typical choice of significance level, in that researchers seem more wary of mistakenly claiming that there *is* an effect (with a significance level of 5% representing a 5% chance of this type of error) than they are of mistakenly claiming that there is *no* effect (with a power level of 80% or 90% representing a 20% or 10% chance of this type of error). However, if a researcher has particular concerns about mistakenly claiming that there is no effect, the power can be set to 95% or 99%. Consequently, the chances of mistakenly claiming no effect when an effect exists will be reduced to 5% or 1%, respectively. For example, suppose a policy-maker is interested in comparing the existing method of booking surgical consultation appointments using the wait lists of individual surgeons with a new method of booking such appointments using a pooled wait list. If the policy-maker wants to reduce the chances of incorrectly claiming that the appointment rates do not differ, the power of the test should be set to a higher level.

Step 4: Choose the Anticipated Effect Size

The effect size is typically chosen to answer the question *What is the smallest anticipated difference in the performance measure between experimental groups?* To address this question, the researcher relies on experts in the subject area of the study, such as clinicians or health policy-makers, to specify what would constitute a meaningful difference. For example, suppose a policy-maker is interested in comparing two methods of booking elective surgery to determine their relative effects on whether a patient undergoes surgery within a recommended time frame. Because the experimental outcome of interest is binary, a natural performance measure would be the proportion of patients who undergo surgery within the recommended time frame, and a corresponding measure of effect size would be the difference in proportions between the two methods of booking surgery.

In this example, the policy-maker might decide that a meaningful difference in the proportion of patients with on-time surgery is 0.10 or larger and that differences less than 0.10 are not meaningful or not worth the effort of switching from one method of booking surgery to another. As such, the researcher would set the effect size at 0.10. Suitable measures of effect size for various experimental outcomes are presented in Chap. 8 and Chap. 9. If a researcher is interested in detecting any difference whatsoever between the experimental groups, then a small effect size is appropriate. On the other hand, if the effect of the intervention must be substantial before a policy-maker would consider replacing an existing policy with a new policy, then a larger effect size should be selected. For example, if the policy-maker is willing to adopt a new policy only if it increases the proportion of on-time surgeries by at least 5%, then the effect size for a difference in proportions should be set no lower than 0.05.

Step 5: Determine the Cluster Characteristics

If the hypothesis is formulated at the individual (i.e., patient) level, characteristics of the cluster (i.e., hospital) will also be required to estimate the number of simulation runs. In the context of health care evaluation, such characteristics may include the number of simulated patients per modeled hospital, the intracluster correlation coefficient, the total time that simulated patients are at risk of an event (i.e., total person-time) for each hospital, and the coefficient of variation. Values for input into formulas used for estimating the number of simulation runs are based on provisional runs of the simulation model, historical data, the literature, or expert opinion. Methods for estimating cluster characteristics are described in detail in Chap. 9.

Step 6: Estimate the Number of Simulation Runs

The number of simulation runs required to test cluster-level hypotheses is estimated from the information obtained in steps 1 to 4, according to formulas presented in Chap. 8. The number of runs required to test individual-level hypotheses is also based on information obtained in steps 1 to 4, as well as information about cluster characteristics obtained in step 5. Formulas for estimating the number of runs to test individual-level hypotheses appear in Chap. 9. The effect size, statistical power, and significance level all influence the number of runs.

In Chaps. 8 and 9, we discuss in detail how changes in these elements affect the number of runs required, but a brief summary is provided here. First, as the effect size decreases, with power and significance level held constant, the required number of runs increases. This makes sense intuitively since a researcher will need more information (a greater number of runs) to detect smaller differences between the experimental groups. Similarly, if the researcher wants the study to have higher power, with effect size and significance level held constant, a larger number of runs will be required. Again, this makes intuitive sense since the researcher requires more information to increase the chances of correctly claiming that there is a difference between experimental groups. Finally, a lower significance level, with effect size and power held constant, also requires a larger number of runs. In this situation, more information is needed to reduce the chances of incorrectly claiming a difference between experimental groups when no difference exists.

Appendix C
Specifications of the Statechart Diagram

The following tables specify the states, transition labels, and events of the Statechart diagram for patient flow. Tables C.1 to C.5 list all the states that patients may occupy in the process shown in Fig. 13.5, a description of their functionality, and their associated events and conditions. Tables C.6 to C.8 list all the events shown in Fig. 13.5 and a description of their occurrences. Table C.9 lists all the functions shown in Fig. 13.5 and a description of their functionality.

B. Sobolev et al., *Health Care Evaluation Using Computer Simulation: Concepts, Methods, and Applications*, DOI 10.1007/978-1-4614-2233-4,

Table C.1 Substates, transitions, and their events and conditions for processing outpatient referrals in the Statechart diagram for patient flow

Substate{descriptor} \function called	Entering transition; event(condition)	Leaving transition; event(condition)
Referral_requested {Represents referral that has been requested}	referral	document
Referral_documented {Represents referral that has been documented}	document	book
Registered_on_list {Represents referral that has been registered on the appointment list}	register	book
On_pooled_list {Represents referral that has been registered on the appointment list under the policy *Pooled list*}	(pooled = true)	
On_individual_list {Represents referral that has been registered on the appointment list under the policy *Individual lists*}	(individual = true)	
On_shortest_list {Represents referral that has been registered on the appointment list under the policy *Shortest list*}	(shortest = true)	
Booked_for_appointment {Represents referral that has been booked for appointment} \book_appointment( )	book, further_tests	appointment
Assessed_at_consultation {Represents referral that has been assessed in clinic} \perform_tests( )"	appointment	further_tests, book_sx

Table C.2 Substates, transitions, and their events and conditions for booking of elective surgeries in the Statecharts diagram for patient flow

Substate{descriptor} \function called	Entering transition; event(condition)	Leaving transition; event(condition)
Registered_on_surgical_wait_list {Represents patient who has been registered on a surgical wait list}	book_sx, further_tests (refuse_to_enter_list = false)	leave_list, death
Prebooked {Represents patient who has been prebooked for surgery under policy *Prebooking*}	(prebooking = true)	further_tests
Listed_with_no_committed_date {Represents patient who has been registered on surgical list with no committed date for operation under policy *Wait-list booking*}	(wait-list booking = true)	further_tests
Preoperative assessment {Represents assessment of patient before surgery}	pre_sx_assessment	
Assessed_in_PAC {Represents patient who has been assessed before surgery in outpatient clinic under policy *All screened*} \perform_tests( )	(all_screened = true)	further_tests
Assessed_in_hospital {Represents patient who has been assessed before surgery in hospital under policy *Some screened*} \perform_tests( )	(some_screened = true and slot_available = false)	further_tests
Not_entered_list {Represents patient who refused to be operated}	book_sx, further_tests (refuse_to_enter_list = true)	
Left_list {Represents patient who was removed voluntarily from surgical wait list}	leave_list	
Deceased {Represents death while waiting for surgery}	death	

Table C.3 Substates, transitions, and their events and conditions for processing inpatient referrals and emergency arrivals, booking inpatient surgeries, and scheduling operating room in the Statechart diagram for patient flow

Substate{descriptor} \function called	Entering transition; event(condition)	Leaving transition; event(condition)
Processing of inpatient referrals		
Referral_requested_and_processed {Represents inpatient referral that has been requested and processed}	referral	assessment, fast_track
Assessed_by_on_call_surgeon {Represents inpatient referral that has been assessed in hospital by the on-call surgeon}	assessment	registration_sx, book_EM
Processing of emergency arrivals		
In_emergency_department {Represents patient that has arrived to the emergency department}	EM_arrival	assessment
Booking of inpatient surgeries		
Registered_on_surgical_queue {Represents inpatient that has been registered in the surgical queue}	registration_sx, unplanned_inpatient	book
Fast_tracked {Represents inpatient that has been fast-tracked for operation}	fast_tracked	book, discharge
Preoperative_assessment {Represents the assessment of inpatient before operation}	pre_sx_assessment	
Assessed_in_hospital {Represents inpatient that has been assessed before operation in hospital}		
Discharged_with_planned_admission {Represents inpatient that has been discharged from hospital with promise to be readmitted}	discharge	book
Operating room scheduling		
On_draft_OR_list {Represents patient that has been placed on the draft operating room list}	book	create_final_OR_list
On_final_OR_list {Represents patient that has been placed on the final operating room list} \plan_discharge( )	book, unplanned_EM, book_EM, reschedule, create_final_OR_list	cancellation, operate

Table C.4 Substates, transitions, and their events and conditions for rescheduling cancellations, surgery, intensive care treatment, ward treatment, and discharge in the Statechart diagram for patient flow

Substate{descriptor} \function called	Entering transition; event(condition)	Leaving transition; event(condition)
Rescheduling of canceled cases		
Cancelled_patient_reasons		
{Represents patient whose surgery has been canceled due to patient reasons}	cancellation	reschedule
Cancelled_hospital_reasons		
{Represents patient whose surgery has been canceled due to hospital reasons}	cancellation	reschedule
Cancelled_more_urgent_arrival		
{Represents patient whose surgery has been canceled due to the arrival of a more urgent patient}	cancellation	reschedule
Surgery		
Operated		
{Represents patient that has been operated}	operate	post_anesth_care
Intensive care treatment		
In_CS_ICU		
{Represents patient recovering in the cardiac surgery intensive care unit}	post_anesth_care (Beds_CS_ICU_available = true)	death, discharge_to_ward
In_Main_ICU		
{Represents patient recovering in the main intensive care unit}	post_anesth_care (Beds_CS_ICU_available = true and EM_patient = true)	death, discharge_to_ward
Management of patients in the ward		
In_ward		
{Represents patient recovering in the hospital ward}	discharge_to_ward	death, readmission_to_ICU, discharge
Discharge of patients		
Discharged_from_hospital		
{Represents patient that has been discharged from the hospital}	discharge	

Table C.5 Substates, transitions, and their events and conditions for allocating resources in the Statechart diagram for patient flow

Substate{descriptor} \function called	Entering transition; event(condition)	Leaving transition; event(condition)
OR_time_revised_and_reassessed {Represents the activity of revising and reassessing the OR time allocated to surgeons} \OR_slot_allocation( )	end_of_year	beginning_of_year
OR_slot_allocated {Represents the activity of allocating the OR time to surgeons} \appointment_slot_allocation( )	beginning_of_year	
Appointment_slot_allocated {Represents the activity of allocating the clinic appointment time to surgeons}		end_of_year

Table C.6 Events and their occurrence for outpatient referrals and booking of elective surgeries in the Statechart diagram for patient flow

State/event	Occurrence
Processing of outpatient referrals	
referral	Every time a patient is referred for surgical consultation
document	Every time the details for a referral are documented
register	Every time a patient is to be registered on the appointment list
book	Every time a patient is booked for consultation
book_sx	Every time a patient is to be booked for operation
Booking of elective surgeries	
pre_sx_assessment	Every time a patient is to be assessed at the preadmission clinic or in hospital
further_tests	Every time further tests are to be performed after preoperative assessment
leave_list	Every time a patient is removed voluntarily from the surgical wait list
death	Every time a patient dies while waiting for the operation
unplanned_inpatient	Every time a patient is to be admitted to hospital because of deteriorating condition
book	Every time a patient is to be placed on the draft operating room list
unplanned_EM	Every time a patient is placed on the final operating room list because of deteriorating condition

Table C.7 Events and their occurrence for processing inpatient referrals and emergency arrivals, booking of inpatient surgeries, and operating room scheduling in the Statechart diagram for patient flow

State/event	Occurrence
Processing of inpatient referrals	
referral	Every time a patient is referred for surgical consultation in hospital
assessment	Every time an inpatient is to be assessed by the on-call surgeon
registration_sx	Every time an inpatient is to be registered for the operation
fast_track	Every time an inpatient is to be fast-tracked for the operation
book_EM	Every time an inpatient is to be booked for the operation as an emergency patient
Processing of emergency arrivals	
EM_arrival	Every time a patient arrives at the emergency department
assessment	Every time an emergency patient is assessed by the on-call surgeon
Booking of inpatient surgeries	
pre_sx_assessment	Every time a patient is assessed in hospital
book	Every time an inpatient is to be booked for operation on the draft operating room list
discharge	Every time an inpatient is discharged with a promise to readmit
Operating room scheduling	
create_final_OR_list	Weekly when the operating room list is finalized
operate	Every time a patient is admitted to operating room

Table C.8 Events and their occurrence for rescheduling of canceled cases, surgery, intensive care treatment, management of patients in the ward, allocation of resources in the Statechart diagram for patient flow

State/event	Occurrence
Rescheduling of canceled cases	
reschedule	Every time an operation is to be rescheduled
Surgery	
post_anesth_care	Every time a patient is to start postanesthesia care
Intensive care treatment	
discharge_to_ward	Every time a patient is to be discharged to hospital ward
death	Every time a death in intensive care unit occurs
Management of patients in the ward	
readmission_to_ICU	Every time a patient is to be readmitted to intensive care unit
discharge	Every time a patient is discharged from hospital
death	Every time a death in hospital ward occurs
Allocation of resources	
beginning_of_year	Once a year to indicate the start of a fiscal year
end_of_year	Once a year to indicate the end of a fiscal year

Table C.9 Functions of cardiac surgical care and their functionality in the Statecharts diagram for patient flow

Function	Functionality
book_appointment( )	Performs the booking of surgical consultation appointments in the outpatient clinic
perform_tests( )	Performs tests for patients requiring further examinations
plan_discharge( )	Performs the management of discharge planning (e.g., patient education and arranging postoperative services)
OR_slot_allocation( )	Performs the annual allocation of available operating room time to surgeons
appointment_slot_allocation( )	Performs the annual allocation of appointment slots to surgeons

Appendix D
Data Dictionaries for Case Studies

In this appendix, we provide the data dictionaries for variables from the analytical data sets used in the simulation studies of the process of surgical care (see Chaps. 14–16). Table D.1 shows the data dictionary for the data sets containing records of simulated patients undergoing elective procedures. The variables in this dictionary contain information on the study population, hospital characteristics, patient attributes, and outcomes. Table D.2 shows the data dictionary for the data sets containing records of simulated patients undergoing urgent procedures. The variables in this data set allowed us to compute the weekly number of inpatient or emergency procedures, which was used for adjustment in regression analyses.

B. Sobolev et al., *Health Care Evaluation Using Computer Simulation: Concepts, Methods, and Applications*, DOI 10.1007/978-1-4614-2233-4,

Table D.1 Data dictionary for the analytical data set for patients undergoing elective procedures

Variable	Description	Type	Categories or values
Hospital level			
runid	Hospital identifier	Categorical	≥1
meth_app	Method of booking surgical consultation appointments	Categorical	1—Individual lists 2—Pooled list 3—Shortest list
meth_pac	Method of managing presurgical screening	Categorical	1—All screened 2—Some screened
meth_sx	Method of booking surgery	Categorical	1—Advance booking 2—Wait-list booking
or_slot	Allocation of OR slots between elective and urgent procedures	Categorical	1—Weekly split 2—Daily split
ap_ct	Clearance time for appointment lists at start of simulation (weeks)	Numeric	1, 2, or 3
el_ct	Clearance time for surgical wait lists at start of simulation (weeks)	Numeric	3, 4, 5, or 6
ur_ct	Clearance time for inpatient surgical queues at start of simulation (weeks)	Numeric	0, 1, or 2
n_ptwt	No. of patients waiting during weeks when no surgical consultation appointments are available	Numeric	≥0
ct	Moving average clearance time for surgical consultation appointments (weeks)	Numeric	≥0
idelay	Indicator for delay of any high-priority elective procedures	Categorical	0—No 1—Yes
icanclow	Indicator for cancellation of high-priority elective or urgent procedures <3.2%	Categorical	0—No 1—Yes
inocanc	Indicator for no cancellations of any high-priority elective procedures	Categorical	0—No 1—Yes
Patient level			
pid	Patient identifier	Categorical	≥1
agegrp	Age group (years)	Categorical	1—<50 2—50 to 59 3—60 to 69 4—70 to 79 5—≥80
sex	Sex	Categorical	0—Male 1—Female
anatom	Coronary anatomy affected	Categorical	1—Left main 2—Multivessel 3—Limited
comor	Comorbidity	Categorical	1—Major conditions* 2—Other conditions† 3—None
ref_date	Referral date	Date	dd/mm/yyyy <blank>—NA‡

(continued)

Table D.1 (continued)

Variable	Description	Type	Categories or values
wl_st_app	Date of registration on wait list for surgical consultation appointment	Date	dd/mm/yyyy <blank>—NA‡
wl_en_app	Date of removal from wait list for surgical consultation appointment	Date	dd/mm/yyyy <blank>—NA‡
wltime_app	Time from referral to appointment for surgical consultation (weeks)	Numeric	≥0 <blank>—NA‡
wl_rm_app	Reason for removal from appointment wait list	Categorical	0—Received appointment 1—Did not attend 90—Still on appointment wait list 99—NA‡
ur_ref	Priority at referral for appointment	Categorical	1—High priority 2—Low priority 99—NA‡
sid	Consultation surgeon identifier	Categorical	1—Surgeon 1 2—Surgeon 2 3—Surgeon 3 <blank>—NA§
wl_st_sx	Date of registration on surgical wait list	Date	dd/mm/yyyy <blank>—NA§
wl_en_sx	Date of removal from surgical wait list	Date	dd/mm/yyyy <blank>—NA§
ord_reg	Order of registration on surgical wait list	Numeric	≥1
wl_proj_sx	Projected date of surgery	Date	dd/mm/yyyy <blank>—NA§
slot_type	Type of OR slot	Categorical	1—Elective 2—Urgent
wtime_sx	Time from registration to surgery (weeks)	Numeric	≥0 <blank>—NA§
wl_rm_sx	Reason for removal from surgical wait list	Categorical	0—Received surgery 1—Died 2—Removed for other reason 3—Canceled from final OR list 5—Unplanned emergency admission 6—Became inpatient 90—Still on surgical wait list 99—NA§

(continued)

Table D.1 (continued)

Variable	Description	Type	Categories or values
sx_date	Date of surgery	Date	dd/mm/yyyy¶
ur_bk	Priority at registration on surgical wait list	Categorical	1—High priority 2—Medium priority 3—Low priority 99—NA§
cancel_date_final	Date of cancellation from final OR list	Date	dd/mm/yyyy <blank>—NA‖
cancel_type _final	Reason for cancellation from final OR list	Categorical	1—Inpatient arrival 2—Unfit for surgery 3—No ICU bed available <blank>—NA‖
cancel_id	Event number for cancellation from final OR list	Numeric	1—First cancellation 2—Second cancellation etc.
reinst_date	Date of reinstatement for surgery	Date	dd/mm/yyyy
ctreg	Clearance time for elective surgery at time of registration (weeks)	Numeric	≥ 0
isxafter	Timing of surgery	Categorical	0—Within recommended time 1—After recommended time
isx	Indicator variable for access to surgery	Categorical	0—No 1—Yes
isxafter	Timing of surgery	Categorical	0—Within recommended time 1—After recommended time

Abbreviations: OR = operating room, NA = not applicable, ICU = intensive care unit

∗Congestive heart failure, diabetes mellitus, chronic obstructive pulmonary disease, rheumatoid arthritis, cancer

†Peripheral vascular disease, cerebrovascular disease, dementia, peptic ulcer disease, hemiplegia, renal disease, liver disease

‡Patient was on surgical wait list before start of study period

§Patient did not receive surgical consultation appointment

¶For patients who underwent surgery

‖Patient was not canceled from final OR list

Table D.2 Data dictionary for the analytical data set for inpatients

Variable	Description	Type	Categories or values
runid	Hospital identifier	Categorical	≥ 1
pid	Patient identifier	Categorical	≥ 1
adm_date	Date of admission to hospital	Date	dd/mm/yyyy
sx_date	Date of surgery	Date	dd/mm/yyyy
dis_date	Date of discharge	Date	dd/mm/yyyy
dis_rm	Reason for discharge	Categorical	0—Received surgery 90—Still waiting
urgent	Priority at surgery	Categorical	0—Emergency 1—High priority 2—Low priority 3—Promise to readmit

Glossary

This glossary defines terms used frequently in this book. When a term may have broader meaning in everyday use, we narrow the definition to the context of simulation modeling in health care.

Access curve A graph depicting the cumulative proportion of patients gaining access to a procedure by time since the procedure was indicated.

Activity In workflow modeling, a set of recurring actions required to achieve the functions of the system.

Adjustment variables Variables entered into a regression model to adjust the effect of the primary study variable for differences between study groups.

Alternative hypothesis A statement of a difference between experimental groups; compare "null hypothesis".

Angiography A diagnostic procedure used to find points of narrowing of the arteries that supply blood to the heart; involves administration of a contrast agent into the blood vessels, followed by radiographic imaging.

Attribute A characteristic of an entity.

Average A statistic that summarizes a set of observations with an expected value.

Binary outcome An outcome that takes one of two possible values.

Booking Assignment of a specific date for service.

Box plot A graph showing the 25th and 75th percentiles, the median or average, and the minimum and maximum values of observations.

Cardiology consultation First step in the process of cardiac care, whereby a general physician or a specialist in another area refers a patient to a cardiologist for assessment of a heart condition.

Case study An inquiry that evaluates a policy within a certain context.

B. Sobolev et al., *Health Care Evaluation Using Computer Simulation: Concepts, Methods, and Applications*, DOI 10.1007/978-1-4614-2233-4,

Clearance time The hypothetical amount of time to serve all patients currently waiting for a service; calculated as the ratio of the existing demand to capacity.

Clock In discrete-event simulation, a variable that controls the advancement of time during the simulation.

Cluster A group of entities with certain characteristics in common that is treated within the experiment as a single unit.

Coding Rules for categorizing data for analysis.

Confidence interval A range of values quantifying the uncertainty of an estimate; a 95% confidence interval will contain the true parameter value 95 times out of 100.

CONSORT Consolidated Standards of Reporting Trials; a set of guidelines for improving the reporting of randomized controlled trials.

Control group Study participants exposed to the existing policy.

Comparison group Study participants exposed to the alternative policy.

Coronary artery bypass grafting Surgical revascularization performed to alleviate chest pain and to reduce the risk of death among patients who have limiting angina that persists despite optimal medical treatment and who have coronary anatomy that is suitable for the procedure.

Data dictionary description of variables related to the study question, including their type and their categories or values.

Degrees of freedom The number of independent sources of variation in data.

Discrete-event simulation A computer program that represents a system's behavior in response to events generated within its states or taking place outside the system.

Discrete-time survival regression Statistical method that measures effect of changes in a study factor on timing of an event in terms of odds ratio for the event occurrence while allowing for adjustment for other variables and the probability of its occurrence in nonoverlapping intervals.

Distribution function A function that links each possible of a random variable with the probability of its occurrence.

Effect size A difference in the summary measure of an outcome between study groups.

Elective surgery A procedure performed to treat a condition for which the risk of immediate morbidity and death is believed to be low; may be postponed to accommodate patients with more urgent needs.

Emergency surgery A procedure performed within hours to avoid death or disability.

Entity In discrete-event simulation, a distinct component of the system represented by an object in a simulation model (e.g., patient in the care process).

Event In discrete-event simulation, a notable occurrence at a particular point in time, which triggers a change in the state of the system.

Event list In discrete-event simulation, a compilation of pending events sorted by event time, usually organized as a priority queue.

Experimental study Testing whether a forced change in study factors results in a change in the outcome.

Full factorial design Experiments with one design point for every possible combination of the values of the experimental factors.

Frequency distribution A summary of occurrences of values for a variable.

Generalizability Validity of the findings from an experiment for other groups of patients.

Health services research The study of the organization, use, and outcomes of health care.

Indicator variable A variable that uses 0 or 1 to represent two categories.

Intervention studies A branch of health services research concerned with evaluating the effects of health care interventions.

Intervention In health care, quality improvement initiative, policy, management system, a set of practice guidelines, prevention program, booking method, service model, or a new treatment, medical device, or product.

Linear regression Statistical method that measures effect of changes in a study factor in terms of a difference between means of continuous outcomes, while allowing for adjustment for other variables.

Logistic regression Statistical method that measures effect of changes in a study factor in terms of an odds ratio for occurrence of a binary outcome while allowing for adjustment for other variables.

Mean The expected value of a distribution.

Median The value of a random variable that divides the distribution into equal parts.

Multiplicity In statistical analysis, numerous statistical inferences from the same data set.

Multiplicity value In UML diagrams, value indicating the number of elements participating in the association.

Null hypothesis A statement of no difference between experimental groups; compare "alternative hypothesis".

Observational studies Comparison of outcomes among groups that happen to have been exposed to different treatments, without any action on the part of the researcher to control factors involved in choosing the treatment.

Odds A ratio of the probability of event to its complement.

Odds ratio A measure of effect size that compares proportions between experimental groups.

One-tailed hypothesis A claim that specifies the direction of a difference between experimental groups; compare "two-tailed hypothesis".

Operationalization The process of defining concepts in terms of measurable observations.

Outcome In health services research, an end point of interest in the delivery of health care.

***p* value** The probability of obtaining observed results if the null hypothesis is true.

Patient population A group of patients defined by their condition or the intervention indicated for their condition.

Performance measure In a simulation study, a quantity describing a system's performance on the basis of observations of experimental outcome.

Preoperative assessment In surgical care, assessment of patient's fitness and risks for undergo surgery.

Process In discrete-event simulation, activities ordered in time.

Proportion The fraction of observations that satisfy a specific criterion.

Randomization Process of assignment to groups ensuring the same chance of being assigned to any group.

Randomized trials Comparison of outcomes among study participants who are randomly assigned by the researcher to one of the experimental groups.

Rate The average number of events over a specified time interval.

Regression model An equation that relates study factors to some function of an experimental outcome.

Significance level A preset value of the probability that a result is due to chance; typically set to 0.05.

Simulation modeling Use of a computer program to produce outcomes of operations of a modeled system.

Standard error A measure of dispersion of a statistical estimate.

Standard deviation A measure of dispersion of data.

State In discrete-event simulation, a set of variables describing the modeled system at a particular point in time.

Statechart A diagram representing the dynamic behavior of a system by specifying transitions between its states in response to events.

Statistic A value estimated from data.

Statistical power The probability of correctly claiming that there is a difference between experimental groups; typically set to 80% or 90%.

Study design A course of action for conducting a study.

Study factors Characteristics of the care setting or the patient that may affect the outcomes of a simulation experiment.

Study flow chart A diagram depicting the number of participants over consecutive steps in the study.

Study question In health care evaluation, a problem stated in the context of the social, political, organizational, behavioral, and economic theories that have influenced the design of health care systems.

Summary measure A quantity summarizing the distribution of an outcome variable in a study group.

Surgical consultation Assessment of patient's need for surgery; in cardiac surgical care.

Two-tailed hypothesis A claim that a difference between the experimental groups may exist, without specifying the direction of the difference.

Type I error The probability of incorrectly claiming there is a difference between experimental groups.

Type II error The probability of incorrectly claiming there is no difference between experimental groups.

Unified modeling language (UML) A standardized modeling language, includes a set of diagrammatic notations for specifying system's functioning.

Unit of analysis The entity for statistical inferences.

Unit of observation The entity for which data are collected.

Unit of randomization The entity assigned to an experimental group.

Urgent surgery A procedure performed to avoid morbidity, but can be postponed for a short time; the need for urgent treatment may cause postponement and rescheduling of elective procedures.

References

1. L. Aharonson-Daniel, R. J. Paul, and A. J. Hedley. Management of queues in out-patient departments: The use of computer simulation. *Journal of Health Organization and Management*, 10(6):50–58, 1996.
2. P. Allison. *Logistic regression using the SAS system theory and application*. SAS Institute, Cary, NC, 1999.
3. P. D. Allison. Discrete-time methods for the analysis of event histories. *Sociological Methodology*, Jossey-Bass, San Francisco, CA, pages 61–98, 1982.
4. I. K. Altinel and E. Usla. Simulation modeling for emergency bed requirement planning. *Annals of Operations Research*, 67(1):183–210, 1996.
5. J. Appleby, S. Boyle, N. Devlin, M. Harley, A. Harrison, L. Locock, and R. Thorlby. Sustaining reductions in waiting times: Identifying successful strategies. Technical report, King's Fund, 2005.
6. A. C. Atkinson and A. N. Donev. *Optimum experimental designs*, chapter Criteria of optimality, pages 106–115. Oxford Science Publications, Oxford, 1992.
7. A. Bagust, M. Place, and J. W. Posnett. Dynamics of bed use in accommodating emergency admissions: Stochastic simulation model. *British Medical Journal*, 319(7203):155–158, 1999.
8. N. T. J. Bailey. A study of queues and appointment systems in hospital out-patient departments, with special reference to waiting-times. *Journal of the Royal Statistical Society*, 14(2): 185–199, 1952.
9. J. Banks. *Discrete-event system simulation*. Prentice Hall, 3rd edition, Upper Saddle River, NJ, 2001.
10. S. Barnoon and H. Wolfe. Scheduling a multiple operating room system: A simulation approach. *Health Services Research*, 3(4):272–285, 1968.
11. R. R. Barton. Designing simulation experiments. In *Proceedings of the 33nd conference on Winter simulation*, pages 47–52. IEEE Computer Society, 2001.
12. J. R. Beck and S. G. Pauker. The Markov process in medical prognosis. *Medical Decision Making*, 3(4):419–458, 1983.
13. C. Begg, M. Cho, S. Eastwood, R. Horton, D. Moher, I. Olkin, R. Pitkin, D. Rennie, K. F. Schulz, D. Simel, and D. F. Stroup. Improving the quality of reporting of randomized controlled trials. The CONSORT statement. *The Journal of the American Medical Association*, 276(8):637–639, 1996.
14. J. C. Benneyan. An introduction to using computer simulation in healthcare: Patient wait case study. *Journal of the Society for Health Systems*, 5(3):1–15, 1997.
15. G. Bertolini, C. Rossi, L. Brazzi, D. Radrizzani, G. Rossi, E. Arrighi, and B. Simini. The relationship between labour cost per patient and the size of intensive care units: A multicentre prospective study. *Intensive Care Medicine*, 29(12):2307–2311, 2003.

B. Sobolev et al., *Health Care Evaluation Using Computer Simulation: Concepts, Methods, and Applications*, DOI 10.1007/978-1-4614-2233-4,

16. D. M. Berwick. The John Eisenberg Lecture: Health services research as a citizen in improvement. *Health Services Research*, 40(2):317–336, 2005.
17. J. Blake and M. Carter. A goal programming approach to strategic resource allocation in acute care hospitals. *European Journal of Operational Research*, 140:541–561, 2002.
18. J. Blake and J. Donald. Mount Sinai Hospital uses integer programming to allocate operating room time. *Interfaces*, 32(3):63–73, 2002.
19. J. T. Blake and M. W. Carter. Surgical process management: A conceptual framework. *Surgical Services Management*, 3(9):31–37, 1997.
20. J. T. Blake and M. W. Carter. Surgical process scheduling: A structured review. *Journal of the Society for Health Systems*, 5(3):17–30, 1997.
21. M. Blanc-Jouvan, A. Mercatello, D. Long, M. P. Benoit, M. Khadraoui, C. Nemoz, M. Gay-darova, J. P. Boissel, and J. F. Moskovtchenko. The value of anesthesia consultation in relation to the single preanesthetic visit. *Annales Franaises d'Anesthsie et de Ranimation*, 18(8):843–847, 1999.
22. J. M. Bland and D. G. Altman. One and two sided tests of significance. *British Medical Journal*, 309:248, 1994.
23. J. M. Bland and D. G. Altman. The logrank test. *British Medical Journal*, 328(7447):1073, 2004.
24. E. Bonabeau. Agent-based modeling: Methods and techniques for simulating human systems. *Proceeding of the National Academy of Sciences of the U.S.A*, 99(3):7280–7287, 2002.
25. D. M. Bond. Pre-anesthetic assessment clinics in ontario. *Canadian Journal of anaesthesia*, 46(4):382–387, 1999.
26. G. Booch. *Object-oriented analysis and design with applications*. Benjamin/Cummings Pub. Co, 2nd edition, 1994.
27. G. Booch, I. Jacobson, and J. Rumbaugh. *The Unified Modeling Language user guide*. Addison-Wesley, 2nd edition, Upper Saddle River, NJ, 2005.
28. G. E. P. Box, W. G. Hunter, and J. S. Hunter. *Statistics for experimenters*. Wiley-Interscience, New York, 1978.
29. C. C. Bozarth and R. B. Handfield. *Introduction to operations and supply chain management*. Pearson Prentice Hall, Upper Saddle River, NJ, 2005.
30. M. Brahimi and D. Worthington. Queuing models for out-patient appointment systems - a case study. *Journal of Operational Research Society*, 42(9):733–746, 1991.
31. S. C. Brailsford, V. A. Lattimer, P. Tarnaras, and J. C. Turnbull. Emergency and on-demand health care: Modelling a large complex system. *Journal of the Operational Research Society*, 55(1):34–42, 2004.
32. A. Burton, D. G. Altman, P. Royston, and R. L. Holder. The design of simulation studies in medical statistics. *Statistics in Medicine*, 25(24):4279–4292, 2006.
33. M. K. Campbell, D. R. Elbourne, and D. G. Altman. CONSORT statement: Extension to cluster randomised trials. *British Medical Journal*, 328(7441):702–708, 2004.
34. J. Caro, S. Guo, A. Ward, S. Chalil, F. Malik, and F. Leyva. Modelling the economic and health consequences of cardiac resynchronization therapy in the UK. *Current Medical Research and Opinion*, 22(6):1171–1179, 2006.
35. W. G. Cochran. *Sampling techniques*. Wiley, 3rd edition, New York, 1977.
36. L. H. Cohn and L. H. Edmunds Jr. *Cardiac Surgery in the Adult*. McGraw-Hill, New York, 2003.
37. T. Colton. *Statistics in medicine*. Little Brown and Company, Boston, 1974.
38. A. X. Costa, S. A. Ridley, A. K. Shahani, P. R. Harper, V. De Senna, and M. S. Nielsen. Mathematical modelling and simulation for planning critical care capacity. *Anaesthesia*, 58 (4):320–327, 2003.
39. K. M. Cottrell. Waiting lists: Some problems of definition and a relative measure of waiting time. *Hospital and Health Services Review*, 76:265–269, 1980.
40. Medical Research Council. A framework for the development and evaluation of RCTs for complex interventions to improve health. www.mrc.ac.uk/utilities/Documentrecord/index.htm?d=MRC003372, 2000.

41. D. R. Cox. *Principles of statistical inference*. Cambridge University Press, Cambridge, 2006.
42. J. L. Cronenwett and R. B. Rutherford. *Decision making in vascular surgery*. Saunders, Philadelphia, 2001.
43. R. G. Cumming, C. Sherrington, S. R. Lord, J. M. Simpson, C. Vogler, I. D. Cameron, and V. Naganathan. Cluster randomised trial of a targeted multifactorial intervention to prevent falls among older people in hospital. *British Medical Journal*, 336(7647):758–760, 2008.
44. B. C. Dangerfield. System dynamics applications to European health care issues. *Journal of the Operational Research Society*, 50:345–353, 1999.
45. H. T. Davies and R Davies. Simulating health systems: Modelling problems and software solutions. *European Journal of Operational Research*, 87:35–44, 1995.
46. R. Davies. An assessment of models of a health system. *Journal of the Operational Research Society*, 36(8):679–687, 1985.
47. F. Dexter and R. D. Traub. How to schedule elective surgical cases into specific operating rooms to maximize the efficiency of use of operating room time. *Anesthesia and Analgesia*, 94(4):933–942, 2002.
48. A. Donabedian. Evaluating the quality of medical care. *Milbank Quarterly*, 83(4):691–729, 2005.
49. A. Donner and N. Klar. *Design and analysis of cluster randomization trials in health research*. Arnold Publishing Co., London, 2000.
50. C. Duguay and F. Chetouane. Modeling and improving emergency department systems using discrete event simulation. *Simulation*, 83(4):311–320, 2007.
51. M. Eccles, J. Grimshaw, M. Campbell, and C. Ramsay. Research designs for studies evaluating the effectiveness of change and improvement strategies. *Quality and Safety in Health Care*, 12(1):47–52, 2003.
52. R. H. Edwards, J. Clague, M. Barlow, P. Clarke, and R. Rada. Operations research survey and computer simulation of waiting times in two medical outpatient clinic structures. *Health care analysis*, 2(2):164–169, 1994.
53. E. G. Estrada. Triage systems. *The Nursing Clinics of North America*, 16(1):13–24, 1981.
54. J. E. Everett. A decision support simulation model for the management of an elective surgery waiting system. *Health Care Management Science*, 5(2):89–95, 2002.
55. V. V. Fedorov. *Theory of optimal experiments*. Academic Press, 12th edition, New York, 1972.
56. A. Figueiras, M. T. Herdeiro, J. Polonia, and J. J. Gestal-Otero. An educational intervention to improve physician reporting of adverse drug reactions: A cluster-randomized controlled trial. *Journal of the American Medical Association*, 296(9):1086–1093, 2006.
57. G. S. Fishman. *Discrete-event simulation modeling, programming, and analysis*. Springer, New York, 2001.
58. J. L. Fleiss. *Statistical methods for rates and proportions*. Wiley, New York, 1973.
59. J. L. Fleiss. *The design and analysis of clinical experiments*. Wiley, New York, 1986.
60. D. Fone, S. Hollinghurst, M. Temple, A. Round, N. Lester, A. Weightman, K. Roberts, E. Coyle, G. Bevan, and S. Palmer. Systematic review of the use and value of computer simulation modelling in population health and health care delivery. *Journal of Public Health*, 25(4):325–335, 2003.
61. J. W. Forrester. *Industrial dynamics*. M.I.T. Press, Cambridge, MA, 1961.
62. R. J. Glynn, M. A. Brookhart, M. Stedman, J. Avorn, and D. H. Solomon. Design of cluster-randomized trials of quality improvement interventions aimed at medical care providers. *Medical Care*, 45(10):S38–S43, 2007.
63. D. H. Goldstein, E. G. VanDenKerkhof, and M. J. Rimmer. A model for real time information at the patient's side using portable computers on an acute pain service. *Canadian Journal of anaesthesia*, 49(7):749–754, 2002.
64. Object Management Group. Unified modeling language 2.0: Superstructure, 2005. www.omg.org.
65. V. Guru, S. E. Fremes, and J. V. Tu. Time-related mortality for women after coronary artery bypass graft surgery: A population-based study. *Journal of Thoracic and Cardiovascular Surgery*, 127(4):1158–1165, 2004.

66. C. Ham, R. Kipping, and H. McLeod. Redesigning work processes in health care: Lessons from the national health service. *The Milbank Quarterly*, 81(3):415–439, 2003.
67. D. M. Hamilton and S. Breslawski. Operating room scheduling. Factors to consider. *Association of Operating Room Nurses Journal*, 59(3):665–680, 1994.
68. C. Haraden and R. Resar. Patient flow in hospitals: Understanding and controlling it better. *Frontiers of Health Services Management*, 20(4):3–15, 2004.
69. D. Harel. Statecharts: A visual formalism for complex systems. *Science of Computer Programming*, 8:231–274, 1987.
70. D. Harel and A. Pnueli. *Logics and Models of Concurrent Systems*, chapter On the Development of Reactive Systems, pages 477–498. Springer-Verlag, New York, 1985.
71. D Harel and M. Politi. *Modeling Reactive Systems with Statecharts: The STATEMATE Approach*. McGraw-Hill, New York, 1998.
72. P. R. Harper and H. M. Gamlin. Reduced outpatient waiting times with improved appointment scheduling: A simulation modelling approach. *OR Spectrum*, 25(2):207–222, 2003.
73. F. E. Harrel, K. L. Lee, D. B. Matchar, and T. A. Reichert. Regression models for prognostic prediction: Advantages, problems and suggested solutions. *Cancer Treatment Reports*, 69: 1071–1077, 1985.
74. R. J. Hayes and S. Bennett. Simple sample size calculation for cluster-randomized trials. *International Journal of Epidemiology*, 28:319–326, 1999.
75. J. J. Heckman. The scientific model of causality. *Sociological Methodology*, 35(1):1–97, 2005.
76. J. B. Homer and G. B. Hirsch. System dynamics modeling for public health: Background and opportunities. *American Journal of Public Health*, 96(3):452–458, 2006.
77. Jr. Hosmer, D. W. and S. Lemeshow. *Applied logistic regression*. John Wiley and Sons, New York, 1989.
78. E. S. Huang, Q. Zhang, S. E. Brown, M. L. Drum, D. O. Meltzer, and M. H. Chin. The cost-effectiveness of improving diabetes care in U.S. federally qualified community health centers. *Health Services Research*, 42(6 Pt 1):2174–2193, 2007.
79. G. Iapichino, L. Gattinoni, D. Radrizzani, B. Simini, G. Bertolini, L. Ferla, G. Mistraletti, F. Porta, and D. R. Miranda. Volume of activity and occupancy rate in intensive care units. Association with mortality. *Intensive Care Medicine*, 30(2):290–297, 2004.
80. I. Jacobson. *Object-oriented software engineering—A use case driven approach*. ACM Press, New York, 1992.
81. S. H. Jacobson, S. H. Hall, and Swisher J.R. *Patient flow: Reducing delay in healthcare delivery*, chapter Discrete-event simulation of health care systems, pages 211–252. Springer US, 2006.
82. G. T. Jun, J. Ward, Z. Morris, and J. Clarkson. Health care process modelling: Which method when? *International Journal for Quality in Health Care*, 21(3):214–224, 2009.
83. G. T. Jun, J. Ward, and P. J. Clarkson. Systems modelling approaches to the design of safe healthcare delivery: Ease of use and usefulness perceived by healthcare workers. *Ergonomics*, 53(7):829–847, 2010.
84. J. B. Jun, S. H. Jacobson, and J. R. Swisher. Application of discrete-event simulation in health care clinics: A survey. *Journal of the Operational Research Society*, 50(2):109–123, 1999.
85. S. J. Katz, H. F. Mizgala, and H. G. Welch. British Columbia sends patients to Seattle for coronary artery surgery. Bypassing the queue in Canada. *Journal of the American Medical Association*, 266(8):1108–1111, 1991.
86. B. Keogh and R. Kinsman. Fifth national adult cardiac surgical database report 2003: Improving outcomes for patients. Technical report, Dendrite Clinical Systems, 2004.
87. B. Kirwan and L. K. Ainsworth. *A Guide to task analysis*. Taylor and Francis, London, 1992.
88. K. J. Klassen and T. R. Rohleder. Scheduling outpatient appointments in a dynamic environment. *Journal of Operations Management*, 14(2):83–101, 1996.
89. L. Kuramoto, B. G. Sobolev, and M. G. Donaldson. On reporting results from randomized controlled trials with recurrent events. *BMC Medica Research Methodology*, 8:35, 2008.

90. M. Lamiri, X. Xiea, A. Dolguia, and F. Grimaud. A stochastic model for operating room planning with elective emergency demand for surgery. *European Journal of Operational Research*, 185(3):1026–1037, 2008.
91. T. A. Lang and M. Secic. *How to report statistics in medicine annotated guidelines for authors, editors, and reviewers*. American College of Physicians, 2nd edition, Philadelphia, 2006.
92. A. M. Law. *Simulation modeling and analysis*. Tata McGraw-Hill, 4th edition, New York, 2007.
93. A. Levy, B. Sobolev, R. Hayden, M. Kiely, M. FitzGerald, and M. Schechter. Time on wait lists for coronary bypass surgery in british columbia, canada, 1991 - 2000. *BMC Health Services Research*, 5(1):1–10, 2005.
94. K. Y. Liang and S. L. Zeger. Longitudinal data analysis using generalized linear models. *Biometrika*, 73(1):13–22, 1986.
95. S. R. Lipsitz, N. M. Laird, and D. P. Harrington. Generalized estimating equations for correlated binary data—Using the odds ratio as a measure of association. *Biometrika*, 78 (1):153–160, 1991.
96. C. M. Macal and M. J. North. Tutorial on agent-based modelling and simulation. *Journal of Simulation*, 4:151–162, 2010.
97. J. M. Magerlein and J. B. Martin. Surgical demand scheduling: A review. *Health Services Research*, 13(4):418–433, 1978.
98. A. R. Mahachek. An introduction to patient flow simulation for health care managers. *Journal of the Society for Health Systems*, 3(3):73–81, 1992.
99. G. Maldonado and S. Greenland. Estimating causal effects. *International Journal of Epidemiology*, 31(2):422–429, 2002.
100. Mathworks. Stateflow. Computer Program, 2007. Version 7.
101. P. Matthey, B. T. Finucane, and B. A. Finegan. The attitude of the general public towards preoperative assessment and risks associated with general anesthesia. *Canadian Journal of anaesthesia*, 48(4):333–339, 2001.
102. C. McIntosh, F. Dexter, and R. H. Epstein. The impact of service-specific staffing, case scheduling, turnovers, and first-case starts on anesthesia group and operating room productivity: A tutorial using data from an Australian hospital. *Anesthesia and Analgesia*, 103(6): 1499–1516, 2006.
103. H. McLeod, C. Ham, and R. Kipping. Booking patients for hospital admissions: Evaluation of a pilot programme for day cases. *British Medical Journal*, 327(7424):1147, 2003.
104. N. Melao and M. Pidd. A conceptual framework for understanding business processes and business process modelling. *Information Systems Journal*, 10(2):105–129, 2000.
105. C. Menzel and R. J. Mayer. *Handbook on architectures of information aystems*, chapter The IDEF family of languages, pages 215–249. Springer, New York, 2006.
106. P. Meredith, C. Ham, and R. Kipping. Modernising the NHS: Booking patients for hospital care: A progress report. Technical report, University of Birmingham, 1999.
107. G. Moens, K. Johannik, T. Dohogne, and G. Vandepoele. The effectiveness of teaching appropriate lifting and transfer techniques to nursing students: Results after two years of follow-up. *Archives of Public Health*, 60(2):115–123, 2002.
108. D. Moher, K. F. Schulz, D. Altman, and CONSORT Group. The CONSORT statement: Revised recommendations for improving the quality of reports of parallel-group randomized trials. *Journal of the American Medical Association*, 285(15):1987–1991, 2001.
109. D. Moher, S. Hopewell, K. F. Schulz, V. Montori, P. C. Gotzsche, P. J. Devereaux, D. Elbourne, M. Egger, and D. G. Altman. CONSORT 2010 Explanation and Elaboration: Updated guidelines for reporting parallel group randomised trials. *Journal of Clinical Epidemiology*, 63(8):e1–37, 2010.
110. S. Z. Mordiffi, S. P. Tan, and M. K. Wong. Information provided to surgical patients versus information needed. *Association of Operating Room Nurses Journal*, 77(3):546–552, 2003.
111. S. L. Morgan and C. Winship. *Counterfactuals and causal inference: Methods and principles for social research*. Cambridge University Press, Cambridge, UK, 2007.

112. N. Motomura, H. Miyata, H. Tsukihara, M. Okada, and S. Takamoto. First report on 30-day and operative mortality in risk model of isolated coronary artery bypass grafting in japan. *Annals of Thoracic Surgery*, 86(6):1866–1872, 2008.
113. T. Murata. Petri nets: Properties, analysis and applications. *Proceedings of the IEEE*, 77(4): 541–580, 1989.
114. M. Murray and D. M. Berwick. Advanced access: Reducing waiting and delays in primary care. *Journal of the American Medical Association*, 289(8):1035–1040, 2003.
115. M. Murray, T. Bodenheimer, D. Rittenhouse, and K. Grumbach. Improving timely access to primary care: casC studies of the advanced access model. *Journal of the American Medical Association*, 289(8):1042–1046, 2003.
116. N. Mustafee, K Katsaliaki, and S. J. E. Taylor. Profiling literature in healthcare simulation. *Simulation*, 86(8):543–558, 2010.
117. R. Nance. *Management science*, chapter On time flow mechanisms for discrete system simulation, pages 59–73. Informs, Hanover, MD, 1971.
118. G. T. O'Connor, S. K. Plume, E. M. Olmstead, L. H. Coffin, J. R. Morton, C. T. Maloney, E. R. Nowicki, D. G. Levy, J. F. Tryzelaar, F. Hernandez, and . Multivariate prediction of in-hospital mortality associated with coronary artery bypass graft surgery. Northern New England Cardiovascular Disease Study Group. *Circulation*, 85(6):2110–2118, 1992.
119. Institute of Medicine.Committee on Quality of Health Care. *To err is human: Building a safer health system*. National Academies Press, Washington, D.C., 2000.
120. A. O'Hagan, M. Stevenson, and J. Madan. Monte Carlo probabilistic sensitivity analysis for patient level simulation models: Efficient estimation of mean and variance using ANOVA. *Health Economics*, 16(10):1009–1023, 2007.
121. J. Papaceit, M. Olona, C. Ramon, R. Garcia-Aguado, R. Rodriguez, and M. Rull. National survey of preoperative management and patient selection in ambulatory surgery centers. *Gaceta Sanitaria*, 17(5):384–392, 2003.
122. J. Pearl. *Causality: Models, reasoning, and inference*. Cambridge University Press, Cambridge, UK, 2000.
123. C. O. Phillips, S. M. Wright, D. E. Kern, R. M. Singa, S. Shepperd, and H. R. Rubin. Comprehensive discharge planning with postdischarge support for older patients with congestive heart failure: A meta-analysis. *Journal of the American Medical Association*, 291(11):1358–1367, 2004.
124. M. Pidd. *Tools for thinking: Modelling in management science*. Wiley, 2nd edition, London, 2003.
125. M. Ramchandani, S. Mirza, A. Sharma, and G. Kirkby. Pooled cataract waiting lists: Views of hospital consultants, general practitioners and patients. *Journal of the Royal Society of Medicine*, 95(12):598–600, 2002.
126. D. Rickles. Causality in complex interventions. *Medicine, Health Care and Philosophy*, 12 (1):77–90, 2009.
127. B. Rosner. *Fundamentals of biostatistics*. Duxbury, 5th edition, Pacific Grove, CA, 1999.
128. R. Y. Rubinstein. *Simulation and the Monte Carlo method*. Wiley, New York, 1981.
129. J. Rumbaugh. *Object-oriented modeling and design*. Prentice Hall, Englewood Cliffs, NJ, 1991.
130. M. Samek. *Practical UML statecharts in C/C++: Event-driven programming for embedded systems*. Elsevier/Newnes, 2nd edition, San Francisco, CA, 2009.
131. H. H. Schmitz and N. K. Kwak. Monte Carlo Simulation of operating-room and recovery-room usage. *Operations Research*, 20(6):1171–1180, 1972.
132. K. F. Schulz, D. G. Altman, D. Moher, and the CONSORT Group. CONSORT 2010 statement: Updated guidelines for reporting parallel group randomised trials. *British Medical Journal*, 340:c332, 2010.
133. S. Schwarz. ASTERIKS - a management game for hospitals. *Journal of the Society for Health Systems*, 3(3):5–14, 1992.
134. W. Shearer, J. Monagle, and M. Michaels. A model of community based, preadmission management for elective surgical patients. *Canadian Journal of anaesthesia*, 44(12):1311–1314, 1997.

135. W. Shen and D. H. Norrie. Agent-based systems for intelligent manufacturing: A state-of-the-art survey. *Knowledge and Information Systems*, 1(2):129–156, 1999.
136. J. H. Silber and S. V. Williams. Hospital and patient characteristics associated with death after surgery—A study of adverse occurrence and failure to rescue. *Medical Care*, 30(7):615–629, 1992.
137. G. W. Snedecor and W. G. Cochran. *Statistical methods*. Iowa State University Press, 6th edition, Ames, IA, 1967.
138. B. Sobolev and L. Kuramoto. Policy analysis using patient flow simulations: Conceptual framework and study design. *Clinical and Investigative Medicine*, 28(6):359–363, 2005.
139. B. Sobolev and L. Kuramoto. *Analysis of waiting-time data in health services research*. Springer, New York, 2008.
140. B. Sobolev and L. Kuramoto. Cluster-randomized design for simulation-based evaluation of complex healthcare interventions. *Journal of Simulation*, 4(1):24–33, 2010.
141. B. Sobolev, P. Brown, D. Zelt, and L. Kuramoto. Waiting time in relation to wait-list size at registration: Statistical analysis of a waiting-list registry. *Clinical and Investigative Medicine*, 27(6):298–305, 2004.
142. B. Sobolev, A. Levy, R. Hayden, and L. Kuramoto. Does wait-list size at registration influence time to surgery? analysis of a population-based cardiac surgery registry. *Health Services Research*, 41:23–49, 2006.
143. B. Sobolev, D. Harel, C. Vasilakis, and A. Levy. Using the statecharts paradigm for simulation of patient flow in surgical care. *Health Care Management Science*, 11(1):79–86, 2008.
144. B. Sobolev, V. Sanchez, L. Kuramoto, A. R. Levy, M. Schechter, and J. M. FitzGerald. Evaluation of booking systems for elective surgery using simulation experiments. *Healthcare Policy*, 3(4):113–124, 2008.
145. B. Sobolev, V. Sanchez, and L. Kuramoto. *Discrete event simulations*, chapter Evaluation of methods for scheduling clinic appointments in surgical service: A statecharts based simulation study, pages 165–185. Sciyo, Rijeka, 2010.
146. F. A. Sonnenberg and J. R. Beck. Markov models in medical decision making: A practical guide. *Medical Decision Making*, 13(4):322–338, 1993.
147. J. E. Stahl, D. Rattner, R. Wiklund, J. Lester, M. Beinfeld, and G. S. Gazelle. Reorganizing the system of care surrounding laparoscopic surgery: A cost-effectiveness analysis using discrete-event simulation. *Medical Decision Making*, 24(5):461–471, 2004.
148. M. D. Stevenson, J. Oakley, and J. B. Chilcott. Gaussian process modeling in conjunction with individual patient simulation modeling: A case study describing the calculation of cost-effectiveness ratios for the treatment of established osteoporosis. *Medical Decision Making*, 24(1):89–100, 2004.
149. R. M. Tappen, J. Muzic, and P. Kennedy. Preoperative assessment and discharge planning for older adults undergoing ambulatory surgery. *Association of Operating Room Nurses Journal*, 73(2):464, 467, 469, 2001.
150. K. Taylor and D. Lane. Simulation applied to health services: Opportunities for applying the system dynamics approach. *Health Services Research and Policy*, 3(4):226–232, 1998.
151. A. Tiwari. Formal semantics and analysis methods for simulink stateflow models. Technical report, SRI International, 2002.
152. W. M. K. Trochim and J. P. Donnelly. *Research methods knowledge base*. Atomic Dog Publishing, 3rd edition, Mason, OH, 2008.
153. O. C. Ukoumunne, M. C. Gulliford, S. Chinn, J. A. Sterne, P. G. Burney, and A. Donner. Methods in health service research. evaluation of health interventions at area and organisation level. *British Medical Journal*, 319(7206):376–379, 1999.
154. W. A. van Klei, P. J. Hennis, J. Moen, C. J. Kalkman, and K. G. Moons. The accuracy of trained nurses in pre-operative health assessment: Results of the open study. *Anaesthesia*, 59 (10):971–978, 2004.
155. C. Vasilakis and L. Kuramoto. Comparing two methods of scheduling outpatient clinic appointments using simulation experiments. *Clinical and Investigative Medicine*, 28(6):368–370, 2005.

156. C. Vasilakis, B. G. Sobolev, L. Kuramoto, and A. R. Levy. A simulation study of scheduling clinic appointments in surgical care: Individual surgeon versus pooled lists. *Journal of the Operational Research Society*, 58(2):202–211, 2007.
157. C. Vasilakis, D. Lecnzarowicz, and C. Lee. Application of Unified Modelling Language (UML) to the modelling of health care systems: An introduction and literature survey. *International Journal of Healthcare Information Systems and Informatics*, 3(4):39–52, 2008.
158. J. Vissers. Selecting a suitable appointment system in an outpatient setting. *Medical Care*, 17 (12):1207–1220, 1979.
159. E. Vittinghoff, D. V. Glidden, and S. C. Shiboski. *Regression methods in biostatistics : Linear, logistic, survival, and repeated measures models*. Springer-Verlag New York Inc., 2005.
160. M. von der Beeck. *Formal techniques in real-time and fault-tolerant systems*, chapter A comparison of Statecharts variants, pages 128–148. Springer, Berlin, 1994.
161. D. A. Wood, K. Kotseva, S. Connolly, C. Jennings, A. Mead, J. Jones, A. Holden, Bacquer D. De, T. Collier, Backer G. De, and O. Faergeman. Nurse-coordinated multidisciplinary, family-based cardiovascular disease prevention programme (euroaction) for patients with coronary heart disease and asymptomatic individuals at high risk of cardiovascular disease: A paired, cluster-randomised controlled trial. *Lancet*, 371(9629):1999–2012, 2008.
162. C. J. Wright, G. K. Chambers, and Y. Robens-Paradise. Evaluation of indications for and outcomes of elective surgery. *Canadian Medical Association Journal*, 167(5):461–466, 2002.
163. V. Zellermeyer. *Report of the Surgical Process Analysis and Improvement Expert Panel*. Ontario Ministry of Health and Long-Term Care, 2005.

Index

B. Sobolev et al., *Health Care Evaluation Using Computer Simulation: Concepts, Methods, and Applications*, DOI 10.1007/978-1-4614-2233-4,

S

MIX
Papier aus verantwortungsvollen Quellen
Paper from responsible sources
FSC® C105338

If you have any concerns about our products,
you can contact us on
ProductSafety@springernature.com

In case Publisher is established outside the EU,
the EU authorized representative is:
Springer Nature Customer Service Center GmbH
Europaplatz 3, 69115 Heidelberg, Germany

Printed by Libri Plureos GmbH
in Hamburg, Germany